ATLAS
Optical Coherence Tomography of Macular Diseases

ATLAS
Optical Coherence Tomography of Macular Diseases

Vishali Gupta MD
Assistant Professor
Department of Ophthalmology
Postgraduate Institute of Medical Education and Research
Chandigarh, India

Amod Gupta MD
Professor and Head
Department of Ophthalmology
Postgraduate Institute of Medical Education and Research
Chandigarh, India

Mangat R Dogra MD
Additional Professor
Department of Ophthalmology
Postgraduate Institute of Medical Education and Research
Chandigarh, India

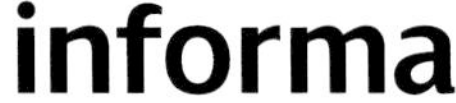
healthcare

New York London

First published in 2004 by Jaypee Brothers Medical Publishers. This edition published in 2011 by Informa Healthcare, London, UK.

Simultaneously published in the USA by Informa Healthcare, 52 Vanderbilt Avenue, 7th Floor, New York, NY 10017, USA.

Informa Healthcare is a trading division of Informa UK Ltd. Registered Office: 37–41 Mortimer Street, London W1T 3JH, UK. Registered in England and Wales number 1072954.

A CIP record for this book is available from the British Library.

Library of Congress Cataloging-in-Publication Data available on application

ISBN-13: 9781841844688

Orders may be sent to: Informa Healthcare, Sheepen Place, Colchester, Essex CO3 3LP, UK
Telephone: +44 (0)20 7017 5540
Email: CSDhealthcarebooks@informa.com
Website: http://informahealthcarebooks.com/

For corporate sales please contact: CorporateBooksIHC@informa.com
For foreign rights please contact: RightsIHC@informa.com
For reprint permissions please contact: PermissionsIHC@informa.com

Preface

For several decades now, the ophthalmologists have exploited the great opportunities that a clear media of the eye provides to examine, study and document the retina in health and disease using a myriad of simple and complex, techniques and technologies including the direct ophthalmoscope, the binocular indirect ophthalmoscope and the slit lamp biomicroscope using contact or non-contact lenses. Development of fundus angiography techniques contributed a great deal in our understanding of the pathogenetic mechanisms and the pathology of the blinding and the benign retinal disease. A great body of work by the ocular pathologists provided the necessary clinicopathological correlates of the retinal disease.

However, as clinicians, we have always viewed retina as a 'surface' and not a 3-dimensional structure, that it actually is, and while we all claimed that on stereoscopic examination we could tell, if the lesion was preretinal, intraretinal or subretinal, it was largely speculative based on our sensitization to the available clinicopathological information.

The emergence of Optical Coherence Tomography (OCT) in the recent years has changed forever, the way we 'look at' or shall we say 'look through' the retina. The OCT provides, in real time, high-resolution cross-sectional images of the macula very similar to obtaining *in vivo* histopathological sections. It represents a major advance in the diagnostics of retinal disease and has found rapid acceptance among the retina specialists.

A while ago, when we started doing the OCT examination along with the clinical and angiographic correlation of our retina patients, we soon realized 'the information' we were missing without the OCT and how the vital inputs it provided, changed the way we practiced 'Retina'. Our excitement of working with this tool, however, was soon dampened by the non-availability of any standard textbook (the only book titled 'Optical Coherence Tomography of Ocular Diseases' by Carmen A Puliafito, Michael R.Hee, Joel S. Schuman and James G. Fujimoto, being out of print) and meant that every new finding on the OCT saw us rushing to the library almost on a daily basis to locate any published reports on the subject.

In this 'Atlas', we have attempted to share our experience of Stratus OCT (Tm) in various macular disorders where we found it helpful in diagnosing and monitoring the response to various therapies and interventions and above all identifying the correct therapeutic approach in a given patient. It finds extensive application in diagnosis, management and follow up of diabetic macular edema, macular hole, taut posterior hyaloid membrane, vitreofoveal traction, idiopathic central serous chorioretinopathy, submacular pathology and many more areas that are divided into 22 chapters. For ease of comprehension, we provide with brief case summaries, fundus photographs, fluorescein angiography and the OCT images and the follow up images for most of the patients that we share with the readers.

We shall like to point out that OCT is not a substitute for a thorough clinical examination, fundus imaging or various angiographic techniques but is a great adjunctive tool to probe the mysteries of retinal disease. It has major limitations in obtaining images through a cloudy media or trying to look at the choroidal pathology. We strongly recommend that to obtain optimum information from the OCT, it be best performed by the clinician himself or herself .

We shall like to acknowledge with thanks the cases of adult foveo-vitreal dystrophy, best disease and photodyanamic therapy of occult choroidal neovascular membrane, provided to us by the courtesy of Dr.Monique Leys, MD, Associate Professor, West Virginia University Eye Institute, USA. We are thankful to Ms. Marianne Whitby , Carl Zeiss Meditec, Dublin, USA for picture of Stratus OCT (Tm) and for all the help she rendered during the preparation of this Atlas. We are also thankful to Carl Zeiss Meditec Inc. and Carl Zeiss India for allowing us to reproduce some of the material from their user's manual that helped us in the preparation of Section One. We shall also like to put on record our appreciation of the untiring Mr.Arun Kapil, our clinical photographer who obtained most of the fundus and angiographic pictures used in this Atlas. Finally, we wish to thank Mr S.S. Saini for his help in editing the manuscript.

Vishali Gupta
Amod Gupta
Mangat R Dogra

Contents

Errata

Incorrect

Correct

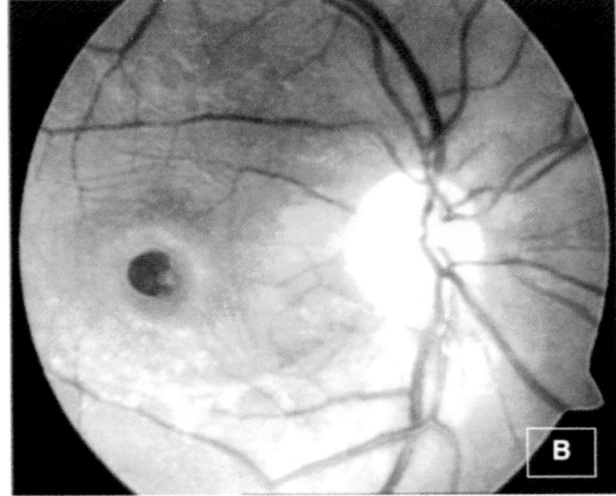

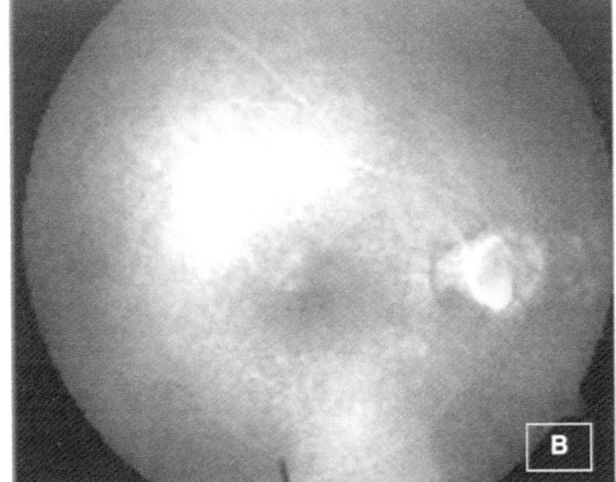

Chapter 7, Page 77, Fig. B

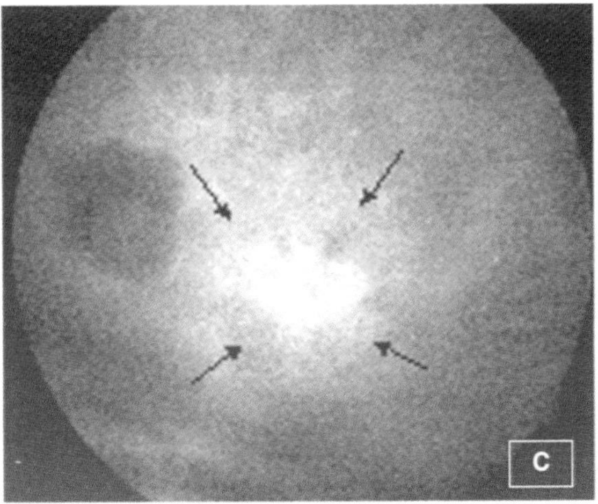

Chapter 11, Page 140, Fig. C

Section One

Introduction to OCT

Chapter 1

Basics of OCT

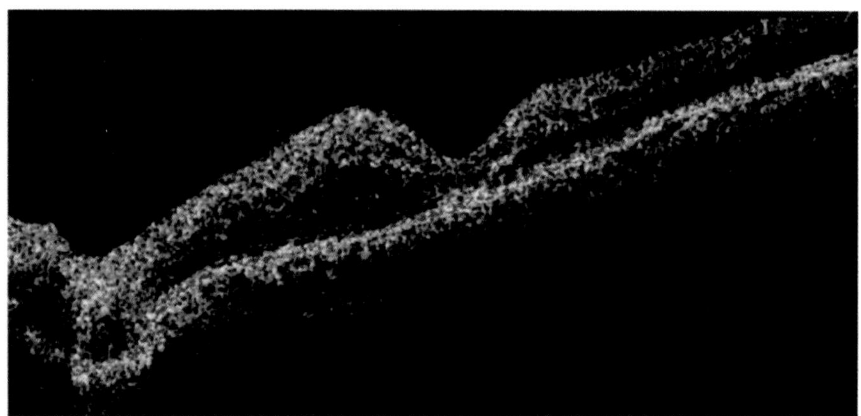

WHAT IS OCT ?

Optical Coherence Tomography (OCT) is a new diagnostic tool that can perform tomography/cross-sectional imaging of biologic tissues with $\leq$10 microns axial resolution using light waves. Since retina is easily accessible to the external light, hence it is especially suited for retinal disorders. This is the first imaging technique that provides information regarding the retinal tomography that is akin to *in vivo* histopathology of the retina. The conventional imaging techniques including fundus photography and fluorescein angiography yield diagnostic information about retinal topography. OCT yields information about retinal tomography that is complementary to the conventional topographic techniques.

Principle

We are all familiar with principle on which ultrasound works where the high frequency sound wave is launched into the eye with the help of a probe. The sound wave is reflected from different boundaries between microstructures. The working principle of OCT is similar to ultrasound with two major differences:

1. It uses light rather than ultrasound. The speed of light is almost a million times faster than sound and this difference allows the measurement of structures with resolution of $\leq$ 10 microns compared to 100-micron scale for ultrasound.
2. Ultrasound needs contact with the tissue under study, whereas OCT does not require any contact.

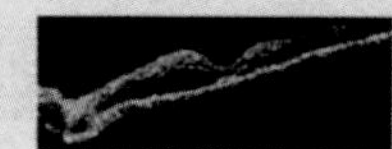

HARDWARE

The essential components of the hardware include:

1. Patient Module
2. Joy Stick
3. Flat Screen Video Monitor
4. Mouse
5. Keyboard
6. DVD-RAM Drive
7. CPU
8. Printer

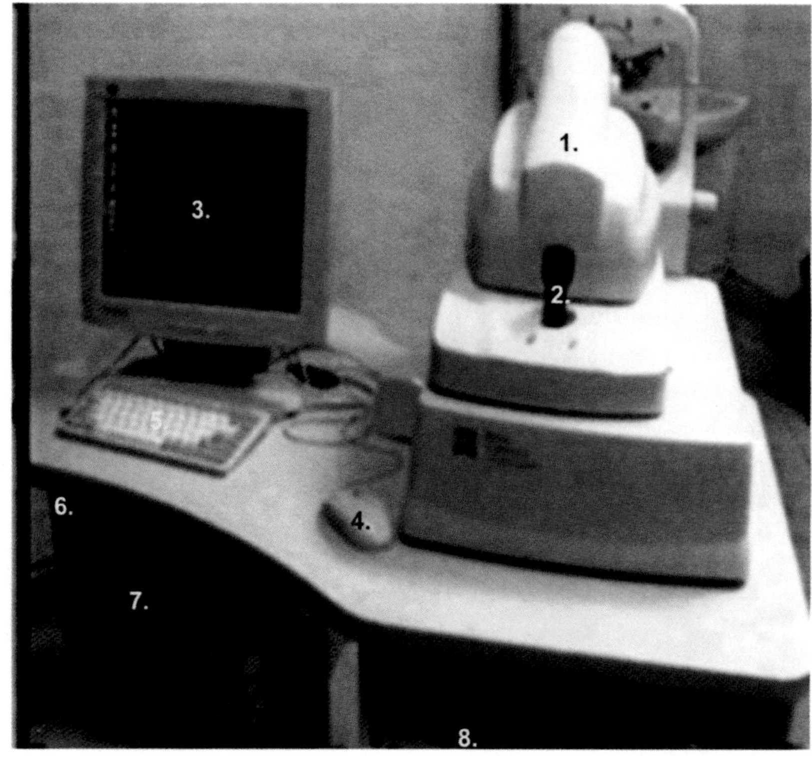

HOW DOES OCT WORK?

It is a non contact, non invasive device where a broad band-width near infrared light beam (820 nm) is projected on to the retina. The light gets reflected from the boundaries between the microstructures and also gets scattered differently from tissues with different optical properties. It then compares the echo time delay of the light that is reflected from the various layers of the retina with the echo time delay of the same wavelength that is reflected from a reference mirror at a known distance. The interferometer then combines the reflected pulses from the retina as well as reflecting mirrors, resulting in a phenomenon known as interference. This interference is then measured by a photodetector, which determines the distance travelled by various echoes by varying the distance to the reference mirror. This finally produces a range of time delays for comparison.

The interferometer integrates several data points over 2 mm of depth to construct a tomogram of retinal structures. It is a real time tomogram using false color scale. Different colors represent the degree of light backscattering from different depths of retina.

The image thus produced has axial resolution of ≤ 10 microns and transverse resolution of 20 microns.

SUGGESTED READINGS

1. Puliafito CA, Hee MR, Schuman JS, Fujimoto JG. Optical Coherence Tomography of Ocular diseases. Slack Inc 1996.
2. Huang D, Swanson EA, Lin CP et al. Optical Coherence tomography. Science 1999;254:1178-81.
3. Hee MR, Izatt JA, Swanson EA et al. Optical Coherence tomography of the human retina. Arch Ophthalmol 1995; 113:325-32.

Chapter 2

Technique of Acquiring OCT

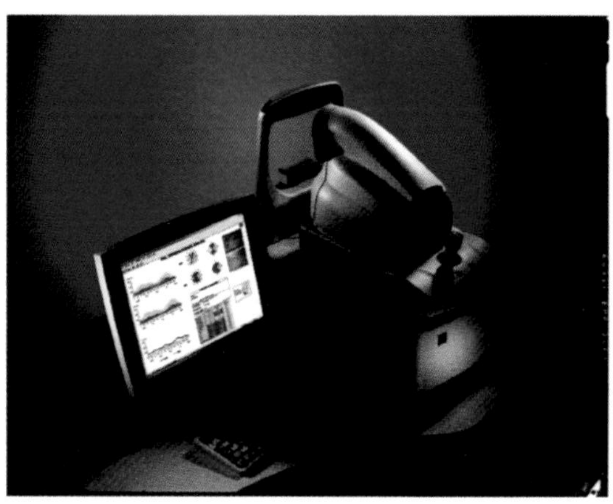

TECHNIQUE

1. *Switch on the system:* This activates all the components and takes about 45 seconds to display 'Start Window'. The menu and toolbar in the Main Window offers various options including **Select Patient, Acquisition Protocol, Analysis Protocol** and so on. You can select the appropriate category and make data entry for new patient (A).
2. *Patient Preparation:* It is preferable to dilate pupil before examination. Small pupils of less than 3 mm may result in images that are truncated or are of poor quality due to lack of image intensity. The patient is asked to look into the 'Internal Fixation' target in the ocular lens with the study eye. In patients with poor vision, the external fixation target can be used. The internal fixation, however, is the preferred method as it is more reproducible.
   For internal fixation, the patient is asked to look inside the ocular lens. When patient looks into the ocular lens, he sees a rectangular field of red with a green light. He is asked to fixate at the green light. The location of internal fixation target can be readjusted as per requirements. The opposite eye of the patient can be covered as this helps the patient to fixate more steadily. With external fixation method, the patient has to use the fellow eye to fixate on the target that is external to the ocular lens.
3. *Obtaining a Scan:* The protocol for scan acquisition can be selected as per requirement. The Scan acquisition window gets activated by a click on the Scan button. The scanner, by default, activates in the fast scan mode, also known as scan alignment mode. This mode is useful for optimizing the alignment and polarization and placement of the scan on the area of interest. Once the alignment is

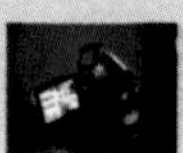

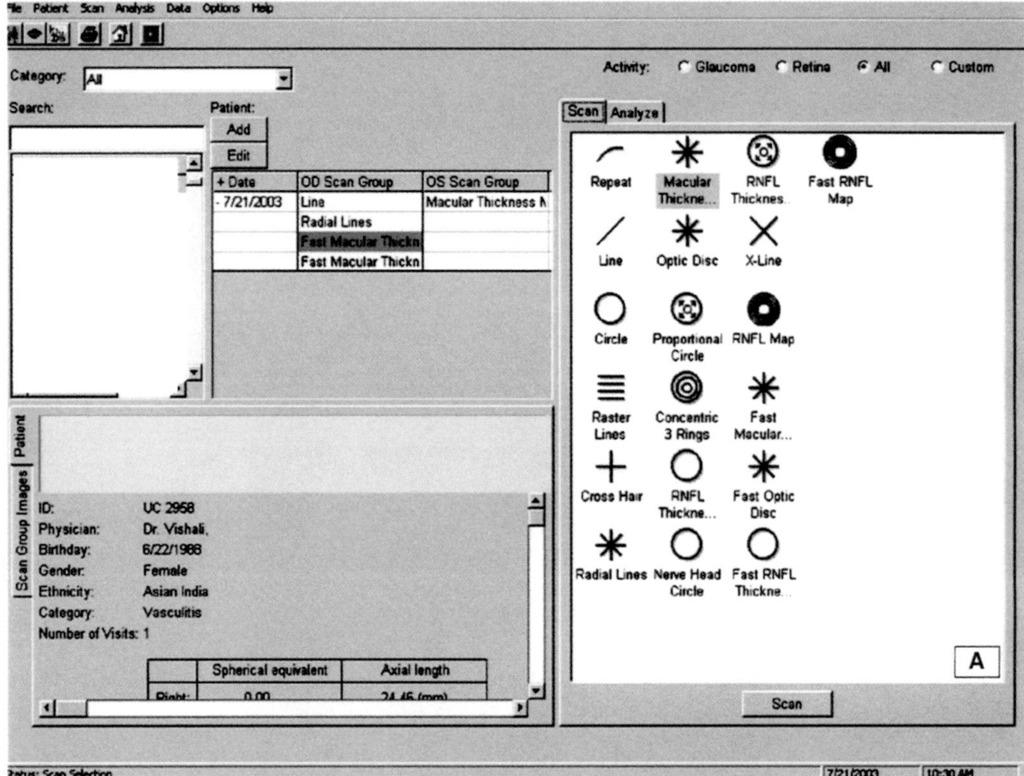

satisfactory, one can click 'Scan Mode' button to change to slow scan mode also known as scan acquisition mode. It is important to note that scanner must be in the slow scan mode to acquire scans. The desired scans can be reviewed, analyzed and saved.

SUGGESTED READING

1. Stratus OCT Model 3000. User Manual Carl Zeiss Meditec Inc. 2002.

Chapter 3

Selection of Scan Protocols

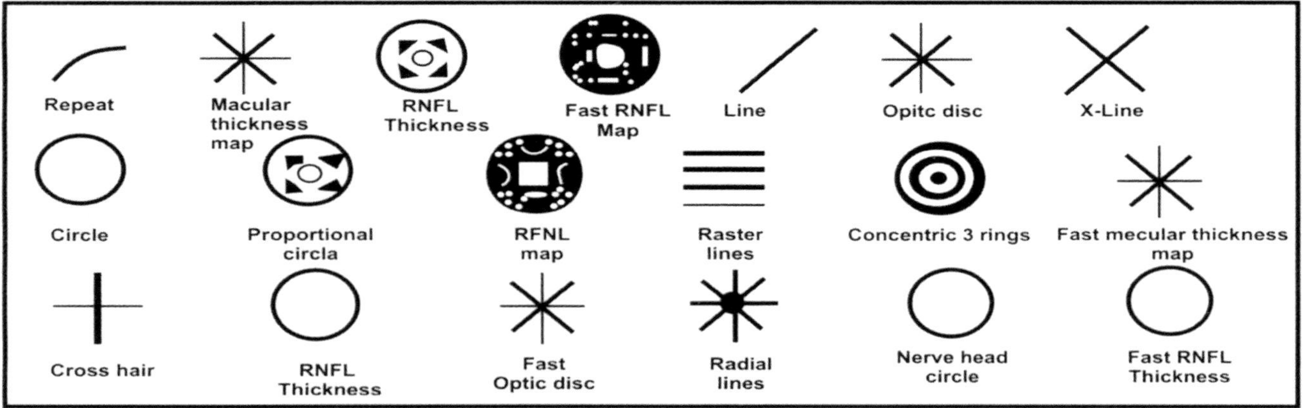

OCT SCAN PROTOCOLS IN MACULA

The Stratus OCT offers 19 scan acquisition protocols designed for examination of the Retina or Glaucoma patients. The protocols that are helpful in macular diseases are:

1. Line
2. Radial lines
3. Macular thickness map
4. Fast macular thickness map
5. Raster lines
6. Repeat

While selecting a protocol, one has to keep in mind the kind of information one wishes to obtain in a given patient. The analysis protocols can be either image processing protocols for quantitative analysis protocol. The image processing protocol can be used with any scan type while the quantitative analysis protocol can be used with certain scan type only. To get the most accurate and meaningful information, one needs to apply the appropriate protocol. Given below is the list of Quantitative Analysis protocols that correlate well with the scan acquisition protocols:

Analysis protocol	*Selection of scan acquisition protocol*
Retinal thickness	any of the protocol, line scan through the macula
Retinal Map	Radial lines, Fast Macular thickness map
Retinal Thickness/Volume	Radial lines, Fast macular thickness map

Scan Protocols Suitable for Macula

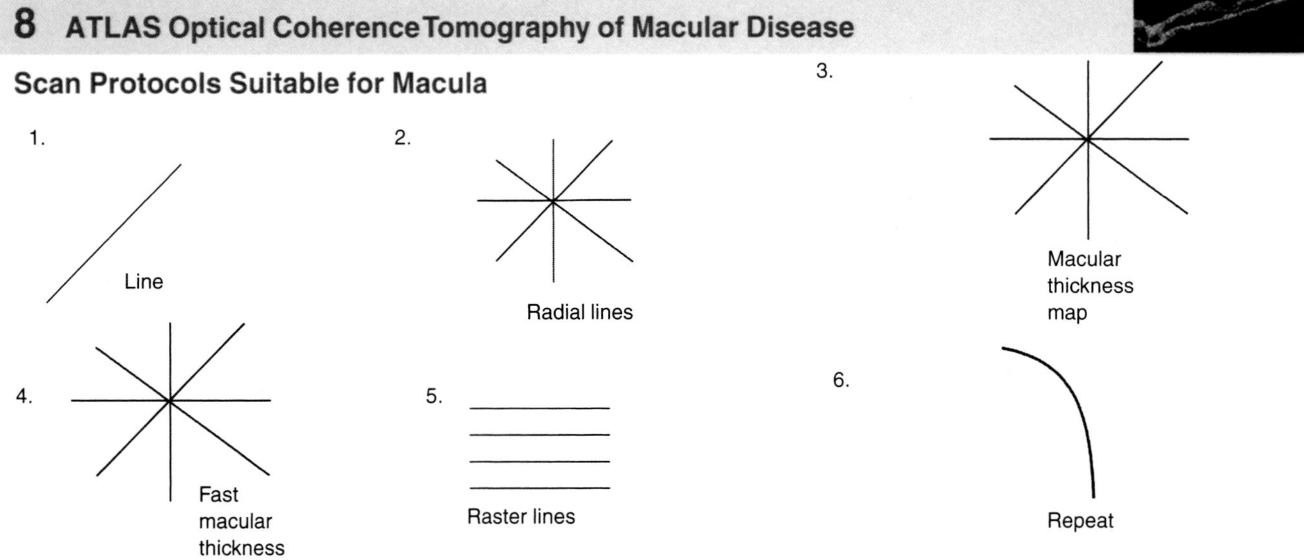

Line Scan

The line scan gives an option of acquiring multiple line scans without returning to main window. The default angle is 0° and the nasal position is defined as 0°. By default, the length of line scan is 5mm (A). The length of the line scan and the angle can be altered (B), though one has to keep in mind that as the scan length increases, the resolution decreases. This protocol enables one to acquire multiple scans of different parameters.

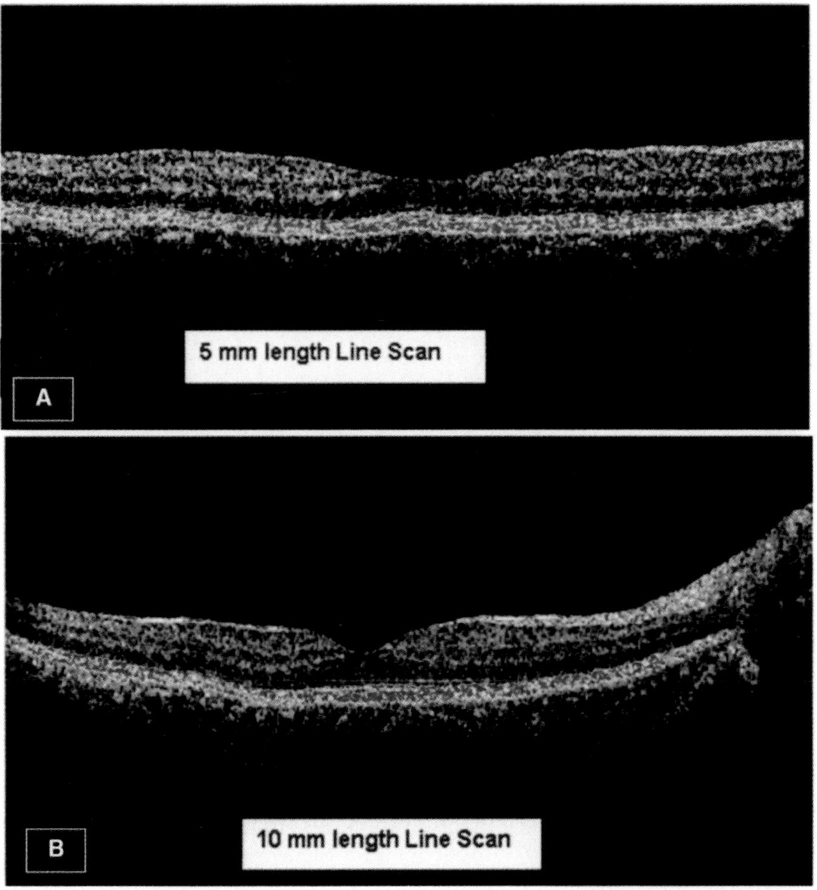

Radial Lines

This scan protocol (A) consists of 6 to 24 equally spaced line scans that can be varied in size and parameters. All the lines pass through a central common axis. The default setting has 6 lines of 6 mm length. However the length of these line scans can be changed by adjusting the size of the aiming circle. The change can be made only before saving the first scan. The radial lines are useful for acquiring Macular scan and retinal thickness/volume analysis

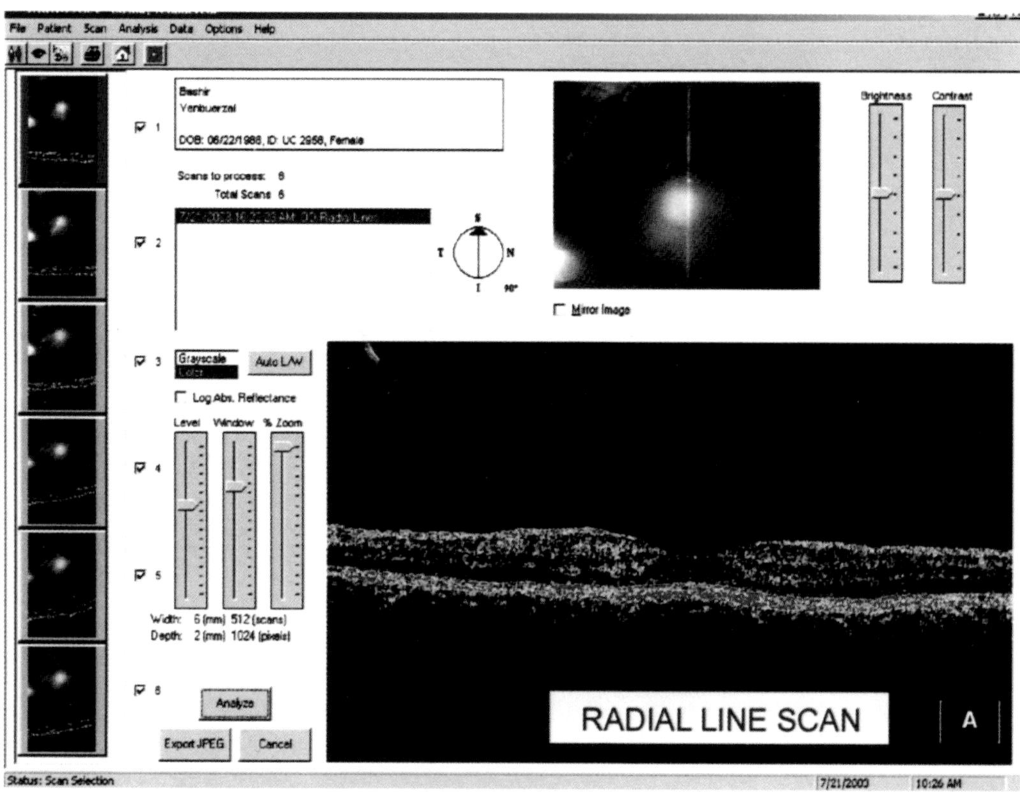

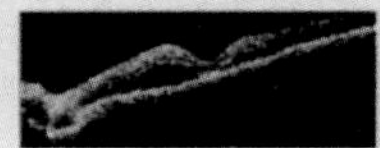

Macular Thickness Map

This is same as radial lines except that the aiming circle has a fixed diameter of 6 mm. The number of lines can be adjusted before saving the first scan. This acquisition protocol helps in measuring the retinal thickness.

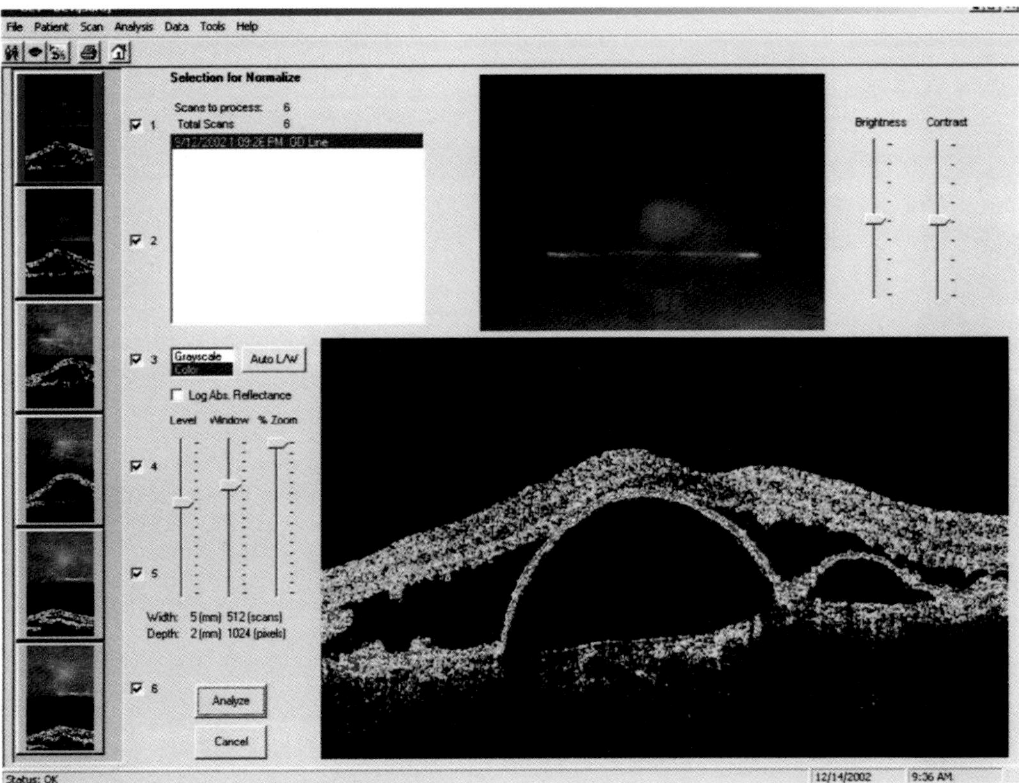

MACULAR THICKNESS MAP

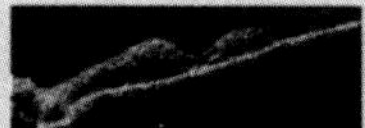

FAST MACULARTHICKNESS MAP

This protocol is designed for use with retinal thickness analysis. When done in both the eyes, it can be used for comparative retinal thickness/Volume analysis. It is a quick protocol that takes only 1.92 seconds to acquire six scans of 6 mm length each. The size and number of scans is fixed in this protocol and cannot be altered.

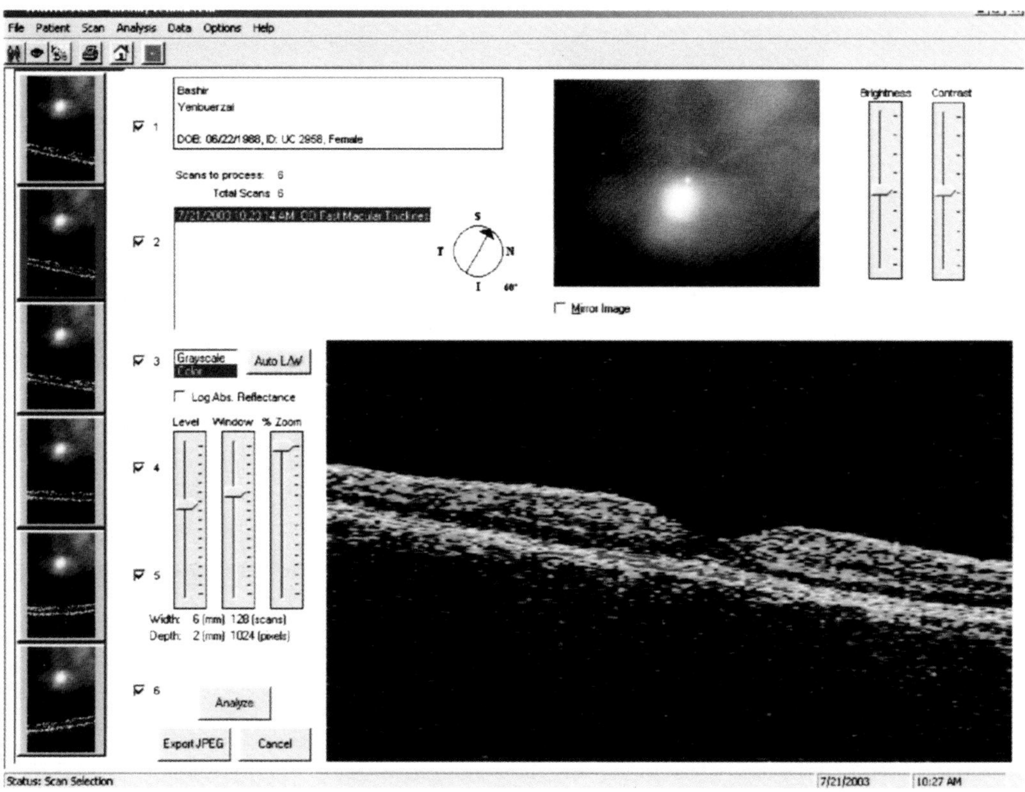

FAST MACULARTHICKNESS MAP

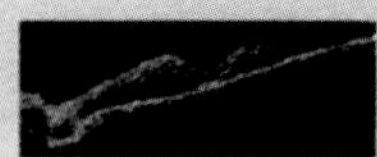

Raster Lines

This protocol provides an option of acquiring series of line scans that are parallel, equally spaced and are 6-24 in number. These multiple line scans are placed over a rectangular region, the area of which can be adjusted so as to cover the entire area of pathology. This is especially useful in conditions like choroidal neovascular membranes where one wishes to obtain scans at multiple levels. The default setting has 3 mm square with 6 lines.

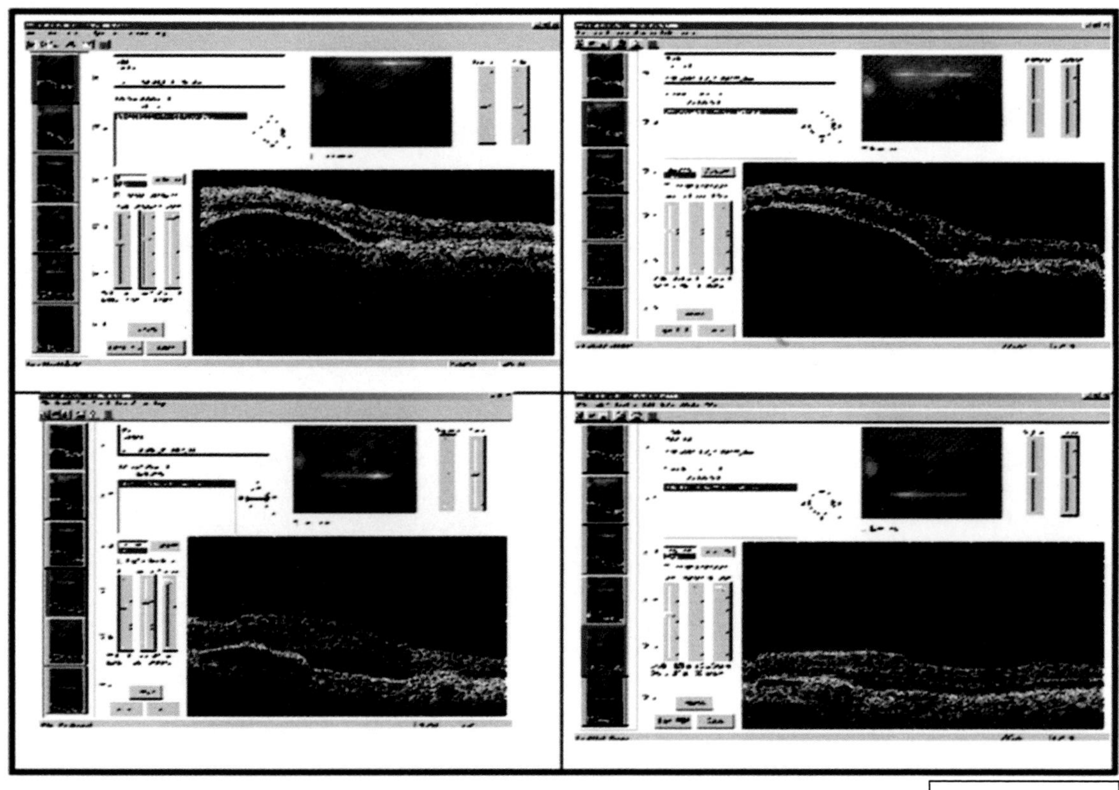

RADIAL LINES

Repeat

Repeat protocol enables one to repeat any of the previously saved protocols using same set of parameters that include scan size, angle, placement of fixation LED (Light emitting diode) and landmark. The system repeats all these parameters giving the same settings as in the previous scan. This protocol is especially helpful when one is monitoring retinal changes. No parameter except placement can be changed.

The landmark can be placed on a point of reference. This helps in reproducibility during repeat scan. The previous image can be displayed for accurate placement of landmark.

SUGGESTED READING

1. Stratus OCT Model 3000. User Manual Carl Zeiss Meditec Inc. 2002

Chapter 4

OCT Scan of Normal Macula

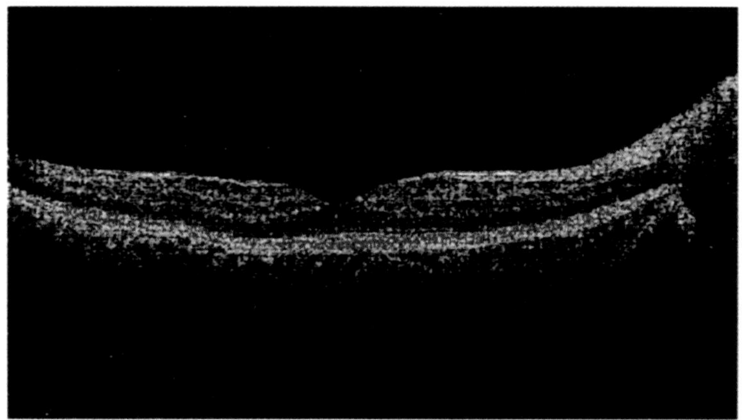

NORMAL MACULA SCAN

On a 10 mm horizontal line scan passing through the foveal center (A) one can clearly demarcate two major landmarks namely optic disc and fovea. The **optic disc** is seen towards the right of the tomogram and is easily identifiable by its contour. The central depression represents the optic head cup and the stalk continuing behind is the anterior part of optic nerve. The **fovea** is seen to the left and is easily identifiable by the characteristic thinning of retinal layers. The vitreous anterior to the retina is non-reflective and is seen as a dark space. The interface between the non-reflective vitreous and backscattering retinal layers is the **vitreo-retinal** interface. The **retinal nerve-fibre layer (NFL)** is highly reflective and increases in thickness towards the optic nerve. The posterior boundary of the retina is marked by a hyper-reflective layer that represents **Retinal pigment epithelium (RPE)** and **choriocapillaries.** The choroid and sclera are not seen well on tomograms as the signal attenuates by the time it reaches these structures. Just anterior to RPE-choriocapillaries complex is a minimally-reflective layer that represents **photoreceptors.** Above this layer of photoreceptors are alternating layers of moderate and low reflectivity that represent different layers of neurosensory retina. The **retinal blood vessels** within the neurosensory retina show backscatter and also cast a shadow behind.

Image Interpretation

There are two ways of interpreting the OCT scan: Objective and Subjective. For the accurate interpretation of the image, one needs to combine both these modalities.

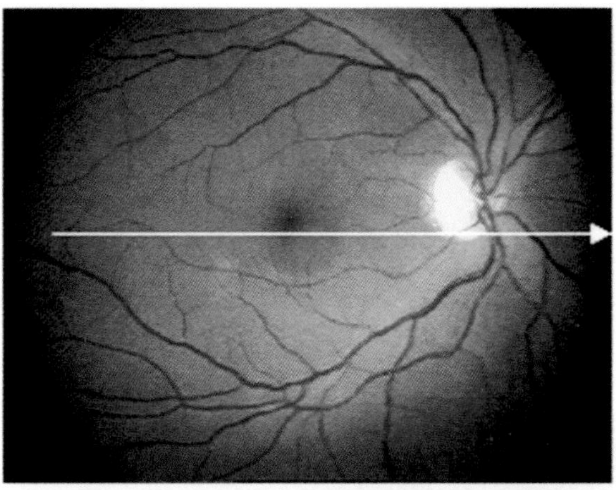

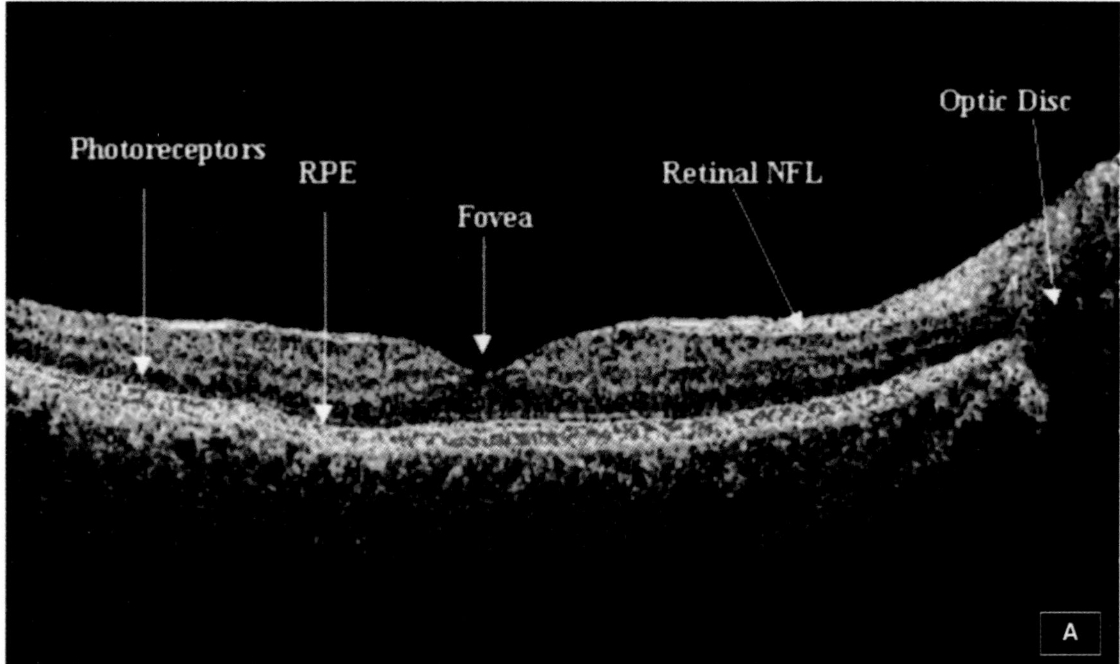

1. **Objective** : We are all familiar with the interpretation of fluorescein angiograms where we categorize the pathology as hypo- or hyper-fluorescent, or ultrasound B scan where images are either hypo- or hyper-echoic. Likewise in OCT scan, we look at the reflectivity pattern of the scanned images. The best way, in our experience, to do this is to select the scan group, select appropriate analysis protocol and go to "Scan selection". This gives a magnified view of the selected image for objective assessment. One can modify the image before studying. In this image, one can make anatomic correlate like 'pigment epithelial detachment' and also study the reflectivity patterns.

   Following lesions are **hyper-reflective:**

   a. *Hard exudates (A):* The hard exudates are seen as hyper-reflective shadows in the neurosensory retina that completely block the reflections from the underlying retina.

   b. *Blood (B):* Blood causes increased scattering. In cases of small and thin hemorrahage, hyper-reflectivity is seen, whereas, if the hemorrhage is thick, it might block the reflections from the underlying structures.

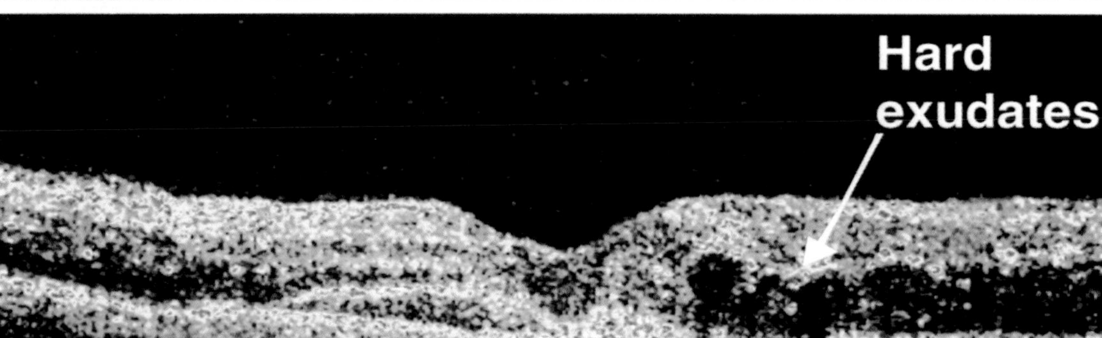

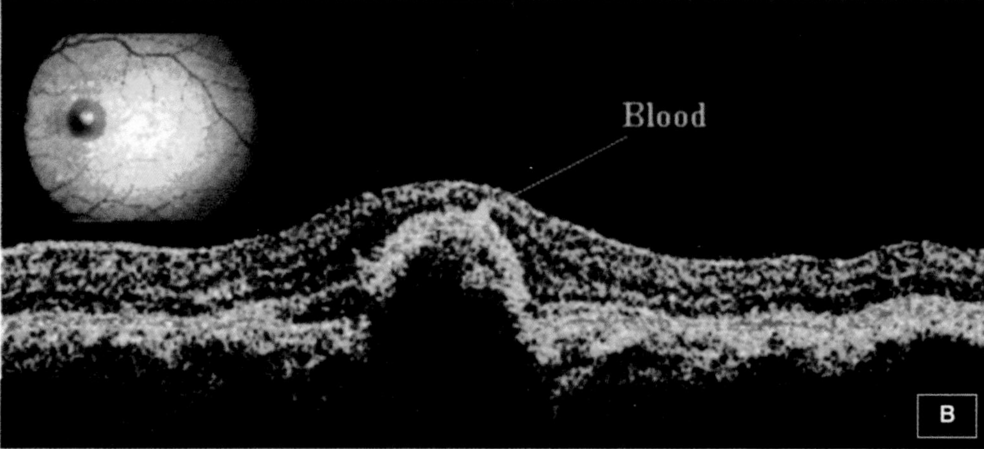

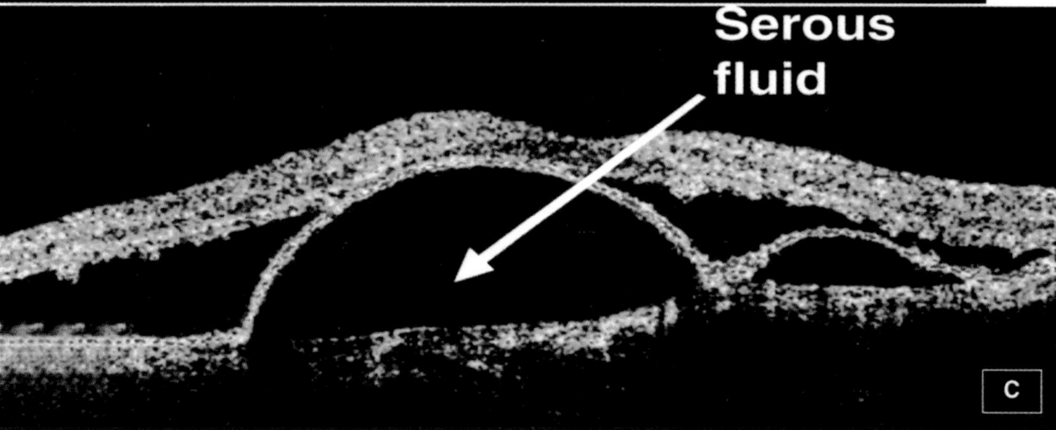

c. *Scars:* All the fibrotic lesions including disciform scars, choroidal rupture scars, healed choroiditis, etc. are hyper-reflective.

Following lesions are **hypo-reflective**:

a. *Serous fluid (C):* Retinal edema is the commonest cause of reduced backscattering and one can actually point out the site of fluid accumulation. The serous fluid that is devoid of any particulate matter produces an optically empty space with no backscattering.

b. *Hypo-pigmented lesions of RPE*

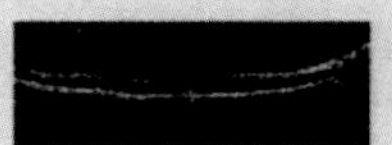

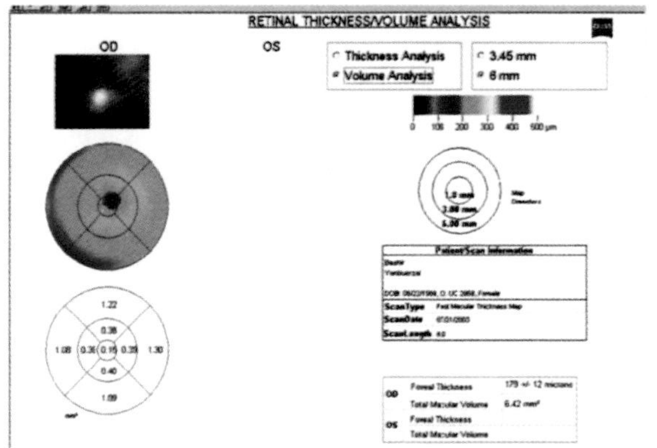

A. Retinal thickness/volume analysis output

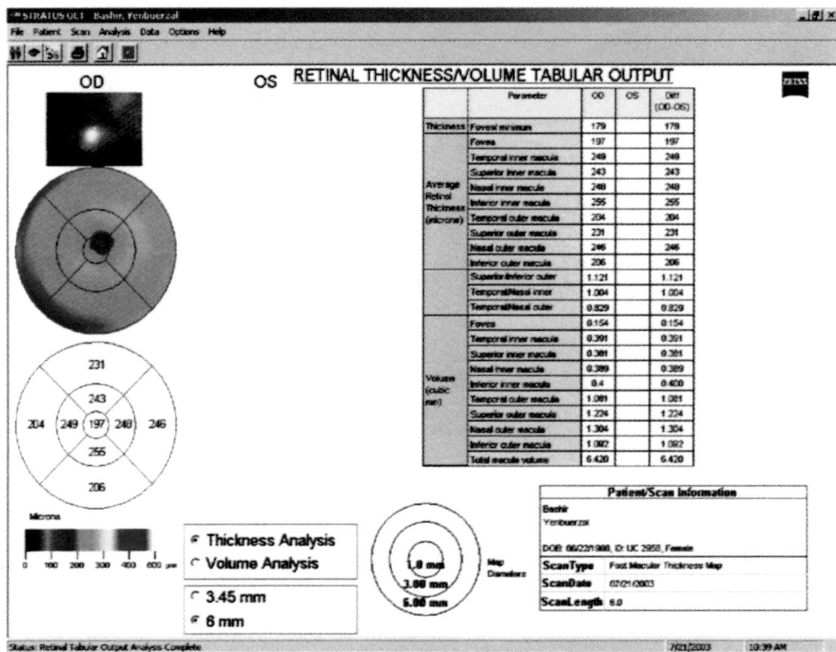

	Parameter	OD	OS	Diff (OD-OS)
Thickness	Foveal minimum	179		179
Average Retinal Thickness (microns)	Fovea	197		197
	Temporal inner macula	249		249
	Superior inner macula	243		243
	Nasal inner macula	248		248
	Inferior inner macula	255		255
	Temporal outer macula	204		204
	Superior outer macula	231		231
	Nasal outer macula	246		246
	Inferior outer macula	206		206
	Superior/Inferior outer	1.121		1.121
	Temporal/Nasal inner	1.004		1.004
	Temporal/Nasal outer	0.829		0.829
Volume (cubic mm)	Fovea	0.154		0.154
	Temporal inner macula	0.391		0.391
	Superior inner macula	0.381		0.381
	Nasal inner macula	0.389		0.389
	Inferior inner macula	0.4		0.400
	Temporal outer macula	1.081		1.081
	Superior outer macula	1.224		1.224
	Nasal outer macula	1.304		1.304
	Inferior outer macula	1.082		1.082
	Total macula volume	6.420		6.420

B. Retinal thickness/volume tabular

One must remember that poor quality scans due to opaque media and refractive errors might be falsely interpreted as hyporeflective. However, hypo-reflectivity in these situations is diffuse resulting in overall attenuation of the scan.

2. *Subjective Analysis:* The software offers the option of both qualitative and quantitative estimation protocols.

Qualitative: Various image modification protocols can be used prior to objective assessment. These protocols include 'Normalize' , 'Align', 'Median Smoothing' and 'Guassian smoothing'. These protocols are essentially image modification protocols and can be used whenever one wishes.

Quantitative

Retinal thickness/Volume (A): This analysis protocol obtains two circular maps for each eye that depict thickness and volume of retina. One has a choice to display either thickness or volume of the retina.

Retinal thickness/Volume Tabular (B): Gives same information as above and also a data table that gives thickness and volume in each quadrant, comparison between the quadrants and between the eyes.

Retinal thickness/Volume Change: This protocol helps to assess the changes in the retinal thickness/ volume between the examinations.

SUGGESTED READINGS

1. Puliafito CA, Hee MR, Schuman JS, Fujimoto JG. Optical Coherence Tomography of Ocular diseases Slack Inc. 1996.
2. Huang D, Swanson EA, Lin CP et al. Optical Coherence Tomography. Science 1999;254:1178-81.
3. Hee MR, Izatt JA, Swanson EA et al. Optical coherence tomography of the human retina. Arch Ophthalmol 1995 ;113: 325-32.
4. Stratus OCT Model 3000. User Manual Carl Zeiss Meditec Inc 2002.

Section Two

OCT Patterns in Various Macular Diseases

Chapter 5

Diabetic Macular Edema

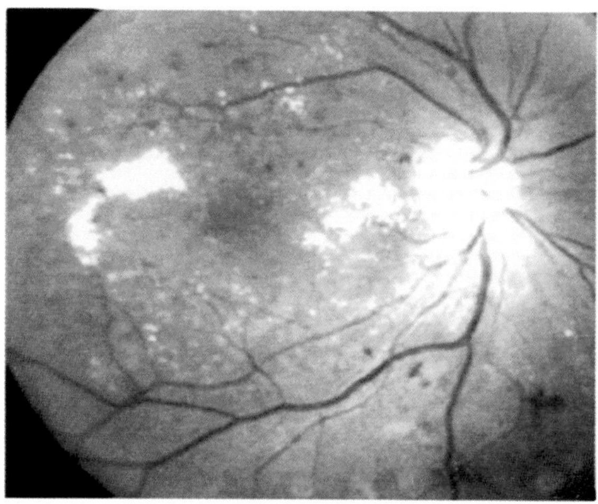

Diabetic macular edema is the most common cause of moderate visual loss in diabetics. The disease is now believed to be multifactorial in origin with a number of systemic factors including hypertension, poor metabolic control of diabetes, dyslipidemia and nephropathy playing a role in its pathogenesis. The macular edema in cases with underlying systemic disorders tends to be diffuse and often recalcitrant to laser photocoagulation. In addition, there is a focal variety of macular edema that is characterized by focal areas of microaneurysmal leak and is usually seen in patients with good systemic control. Since the edema is multifactorial in origin, it produces several manifestations at the ultra structural levels within the retinal layers. The conventional two-dimensional imaging techniques including fundus photographs and fluorescein angiography give a topographic view of the retina that helps in delineating the treatable lesions but are not able to depict the changes occurring within the retinal layers. OCT provides an insight into the underlying retinal layers that yields very useful information. The reduced backscattering is seen mostly in the outer retinal layers and corresponds to intraretinal fluid accumulation. Cystoid macular edema is represented by decreased intraretinal reflectivity and closely resembles the histopathology description. The hard exudates appear as areas of increased reflectivity with a trail of shadow behind. In addition, OCT is also able to diagnose macular traction, taut posterior hyloid membrane, serous detachment under the fovea and lamellar macular holes in these eyes.

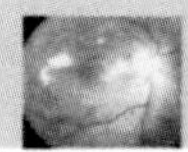

ROLE OF OCT IN DIABETIC MACULAR EDEMA

A. Defining the Disease Pattern

In our experience, we found that diabetic macular edema had 5 distinct patterns that could be defined on OCT alone. These were:
1. Sponge-like retinal thickness
2. Cystoid macular edema
3. Subfoveal serous retinal detachment
4. Foveal tractional retinal detachment
5. Taut posterior hyloid membrane.

B. Longitudinal Tracking of Tissue Alteration following An Intervention

OCT is a very useful tool in monitoring response to any intervention very closely. This indeed gives an ultrastructural detail of the changes taking place within the retinal layers. OCT also helps in quantifying the retinal thickness. One can measure central foveal thickness in microns and measure the retinal volume. In addition, retinal mapping also gives quadrant-wise information about retinal thickness. The quantification makes it easier to monitor the response to therapy.

C. Defining Indications for Pars Plana Vitrectomy

We found OCT to be a very reliable tool in defining the indications for pars plana vitrectomy in diabetic macular edema. In our experience, patterns 4 and 5, i.e. foveal tractional detachment and Taut Posterior Hyloid Membrane were the definite indications of surgery while patterns 2 and 3, i.e., cystoid macular edema and subfoveal serous detachment were relative indications where PPV was indicated only if the cystoid or edema serous detachment was a result of co-existing mechanical traction.

A. PATTERNS OF DIABETIC MACULAR EDEMA ON OCT

By conventional techniques of retinal examination, we see diabetic macular edema as a two dimensional pathology. By looking at the surface of the retina alone, we try to conceptualize the structural changes in the underlying tissues. The OCT almost gives the *in vivo* histopathology of the retinal layers that helps in the better disease understanding and pathogenesis. OCT is a useful tool in monitoring response to an intervention in clinically significant macular edema (CSME). It gives quantitative information regarding the tissue thickness in the follow-up of CSME. Thus, OCT helps in better decision-making. Following series of cases illustrate as to how OCT in addition to the fluorescein angiography helped us in the management of CSME patients.

Patterns of diabetic macular edema. In our experience there are 5 different patterns of diabetic macular edema on OCT. These are:
1. *Sponge like thickening of retinal layers:* This was mostly confined to the outer retinal layers due to backscattering from intraretinal fluid accumulation.

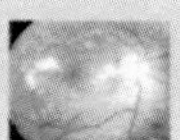

Case 5.1: CSME with Sponge-like Thickening

Case Summary

A 52-year-old Indian type II diabetic was seen with non-proliferative diabetic retinopathy both eyes with significant macular edema right eye (A). The visual acuity in this eye was 20/100. Fluorescein angiography (B) revealed microaneurysms with late leakage consistent with macular edema.

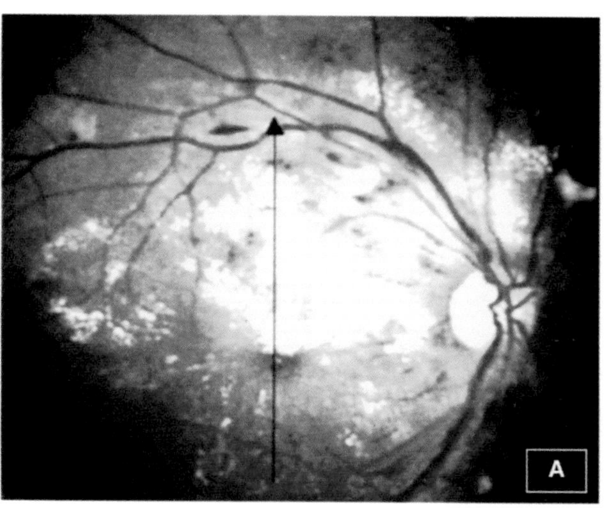

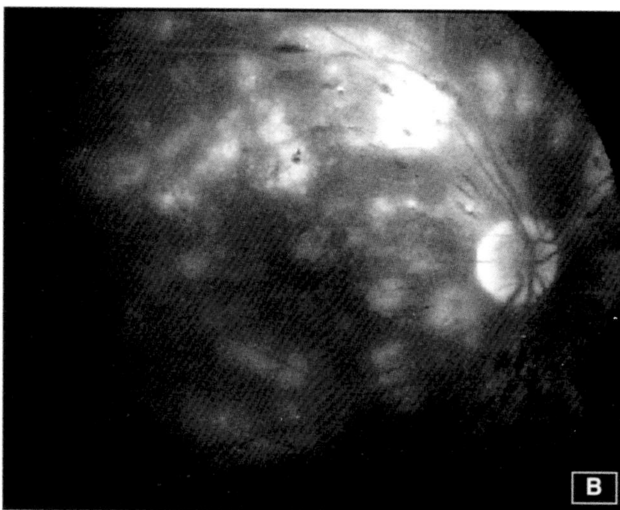

Optical Coherence Tomography

A vertical OCT Scan (C) revealed macular thickening with reduced optical backscatter due to accumulation of fluid in the outer retinal layers. The circinate rings of hard exudates (arrows) were seen as hyper-reflective lesions within the retinal layers with shadowing effect.

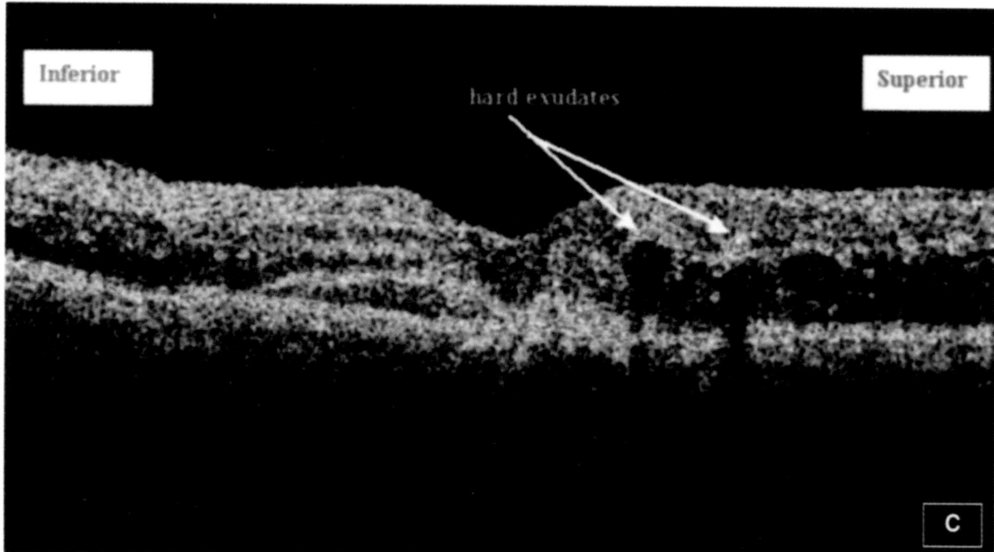

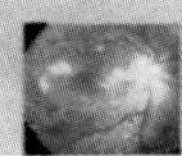

Case 5.2: CSME with Sponge-like Thickening

Case Summary

A 50-year-old Indian type II diabetic was seen with non-proliferative diabetic retinopathy both eyes with significant macular edema left eye (A). The visual acuity in this eye was 20/20. Fluorescein angiography (B) revealed microaneurysms with late leakage consistent with macular edema.

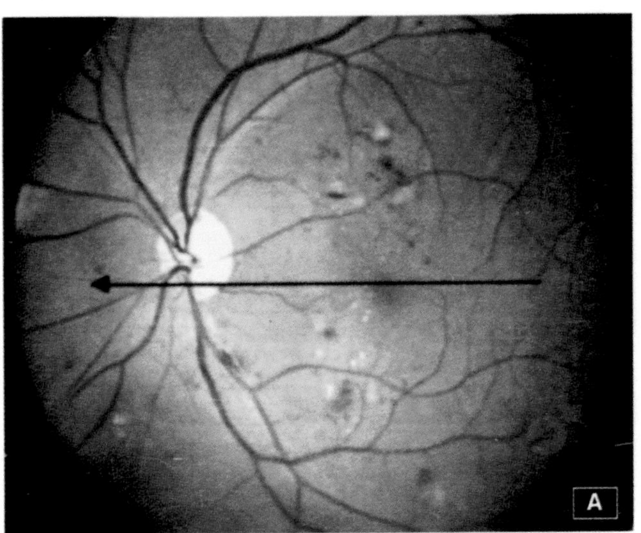

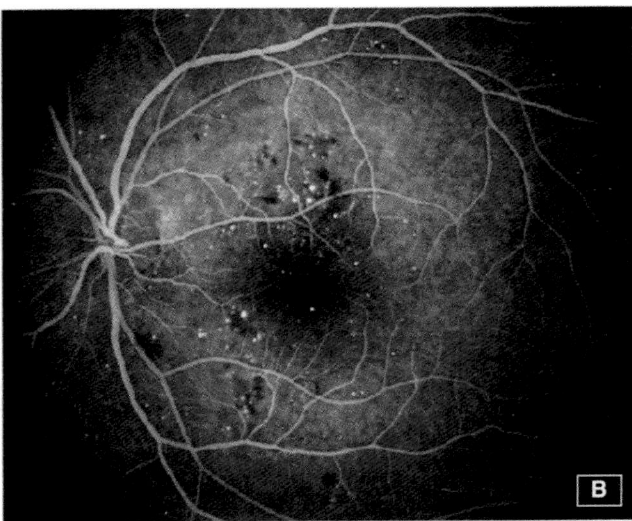

Optical Coherence Tomography

OCT (C) revealed sponge-like thickening of the fovea with hyporeflectivity from outer retinal layers suggesting intraretinal fluid accumulation seen mostly temporal to the fovea. The foveal contour was normal. The hyper-reflective shadows seen within the retinal layers (arrows) were from hard exudates.

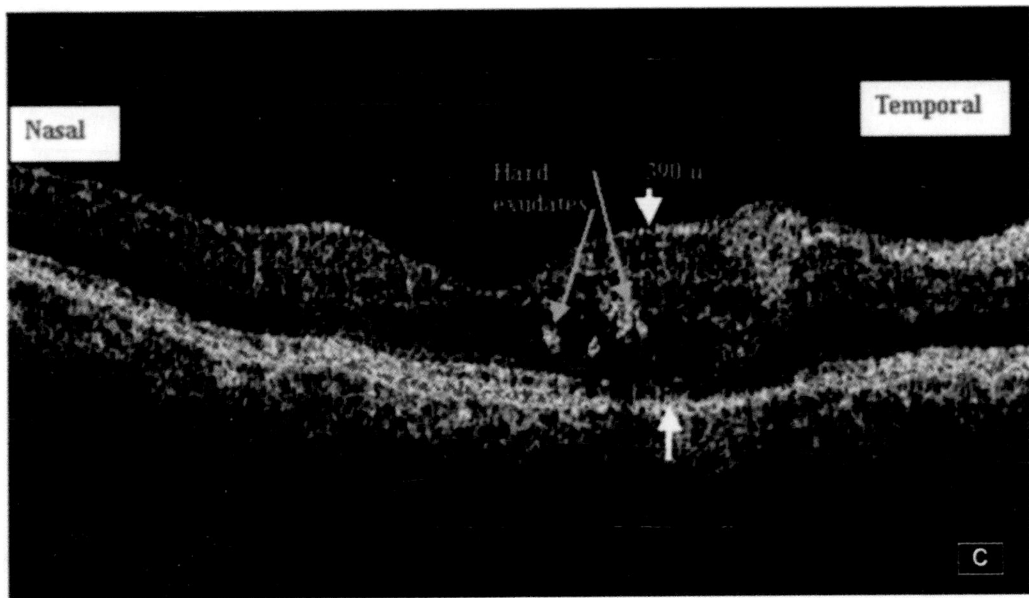

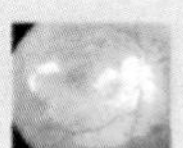

2. *Large cystoid spaces involving variable depth of the retina with intervening septae:* The cystoid spaces are initially confined to the outer retina mainly, but in long standing cases, these cysts fuse to involve almost entire length of the retina.

Case 5.3: CSME with Cystoid Macular Edema

Case Summary

A 54-year-old woman with 20 years history of Non-Insulin-Dependent-Diabetes Mellitus (NIDDM) was examined. Her best-corrected vision in the right eye was 20/200. Fundus showed CSME (A). Fluorescein angiography showed late leakage (B).

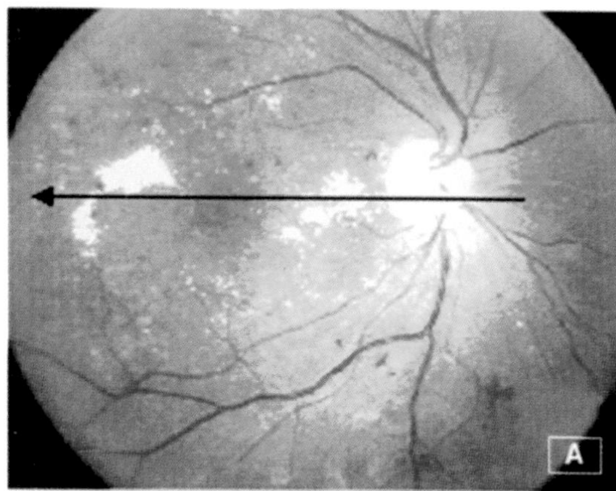

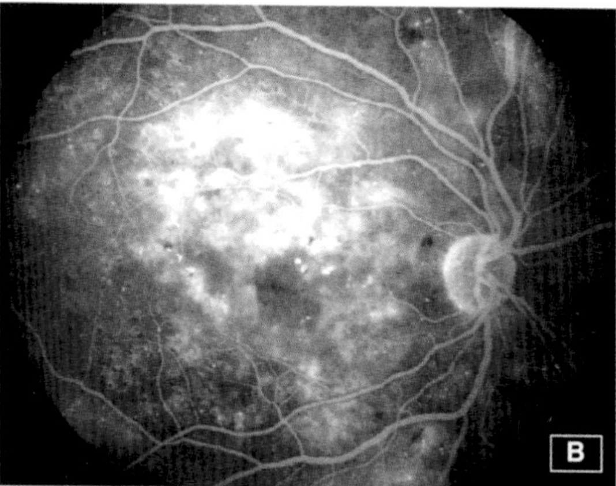

Optical Coherence Tomography

OCT line scan through the fovea (C) showed macular thickening with two nearly full- thickness cystoid spaces under the fovea with intervening septae. The cysts in the adjoining retina were smaller in size and were arranged mainly in the outer retinal layers

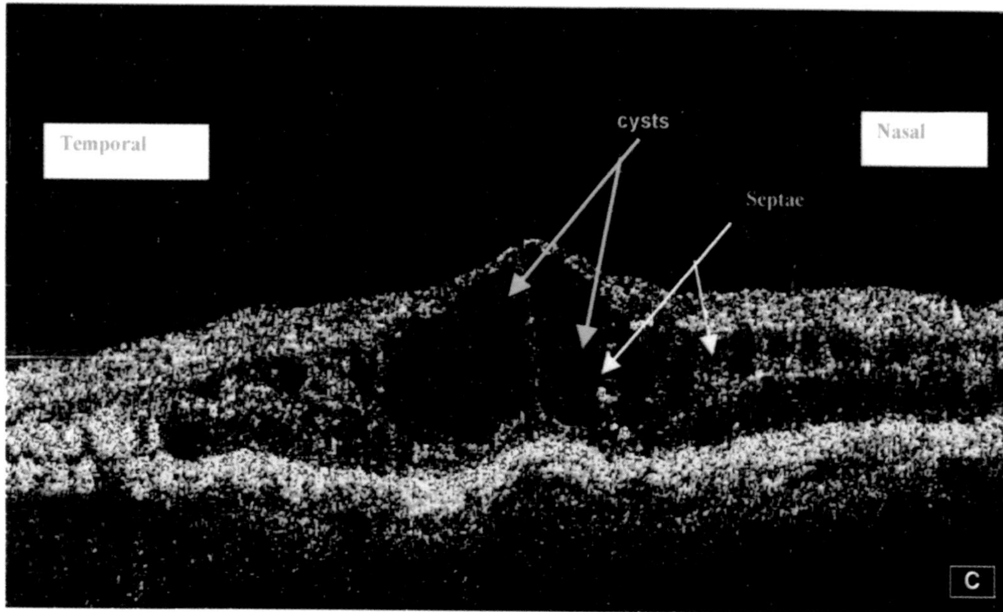

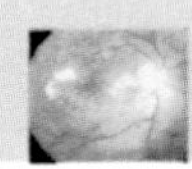

Case 5.4: CSME with Cystoid Spaces

Case Summary

A 38-year–old diabetic woman was seen with non-proliferative diabetic retinopathy with cystoid macular edema (A). Fluorescein angiography revealed diffuse leakage with cystoid spaces in the late phase (B).

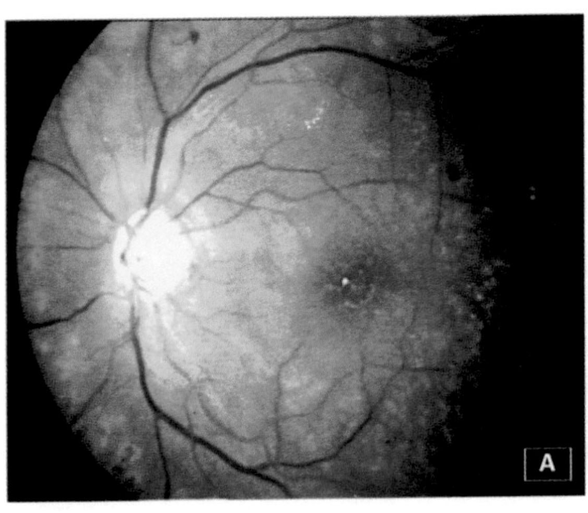

A

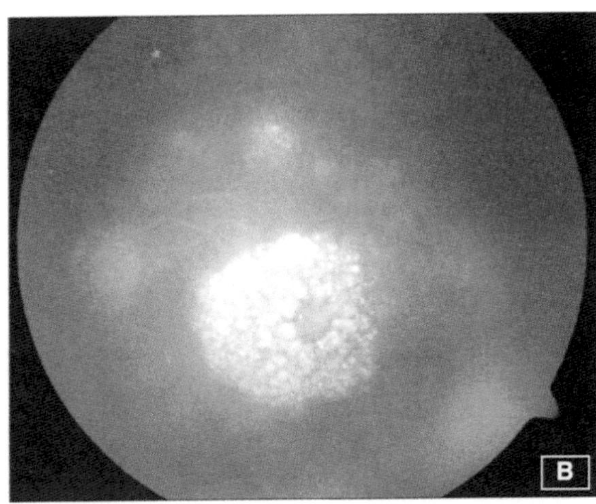

B

Optical Coherence Tomography

Macular thickness OCT scan through various angles confirmed the cystoid spaces with intervening septae (C and D).

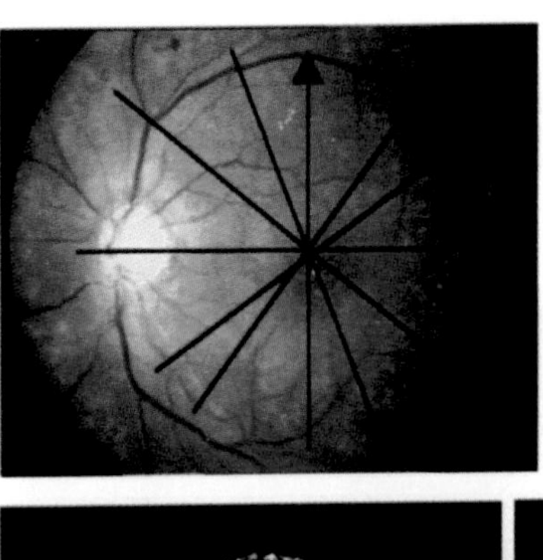

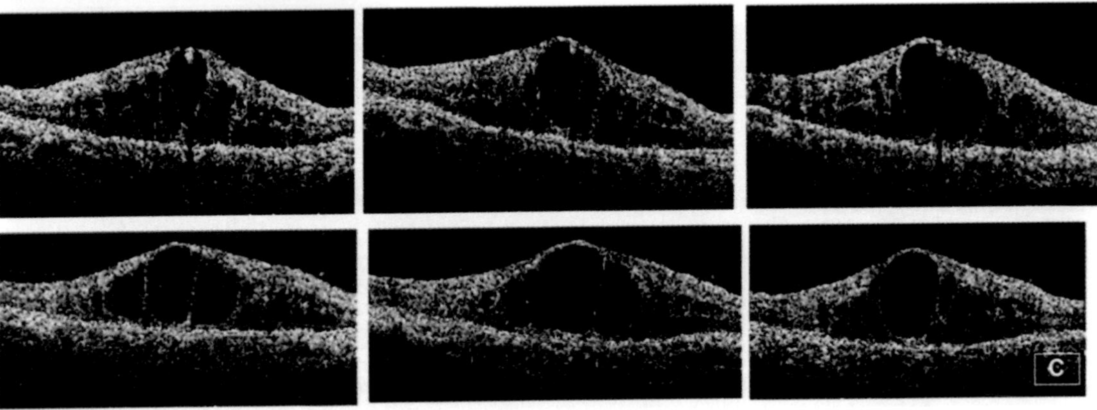

C

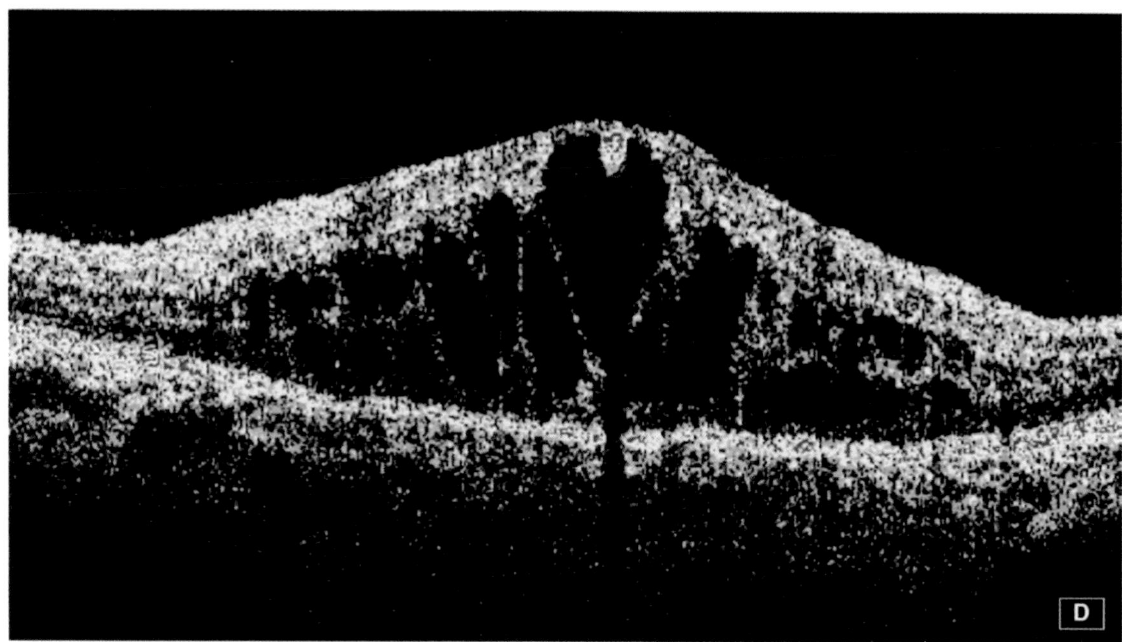

3. *Subfoveal Serous detachment.*

Case 5.5: CSME with Subfoveal Serous Retinal Detachment

Case Summary

A 50-year-old man was seen with non-proliferative diabetic retinopathy and macular edema (A). He had received two sessions of grid laser photocoagulation. His best-corrected visual acuity was 20/200 in the right eye. Fluorescein angiography of the right eye revealed microaneurysms with leak in the late phase (B).

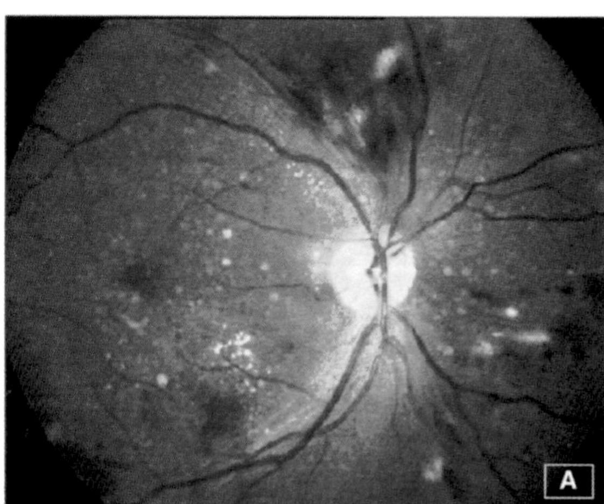

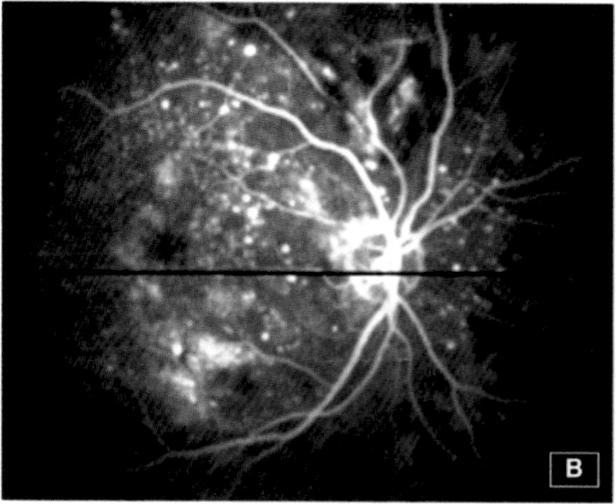

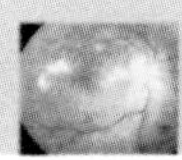

Optical Coherence Tomography

OCT (C) revealed increased macular thickening of 480 microns in the foveal center with hyporeflective areas corresponding to cysts in the retina. In addition, there was an area of hyporeflectivity in the subfoveal region consistent with subfoveal serous retinal detachment (arrow).

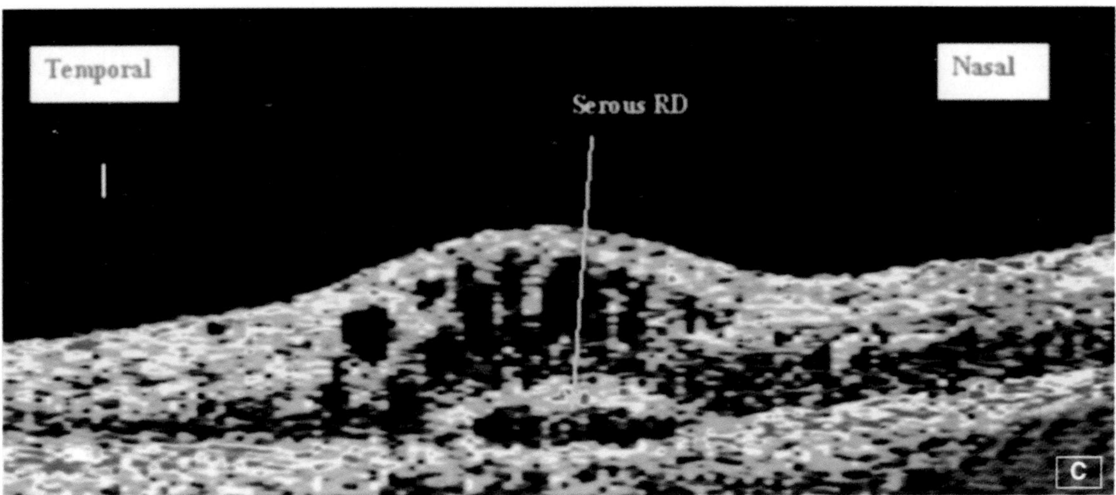

Case 5.6: Laser Induced Serous Retinal Detachment

Case Summary

A 46-year-old woman was seen with proliferative diabetic retinopathy and macular edema (A). Her best-corrected visual acuity was 20/20 in the left eye. Fluorescein angiography of the left eye revealed microaneurysms in the early phase that showed leak in the late phase and neovascularization elsewhere (NVE) (B).

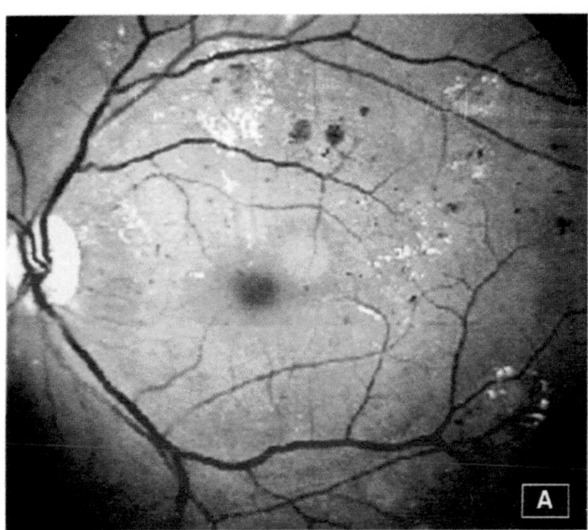

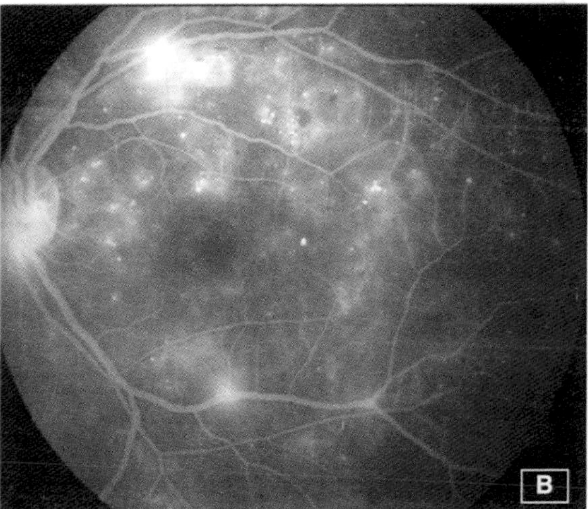

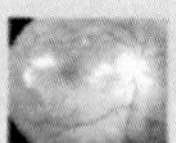

Optical Coherence Tomography

Horizontal line OCT scan through the foveal center (C) showed 'sponge-like retinal thickening' (pattern 1, sponge-like) with reduced backscatter from the outer retinal layers. No serous detachment was seen at this stage.

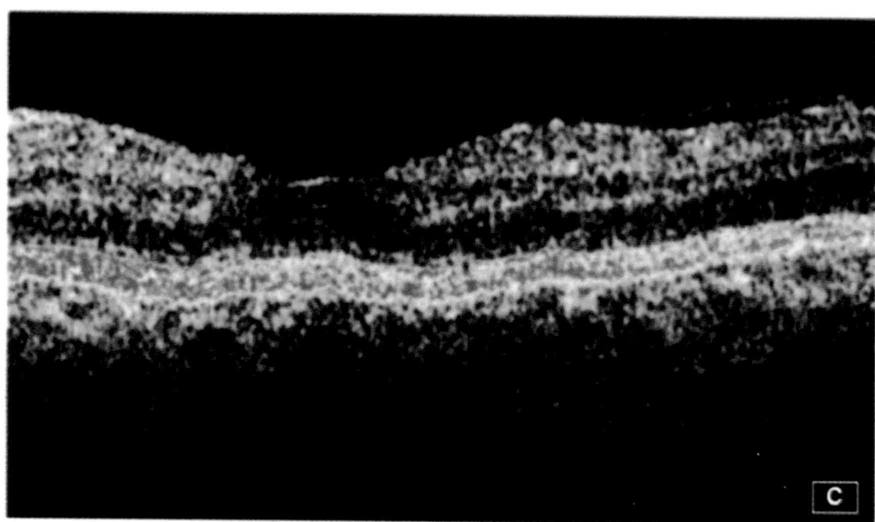

The patient received focal laser photocoagulation and panretinal photocoagulation (PRP) beginning in the nasal retina. The PRP was completed in three sittings done at an interval of one week. Following PRP, her vision was reduced to 20/60. Repeat OCT scan showed increased retinal thickness measuring 390 microns in the foveal center with hyporeflective areas corresponding to the retinal cysts with intervening septae and serous foveal detachment (patterns 2 and 3) (D). The posterior hyaloid membrane (PHM) was seen anteriorly that was attached to the foveal center.

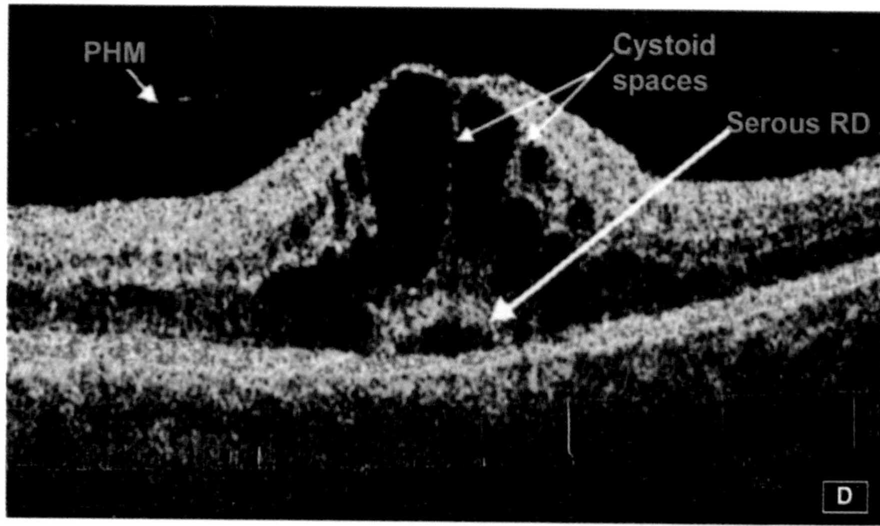

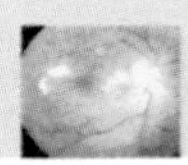

4. *Tractional detachment of fovea*
   Foveo-vitreal traction may result in detachment of the fovea. This can be diagnosed easily on OCT. This is an indication for pars plana vitrectomy to release the traction. Laser photocoagulation may only worsen the macular edema in such eyes.

Case 5.7: CSME with Tractional Foveal Detachment

Case Summary

A 65-year-old man was seen with non-proliferative diabetic retinopathy and macular edema (A). He had received grid laser 6 months ago with worsening of macular edema. His best-corrected visual acuity was 20/200 in the right eye. Fluorescein angiography of the right eye revealed microaneurysms with leak in the late phase (B). *Clinically we failed to visualize a foveo-vitreal traction.*

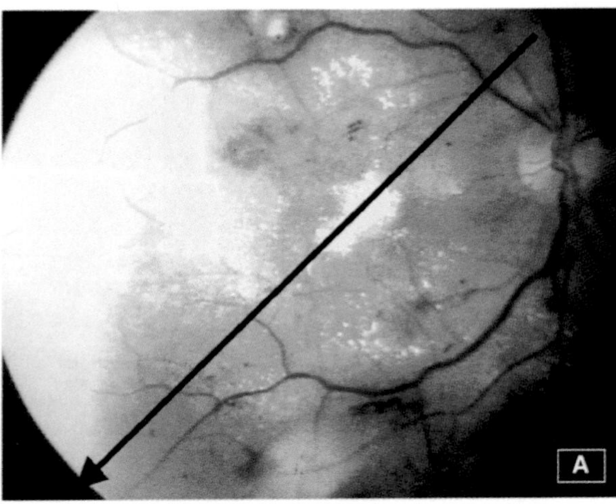
A

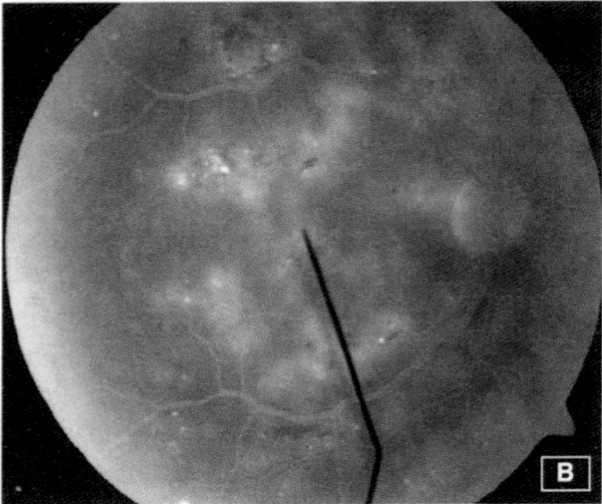
B

Optical Coherence Tomography

OCT line scan through 45 degrees (C) showed increased retinal thickening with vitreoschisis, i.e. splitting of posterior vitreous phase into two lamellae. The posterior lamina of vitreoschisis caused focal traction on the fovea resulting in underlying tractional retinal detachment. Laser photocoagulation of macula in this setting would surely worsen the detachment and the macular edema.

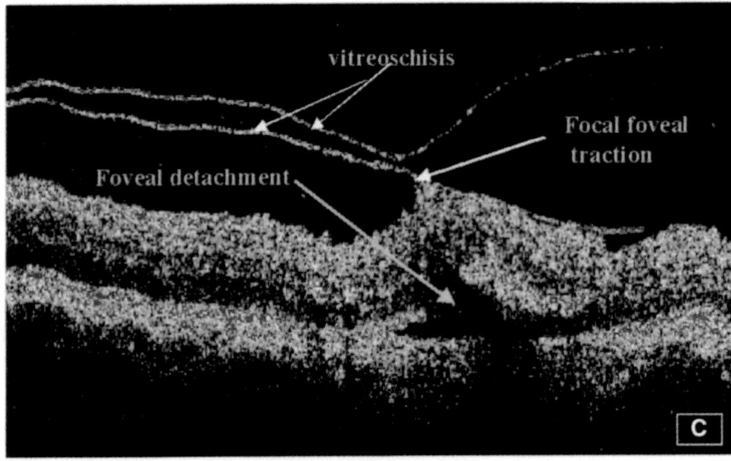

C

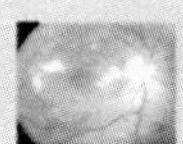

5. *Taut posterior hyloid membrane (TPHM):* TPHM may result in recalcitrant macular edema with foveal detachment that can be diagnosed easily on OCT, even when subclinical. In advanced cases, it can be diagnosed clinically as taut, shiny, glistening membrane with retinal striae on biomicroscopic retinal examination. CSME with TPHM is generally non- responsive to laser and an indication for pars plana vitrectomy. *OCT helps in identification of TPHM that may not be apparent clinically.*

Case 5.8: CSME with Clinically Unapparent TPHM.

Case Summary

A 45-year-old man with type II diabetes of 14 years duration was seen with proliferative diabetic retinopathy and macular edema (A). He had unsuccessfully received 3 sessions of grid laser photocoagulation. His best-corrected visual acuity was 20/300 in the left eye. Fluorescein angiography of the left eye revealed microaneurysms with leak in the late phase with neovascularization elsewhere (NVE) (B).

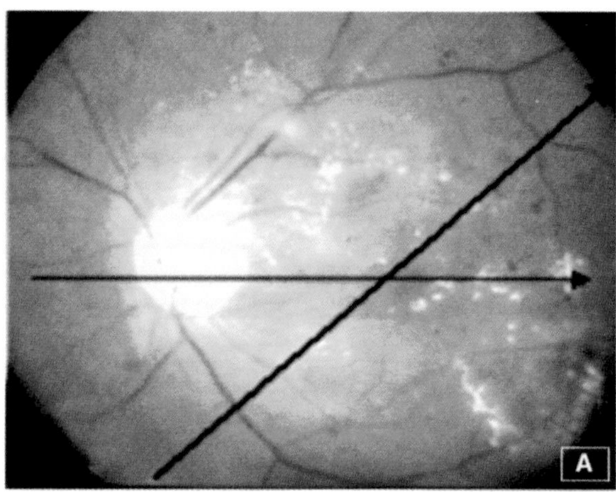

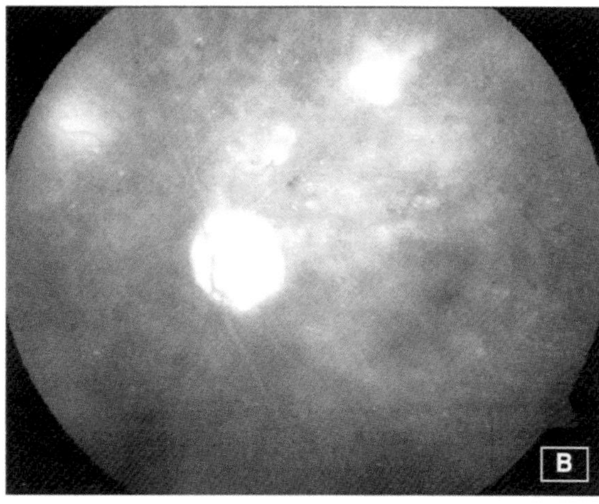

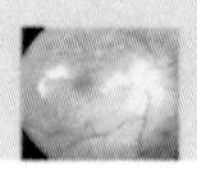

Optical Coherence Tomography

OCT line scan (C and D) showed increased retinal thickening in the center of macula measuring 720 microns with Taut posterior hyloid membrane (TPHM)(arrow) and underlying foveal retinal detachment.

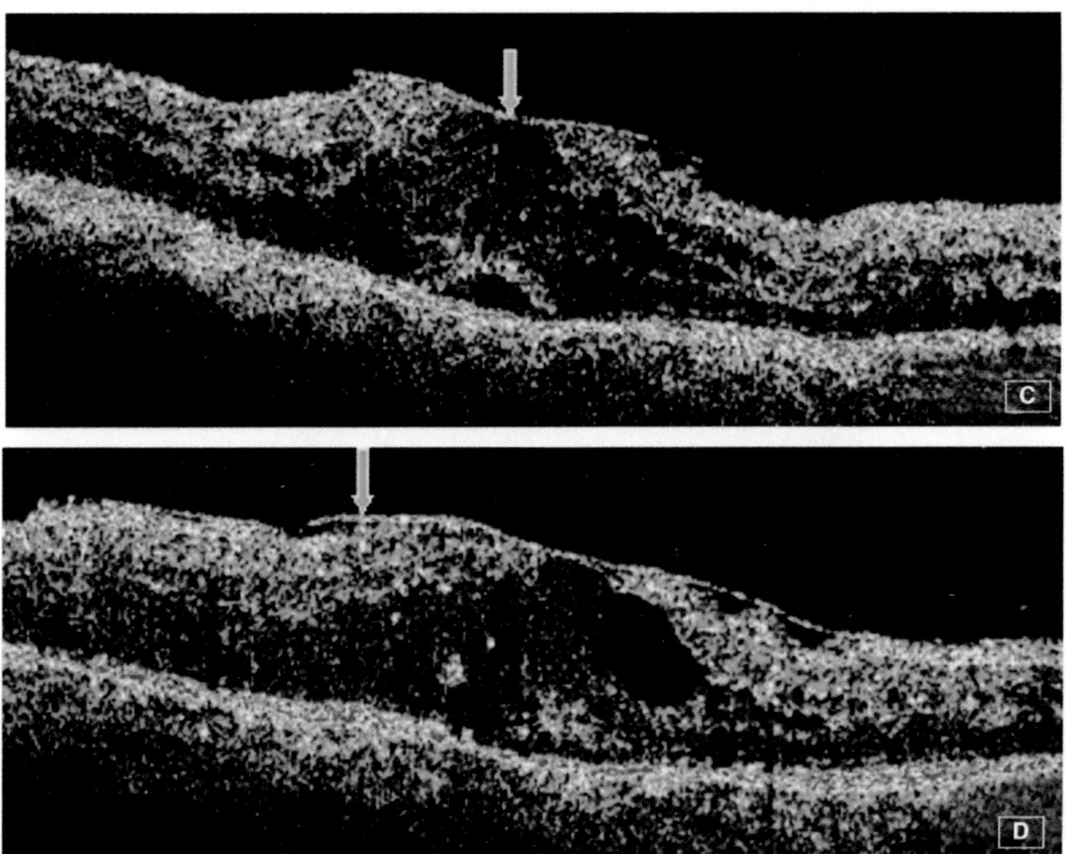

B. MANAGEMENT AND LONGITUDINAL TRACKING OF TISSUE CHANGES IN DIABETIC MACULAR EDEMA ON OCT

Case 5.9: OCT Following Focal Laser Photocoagulation

Case Summary

A-50-year-old Type II diabetic man was seen with clinically significant macular edema in the right eye (A) that showed areas of focal leakage on fluorescein angiography (B). The patient underwent laser photocoagulation for the same.

Optical Coherence Tomography

Vertical OCT line scan (C) showed increased retinal thickness measuring 290 microns with reduced backscattering due to intraretinal fluid accumulation and hyper-reflective hard exudates.

Three months following laser photocoagulation, his macular edema showed resolution with few residual hard exudates (D). Repeat OCT scan (E) showed normal foveal contour with retinal thickness reduced to 180 microns in the foveal center. The superior retina showed reduced backscattering from the outer retinal layers. The hard exudates were seen as hyper-reflective shadows.

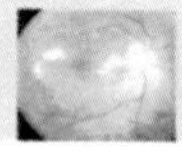

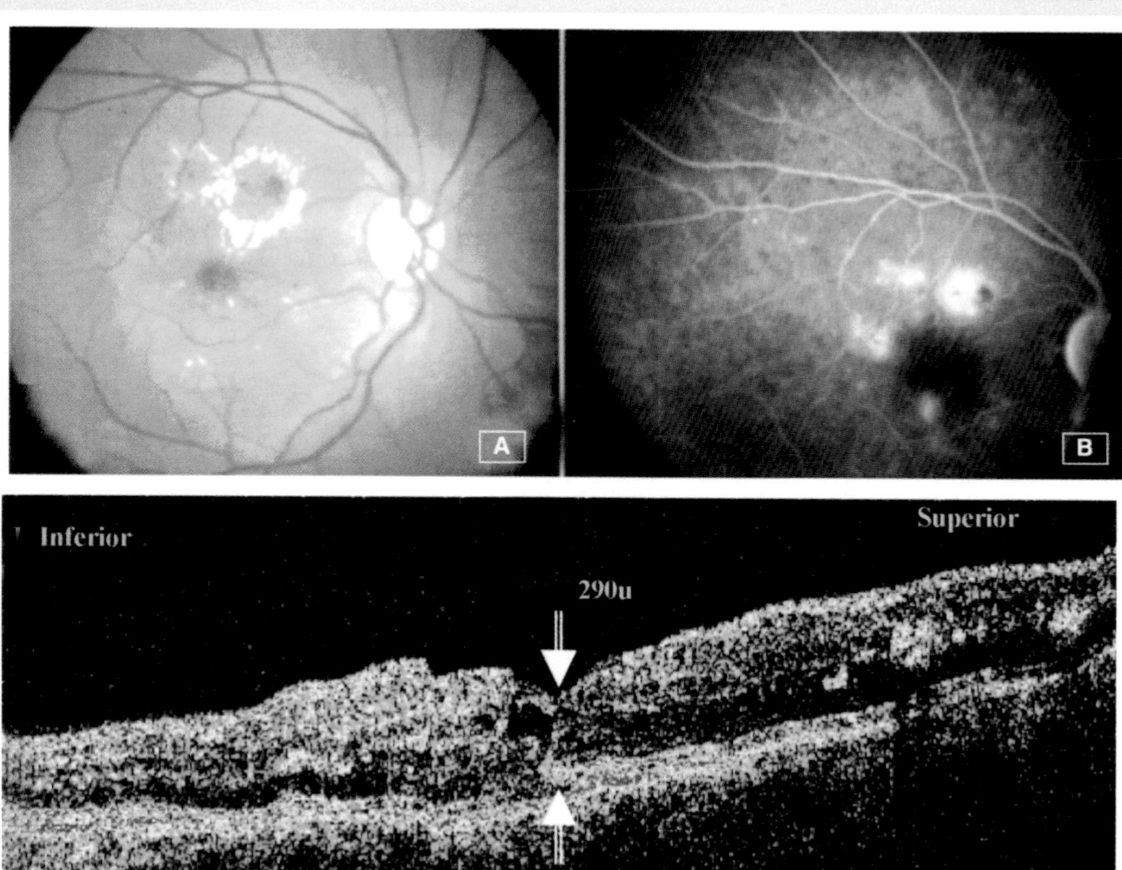
A
B
Inferior
Superior
290u
C

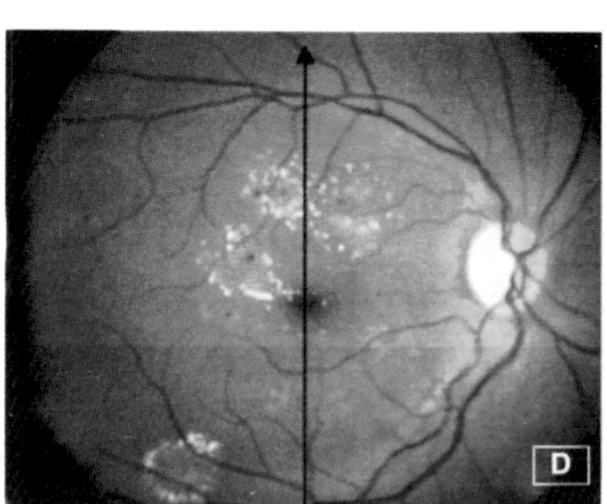
D

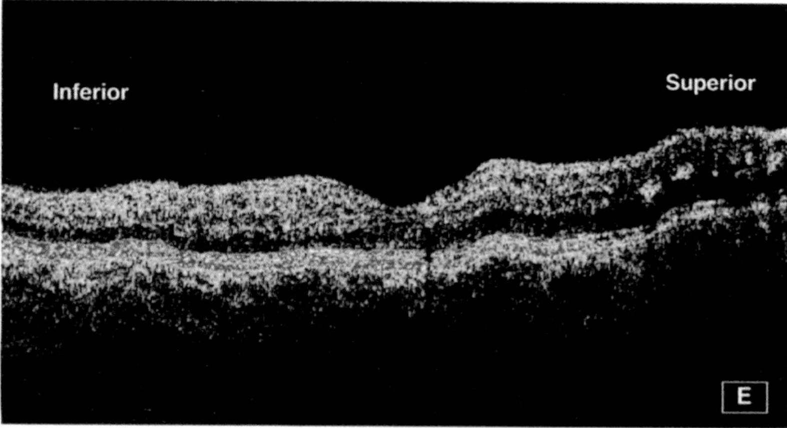
Inferior
Superior
E

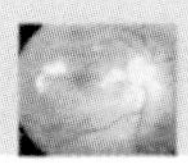

Case 5.10: Focal Laser Photocoagulation Induced Subfoveal Serous Retinal Detachment

Case Summary

A 46-year-old man with type II diabetes was seen with CSME in the left eye (A). His best-corrected visual acuity was 20/30.

Optical Coherence Tomography

OCT line scan through the fovea (B) showed the central retinal thickness measuring 232 microns with reduced backscatter from the outer retinal layers and hyper-reflective hard exudates.

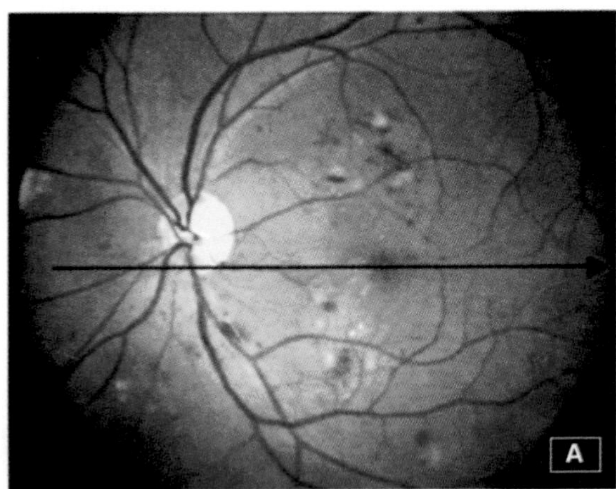

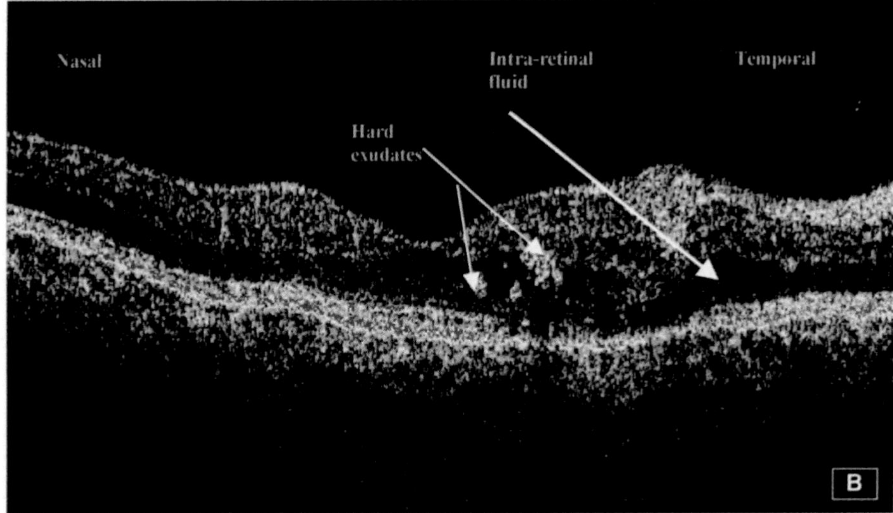

The patient received focal laser photocoagulation of the microaneurysms in this eye. Six weeks later, his visual acuity in this eye was 20/40 (C). Repeat OCT scan (D) showed retinal thickness increased to 650 microns with subfoveal serous retinal detachment and overlying cystoid spaces in the inner retina.

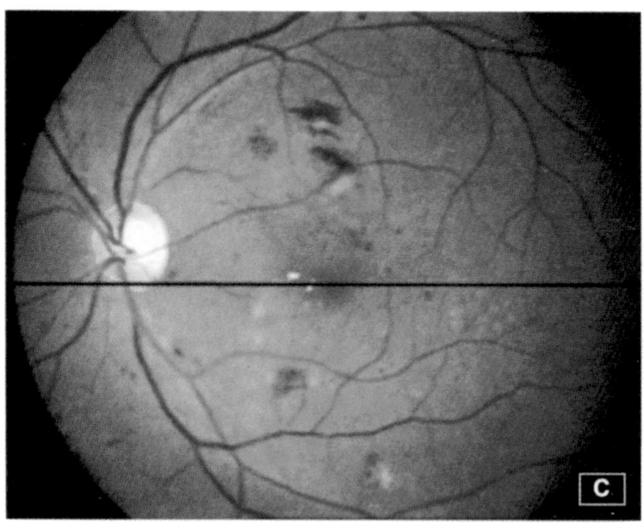

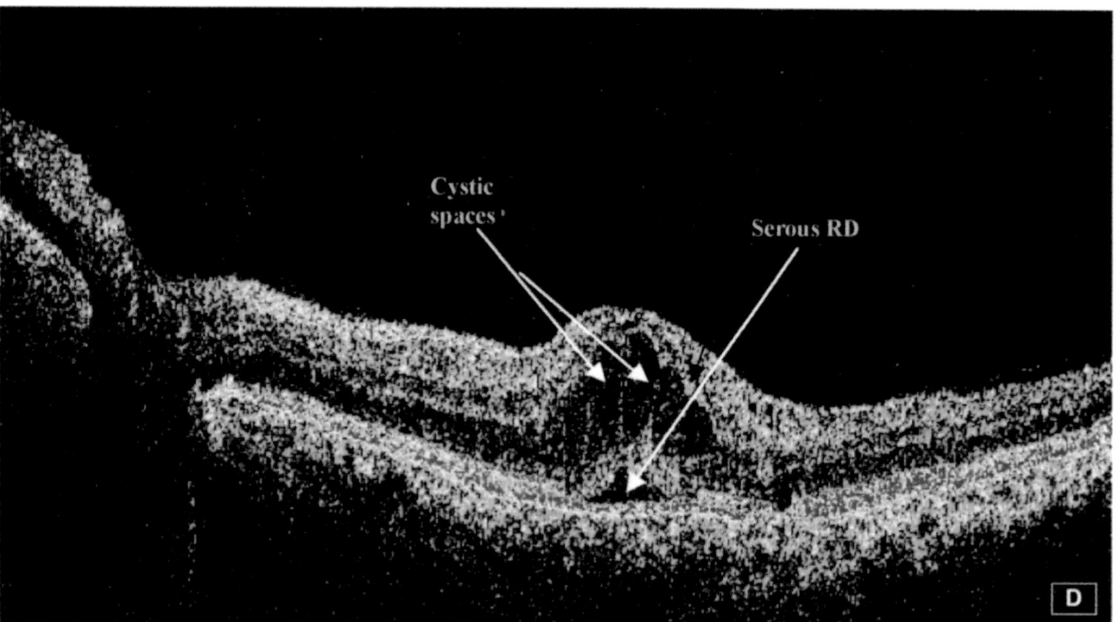

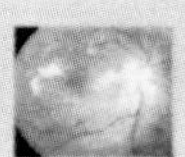

Case 5.11: OCT Guided Pars Plana Vitrectomy for Taut Posterior Hyloid Membrane (TPHM)

Case Summary

A 52-year-old man was seen with recalcitrant CSME in the left eye that had not responded to multiple sessions of grid laser photocoagulation (A). His best-corrected visual acuity was 20/100 in this eye. Fluorescein angiography (B) revealed diffuse leak from microaneurysms and capillary bed with leak from NVE along the upper temporal arcade.

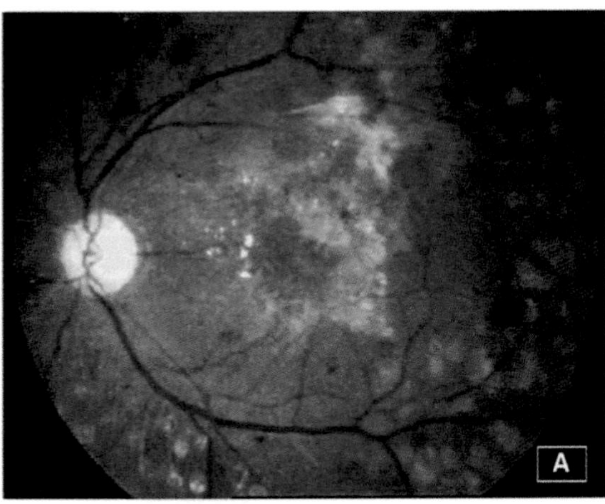

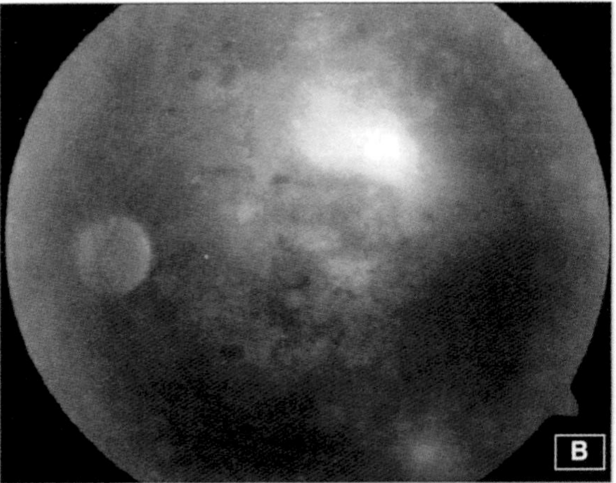

Optical Coherence Tomography

OCT (C) showed loss of foveal contour with increased retinal thickening in the center of macula measuring 610 microns with a hyper-reflective membrane at the vitreoretinal interface suggesting a taut posterior hyloid membrane (TPHM) (arrow) causing foldings of underlying retina probably representing internal limiting membrane folds. The neurosensory retina showed hyporeflective areas suggestive of cysts in the retina that could be probably caused by traction by TPHM.

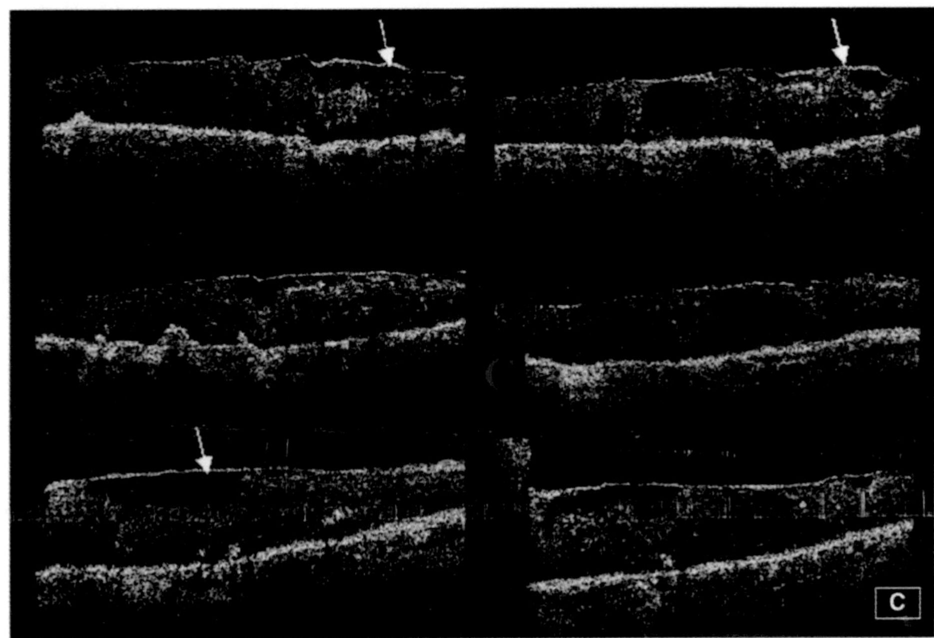

The retinal thickness map analysis showed a thickening of 470 microns in the foveal center (D).

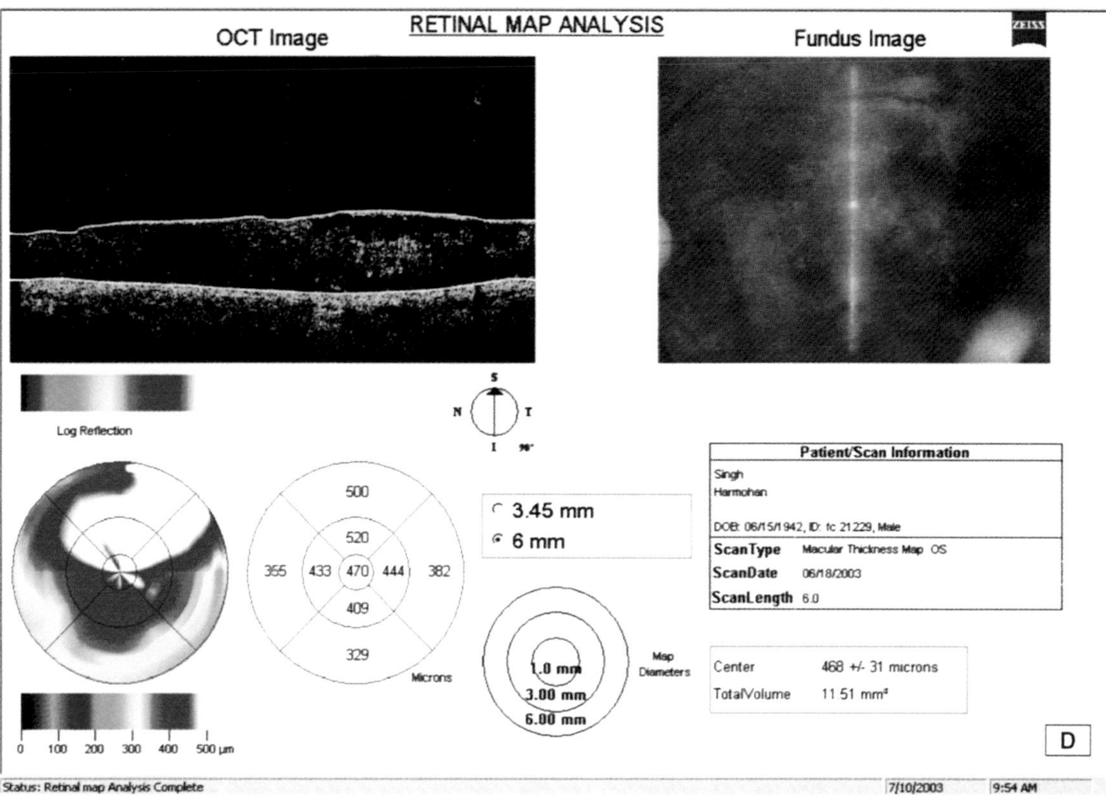

Based on OCT findings, the patient was elected to undergo pars plana vitrectomy in this eye. Four days after surgery, his visual acuity improved to 20/80 (E). Repeat OCT scan (F) showed no hyper-reflective membrane at the vitreo-retinal interface though the retinal folds and cysts were persistent. Thus, in this patient, TPHM was contributing significantly to the persistent macular edema that had failed to respond to the conventional laser photocoagulation.

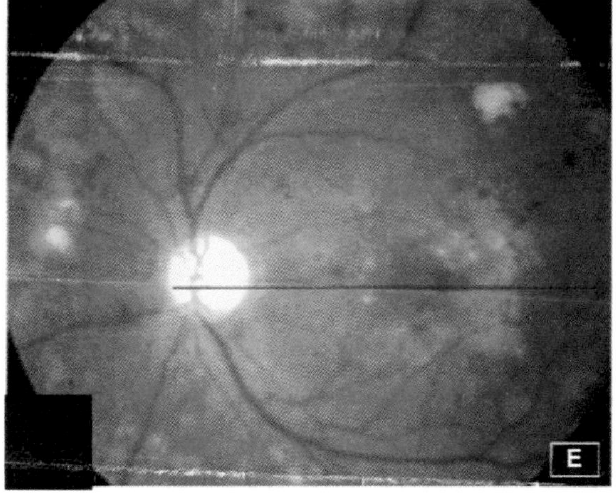

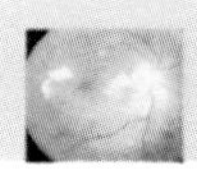

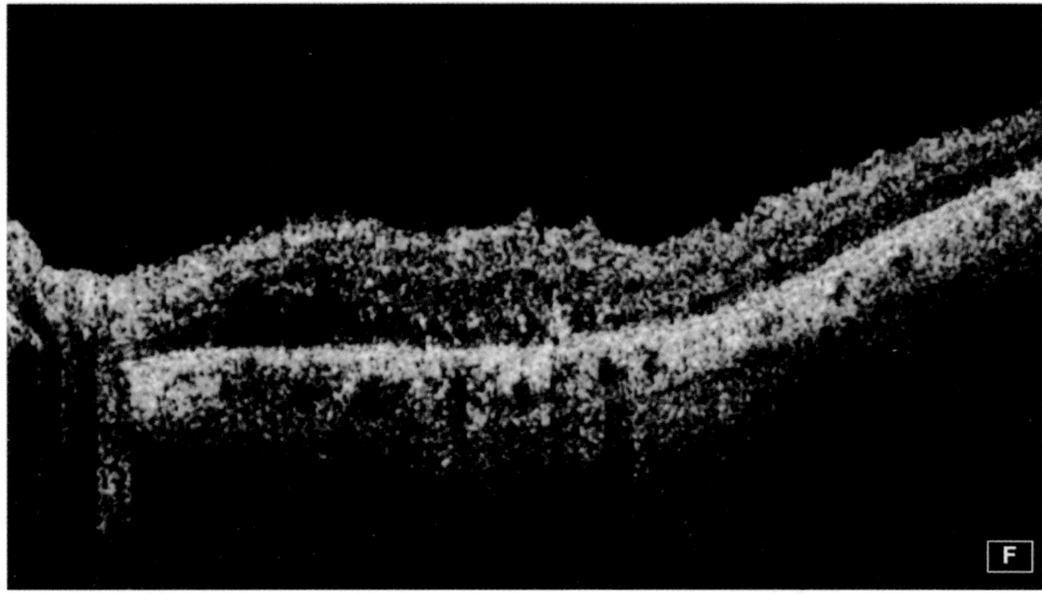

The retinal map thickness chart 4 days postoperatively showed central foveal thickness reduced to 331 microns (G).

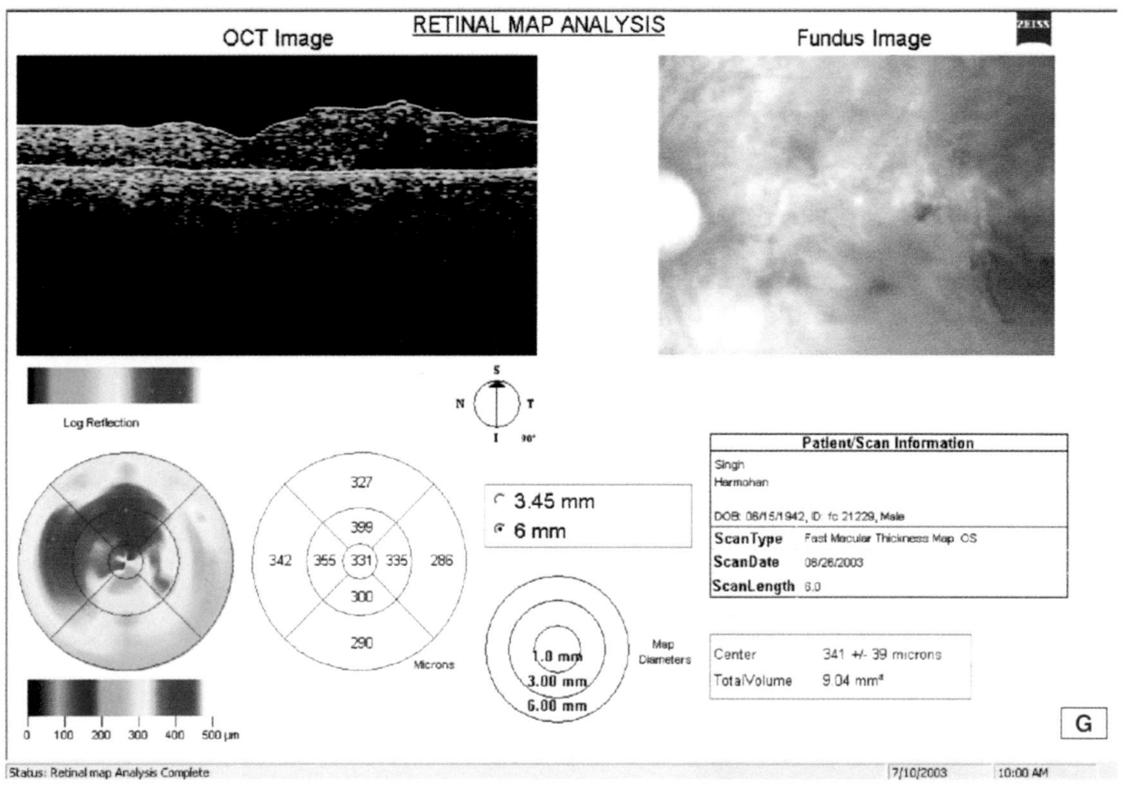

Two weeks postoperatively, his best corrected visual acuity was 20/60 (H). Repeat OCT scan (horizontal) showed the normal foveal contour with no hyloid causing retinal traction and resolution of retinal folds (I). Retinal mapping done 2 weeks postoperatively showed a central retinal thickness measuring 233 microns. **Thus, in this patient OCT played a crucial role in deciding an appropriate management strategy**.

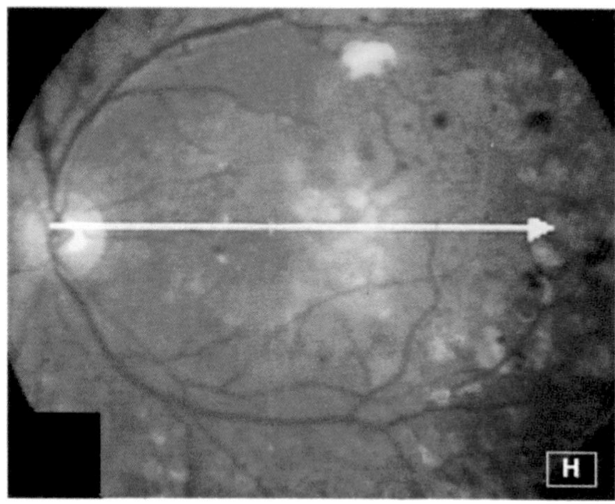

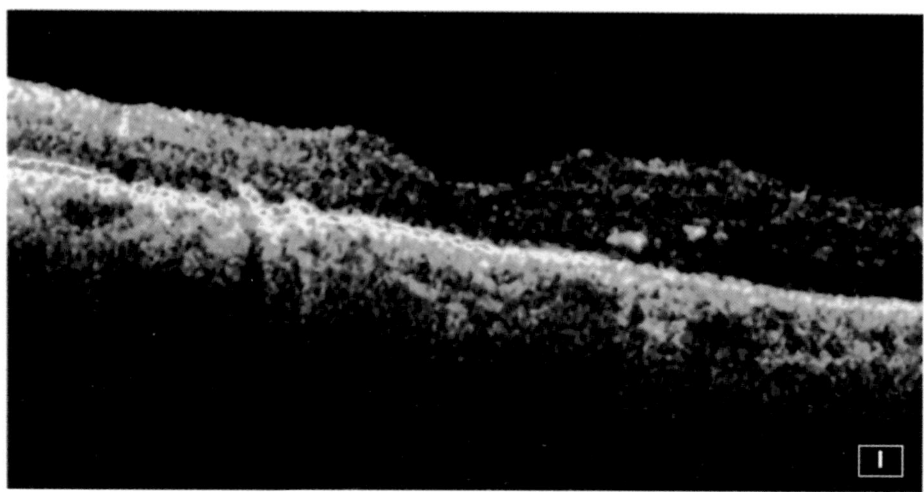

Case 5.12: Intravitreal Triamcinolone Acetonide in Diabetic Macular Edema

Case Summary

A 52- year-old man with non-insulin-dependent diabetes mellitus of 20 years duration was seen with recalcitrant CSME in the left eye that had not responded to multiple sessions of grid laser photocoagulation (A). His best-corrected visual acuity was 20/200 in this eye. Fluorescein angiography revealed diffuse leak from microaneurysms with irregular foveal avascular zone (B).

Optical Coherence Tomography

OCT showed loss of foveal contour with retinal thickness measuring 560 microns in the foveal center. OCT also demonstrated cystic spaces within the retinal layers (C).The patient elected to receive intravitreal triamcinolone acetonide 4 mg. Follow-up scan at 3 weeks showed reduction in the foveal thickness to 273

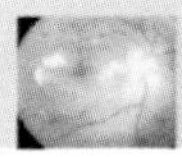

microns and the visual acuity improved to 20/80 (D). The microaneurysms now could be better delineated on fluorescein angiography for which supplement photocoagulation was done. Follow-up OCT at 8 weeks and then at 12 weeks showed further improvement in visual acuity to 20/30.OCT demonstrated return of foveal contour, disappearance of retinal cysts with reduction in macular edema (E,F).

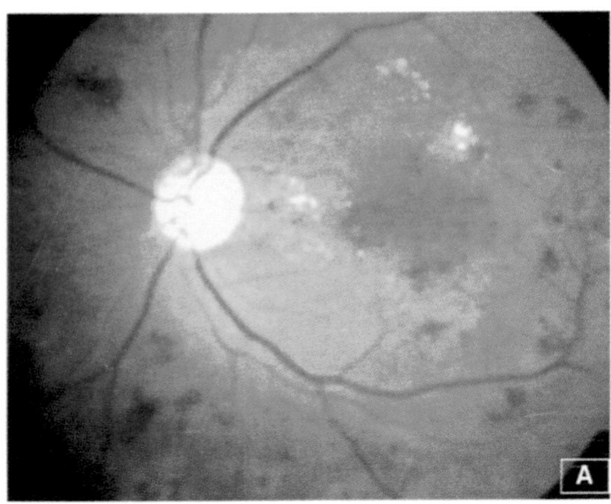

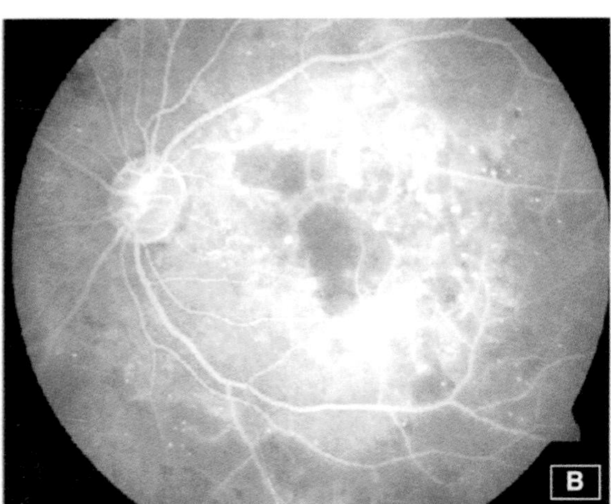

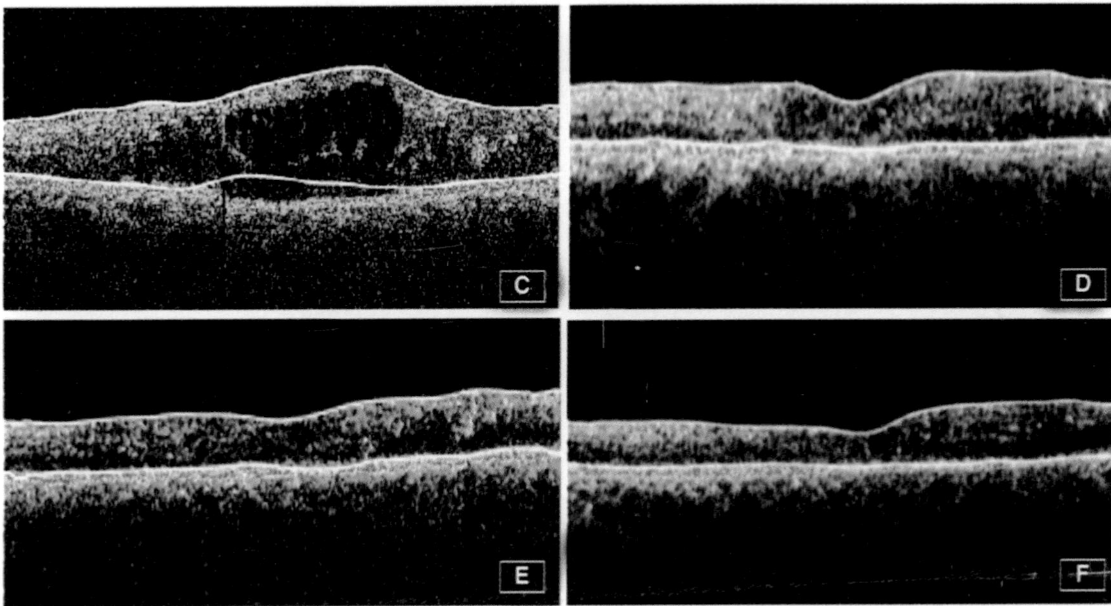

C.OCT GUIDED INDICATIONS OF PARS PLANA VITRECTOMY

Case 5.13: OCT Guided Pars Plana Vitrectomy for Subfoveal Serous Retinal Detachment

Case Summary

A 39-year old man had proliferative diabetic retinopathy and CSME with nasal traction in the left eye (A). His best-corrected visual acuity was 20/200 in this eye. Fluorescein angiography (B) revealed leak from NVD and NVE.

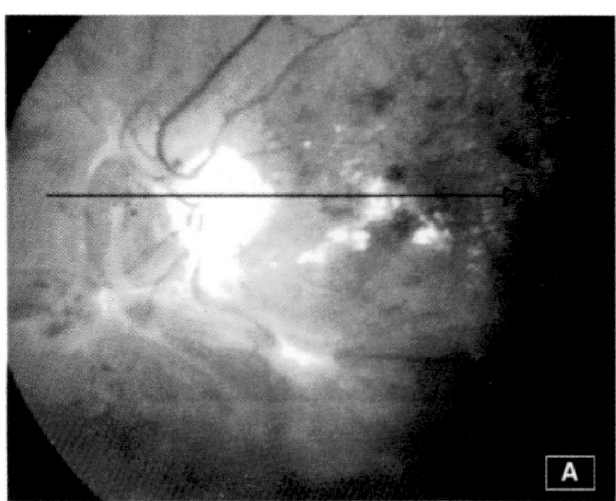

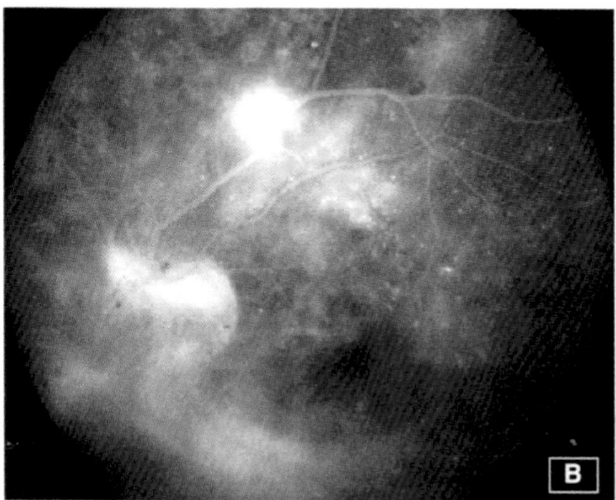

Optical Coherence Tomography

OCT line scan through the foveal center showed loss of foveal contour with retinal thickness measuring 360 microns through the foveal center. There was associated serous retinal detachment under the fovea (C).

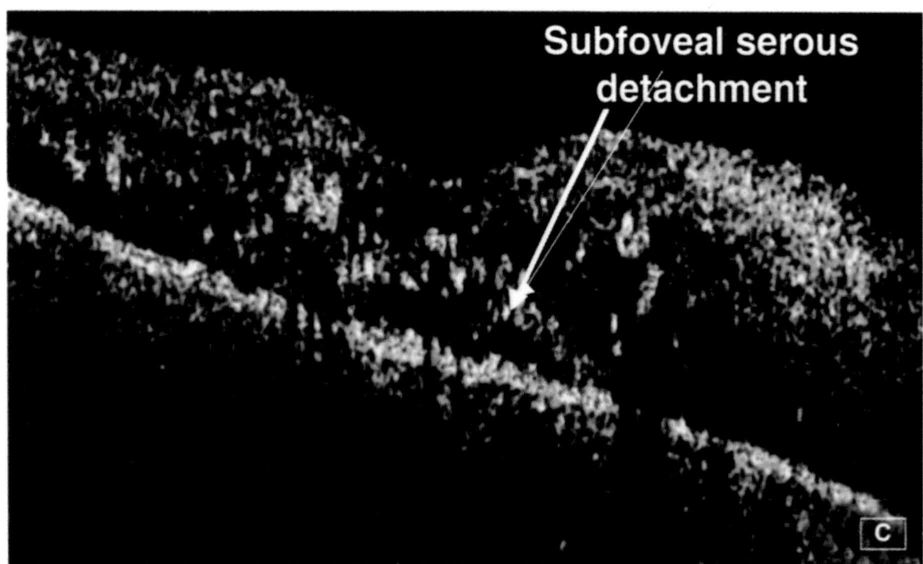

The patient underwent pars plana vitrectomy (PPV). Three months later, his visual acuity had improved to 20/30 with resolution of CSME (D, E).

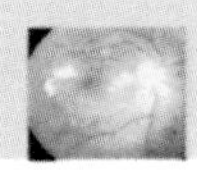

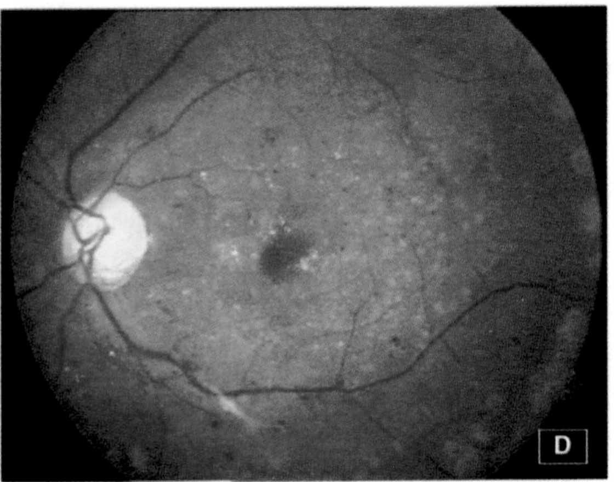

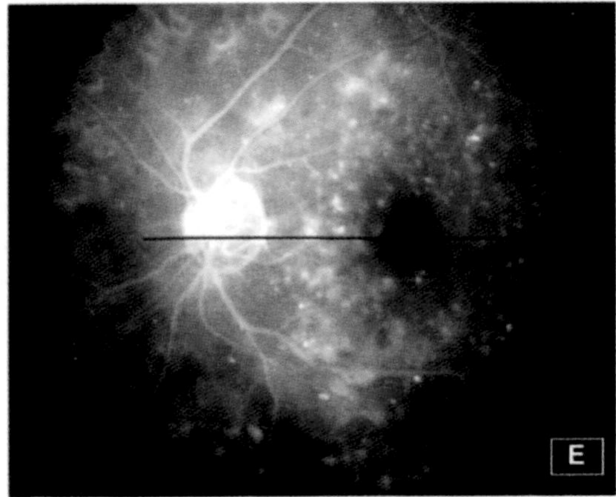

Repeat OCT scan done 3 months later showed reduced foveal thickness in the center measuring 270 microns with resolution of serous retinal detachment (F) and persistence of residual fluid nasal to the fovea. **In this patient, the clinical examination had shown an extramacular tractional detachment, conventionally not an indication for PPV. However, OCT scan showed an associated serous macular detachment, possibly induced by extramacular traction that resolved immediately on removal of traction by PPV. The OCT played a major role in defining an indication for PPV.**

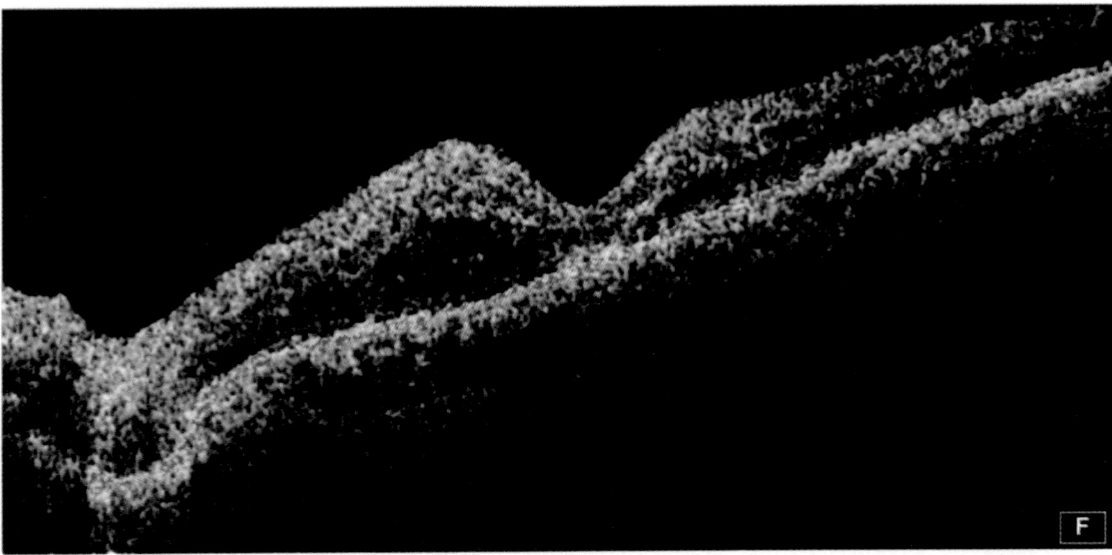

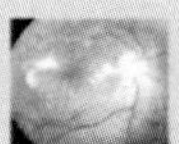

Case 5.14: Pars Plana Vitrectomy for Taut Posterior Hyloid Membrane

Case Summary

A 42-year-old Type II diabetic woman was seen with proliferative diabetic retinopathy with CSME (A). She underwent PRP for the same, following which her pre-retinal blood reduced but she developed recalcitrant CSME with taut posterior hyloid membrane (TPHM) that didn't respond to grid laser photocoagulation (B).

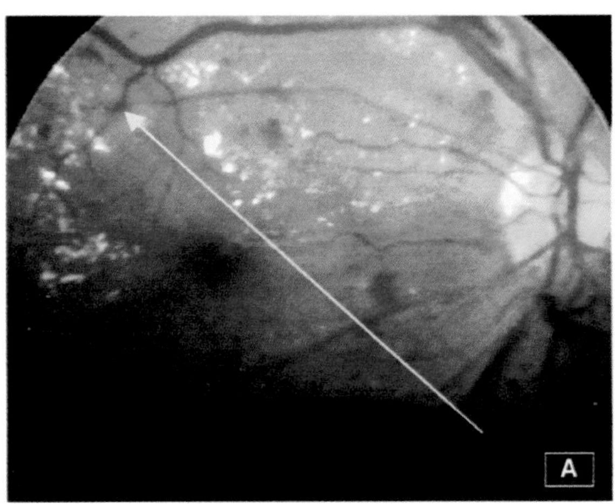

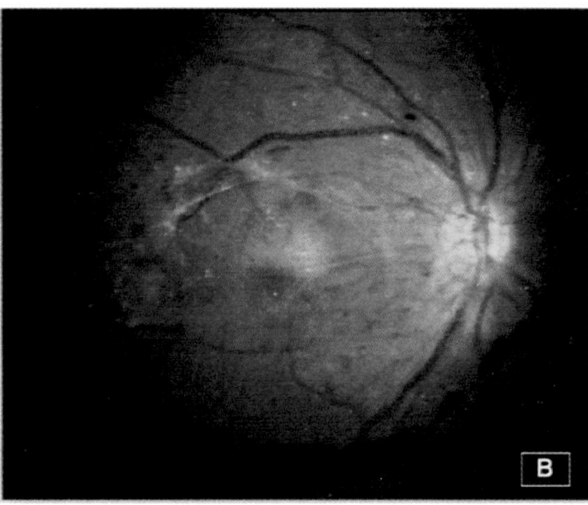

Optical Coherence Tomography

OCT R/E (C) showed loss of foveal contour with retinal thickness measuring 740 microns in the foveal center.The neurosensory retina showed the presence hyporeflective spaces suggestive of cystoid macular edema. Another hyporeflective area under the fovea was suggestive of serous retinal detachment. The posterior hyloid membrane was attached to the foveal center probably resulting in foveal traction.

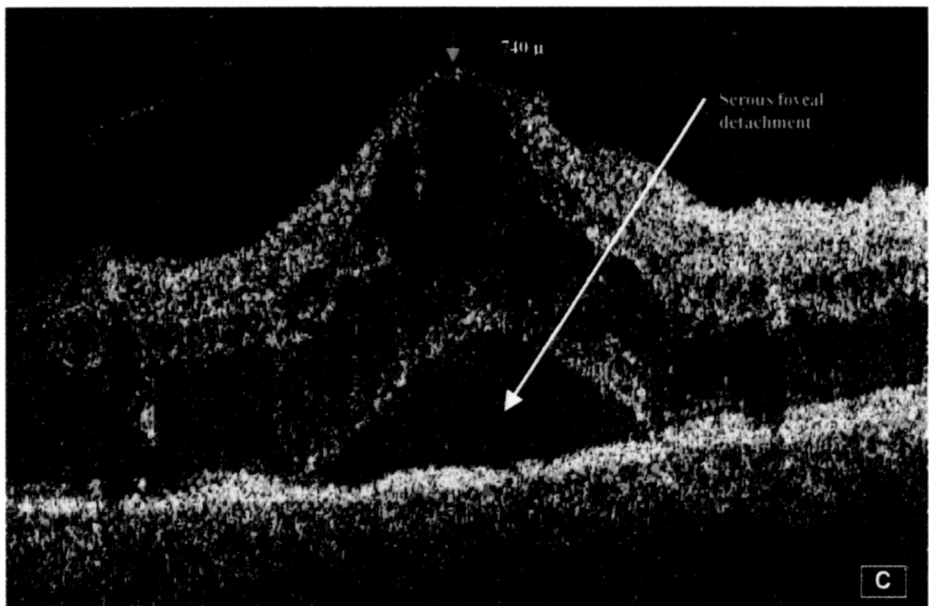

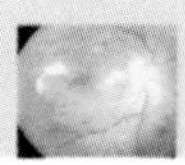

Patient underwent R/E pars plana vitrectomy. Two months later, her visual acuity had improved to 20/40 with resolution of CSME (D). Repeat OCT showed resolution of retinal thickening and CME (E). The central foveal thickness was reduced to 270 microns and there was persistence of serous retinal detachment as well as hyporeflectivity in the outer retinal layers suggestive of fluid.

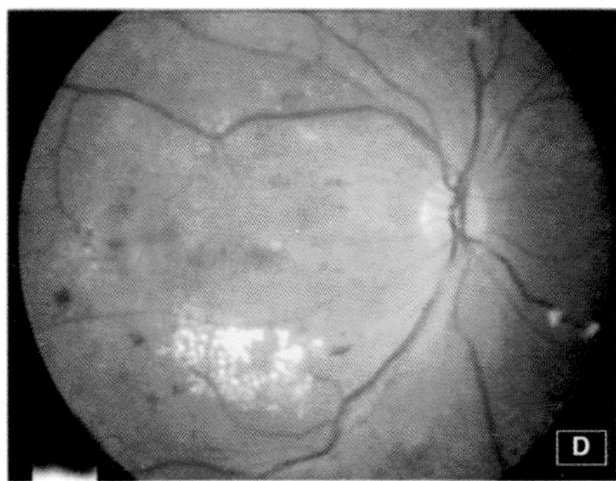

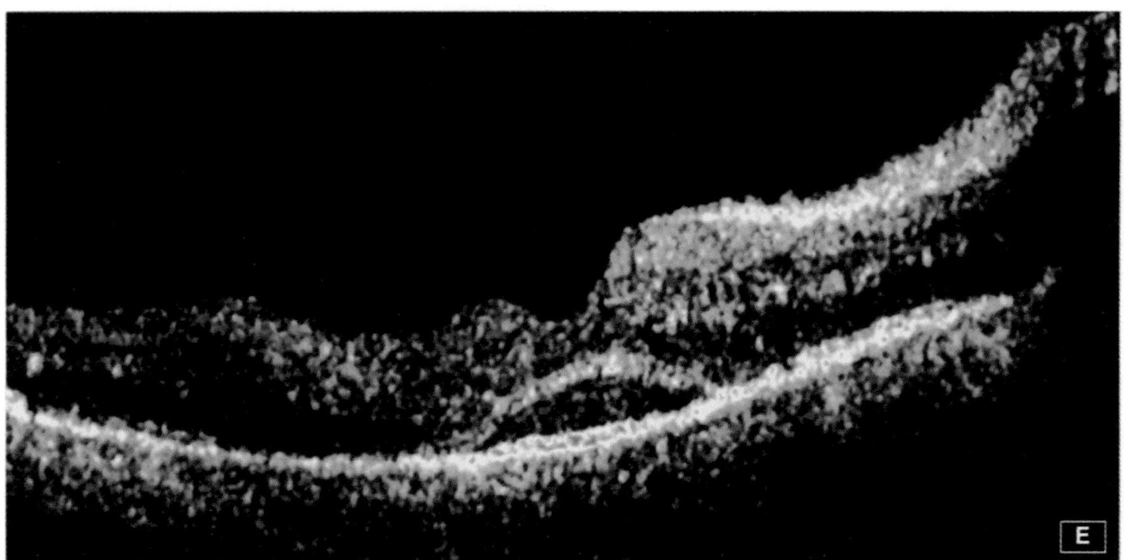

Over the next 7 months, the macular edema reappeared with the reappearance of cystoid spaces, increase in serous detachment and the presence of hyper-reflective membrane on the retinal surface (F, G). The patient was also diagnosed to have nephropathy and was advised for the management for the same. She was found to be metabolically unstable that could have resulted in deterioration as was documented on OCT. This case illustrates that diabetic macular edema is multifactorial in etiology and all the aspects need to taken care of in the management of these patients.

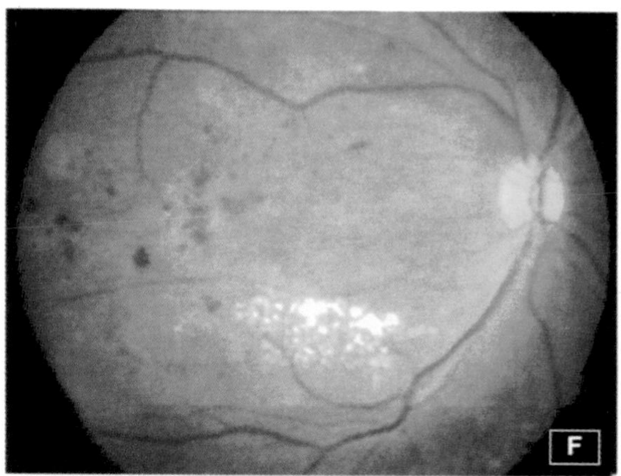

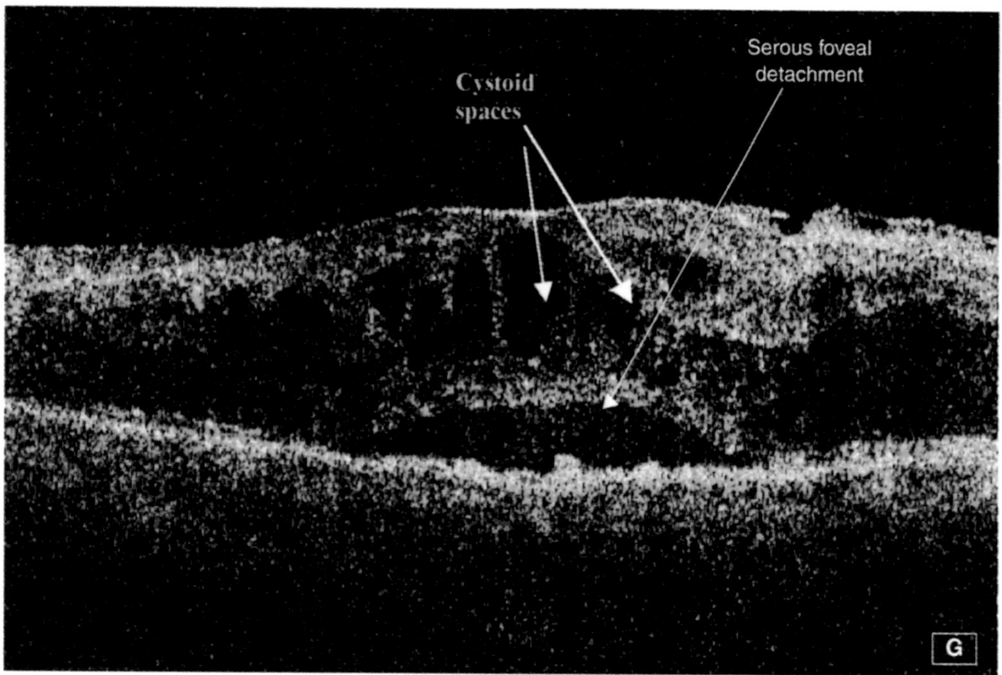

CONCLUSIONS

From these cases, it becomes apparent that OCT has a definitive role to play in the routine management of diabetic macular edema. In many of these patients, the decision regarding the management strategy was based on OCT findings that mostly complemented fluorescein angiography. Pattern 1, i.e. sponge-like thickening was an indication for focal/grid laser photocoagulation. Pattern 2, i.e. cystoid macular edema shows a good response to intravitreal triamcinolone acetonide where OCT helps in close monitoring following the injection. Pattern 3, i.e. subfoveal serous retinal detachment could be laser induced or caused by associated traction, the latter being an indication for PPV. Patterns 4 and 5, i.e. tractional foveal detachment and TPHM either alone or in conjunction with patterns 2 and 3 constitute an indication for surgical intervention.

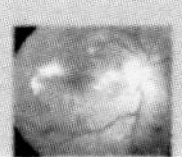

SUGGESTED READINGS

1. Massin P, Duguid G, Erginay A, Haouchine B, Gaudric A. Optical coherence tomography for evaluating diabetic macular edema before and after vitrectomy. Am J Ophthalmol 2003; 135 : 169-77.
2. Goebel W, Kretzchmar-Gross T. Retinal thickness in diabetic retinopathy: A study using optical coherence tomography (OCT).Retina 2002; 22 : 759-67.
3. Hee MR, Puliafito CA, Duker JS et al. Topography of diabetic macular edema with optical coherence tomography. Ophthalmology 1998 ; 105: 360-70.
4. Otani T, Kishi S, Maruyama Y. Patterns of diabetic macular edema with optical coherence tomography. Am J Ophthalmol. 1999 127 : 688-93.

Chapter 6

Idiopathic Central Serous Chorioretinopathy (ICSC)

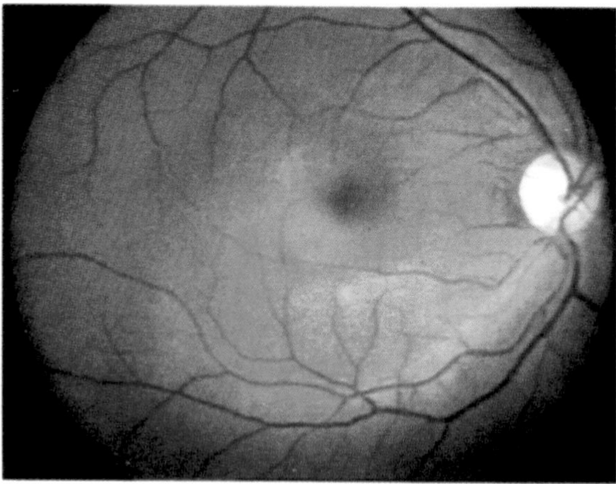

Idiopathic Central Serous Chorioretinopathy (ICSC) is typically a disease of young and middle aged males that is characterized by the accumulation of fluid between the neurosensory retina and Retinal Pigment Epithelium (RPE).The disease is more common in patients with Type A personalities. There may be associated pigment epithelial detachment (PED) seen in some cases. Fluorescein angiography helps in the diagnosis and has well described patterns, i.e.

Expanding Dot sign: The fluorescein diffuses out of the choriocapillaris as a round spot of hyperfluorescence that corresponds to the size of RPE. The hyperfluorescent dot increases in the late phase with diffusion of the dye.

Smock-stack sign: In less than 10% of the cases, the dye streams upward to form umbrella pattern of fluorescein staining.

OCT IN ICSC

A. OCT Patterns in Typical ICSC

Like fluorescein angiography, OCT also shows certain characteristic features in typical ICSC including:

1. *Serous retinal detachment:* This is characterized by the elevation of neurosensory retina due to fluid accumulation between the RPE and neurosensory retina. This fluid was seen to get absorbed in 4-8 weeks leaving no residual changes behind.

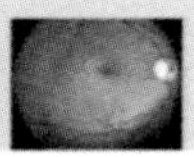

2. *Serous retinal detachment with pigment epithelial detachment:* Contrary to the popular belief that PED was an uncommon feature of ICSC, OCT depicted PED in almost all cases of ICSC. As would be shown in the following cases, the PED in these patients corresponded to the point of leak seen on fluorescein angiography. The PED was very slow to regress and in few patients it was persistent even after a year following the initial episode.

B. OCT in Diagnosing Complications of ICSC

ICSC could be complicated by choroidal neovascular membrane, subretinal fibrin, RPE rip or neurosensory atrophy of the fovea. All these features can be accurately depicted on OCT that helps not only in making early diagnosis and management but also in prognosticating the outcome in these patients.

C. OCT in Atypical ICSC

1. *Small PEDs:* In few patients, PED may be very small that cannot be diagnosed on conventional techniques of fundus examination. We found OCT to be a very useful tool in diagnosing small PED in such cases and to differentiate it from other lesions including macular cysts. In cases where serous detachment is very small, OCT is very sensitive in depicting small changes of neurosensory retina. OCT also helps in differentiating pigment epithelial detachment from serous detachment.
2. *Chronic ICSC:* Long standing ICSC shows flask-shaped mottled areas of depigmentation. Fluorescein angiography shows mottled areas of hyperfluorescence that fade during late phase of angiograms. These cases may at times be misdiagnosed due to lack of suspicion. OCT is helpful in these cases by depicting PEDs that persist even though the associated serous fluid is minimal or absent. We, in our experience, found that the RPE in these patients was irregular and thrown into folds with minimal fluid beneath it. These changes in RPE could represent either resolving PED or more likely, the 'sick-RPE', thus indicating that the sick RPE is probably responsible for chronicity of the disease.
3. *ICSC in elderly:* It is a well established fact that ICSC can occur in the elderly patients above 50 years of age where the presentation might be atypical. Also the differential diagnosis at this age would include Age related macular degeneration, metastatic deposits, etc. OCT helps in differentiating these diseases from ICSC. Because of the sharp demarcation between the neurosensory retina and serous fluid, OCT helps in confirming the existence of subretinal fluid that can differentiate ICSC from other RPE and choriocapillary abnormalities.

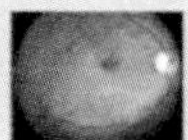

OCT PATTERNS INTYPICAL ICSC

Pattern 1: Serous Retinal Detachment

Case 6.1: ICSC with Serous Retinal Detachment

Case Summary

A 51-year-old woman was seen with complaints of diminished vision in her right eye of 2 months duration. Her best corrected visual acuity was 20/40 in this eye. Fluorescein angiography showed expanding dot sign, thus confirming the diagnosis of ICSC (A).

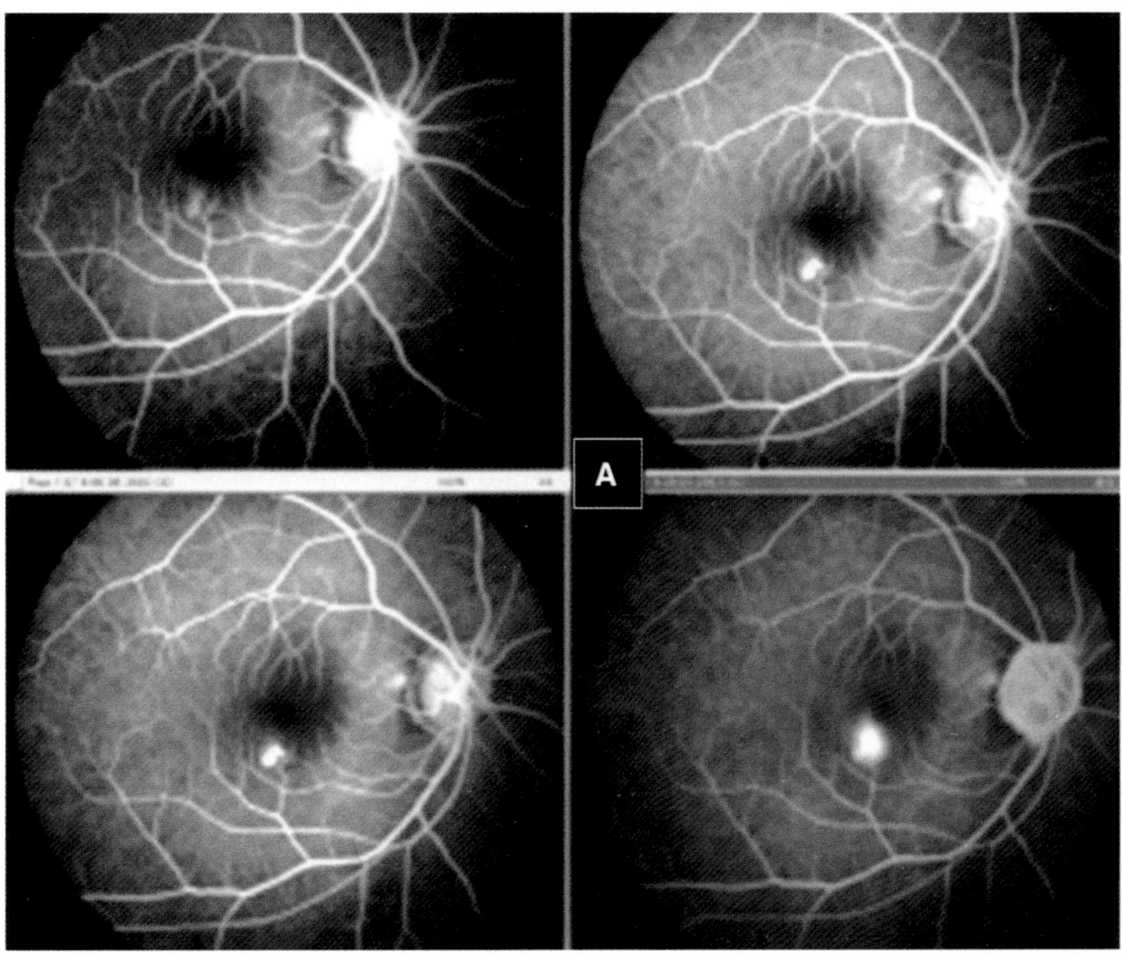

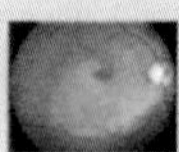

Optical Coherence Tomography

A horizontal line scan through the fovea showed elevation of neurosensory retina with an optically clear space underneath that corresponded to the presence of serous fluid under the fovea (B).

Follow-up Examination

Over a follow-up of 6 weeks, patient felt better, the visual acuity was improved to 20/25. Repeat OCT showed resolution of serous fluid with return of foveal contour to normal (C).

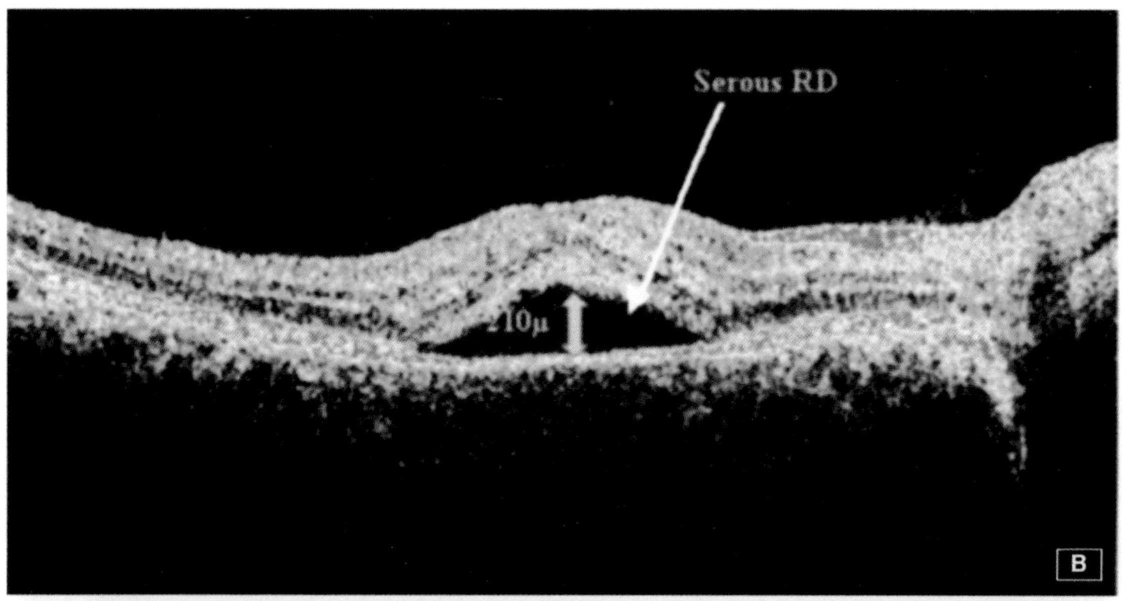

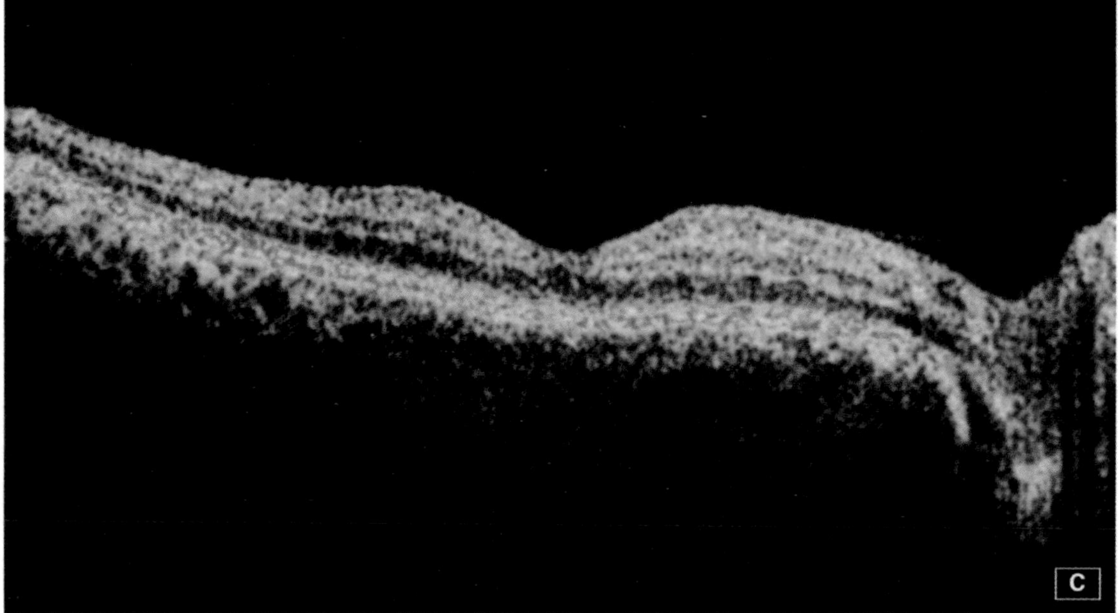

Pattern 2: ICSC with Multiple Pigment Epithelial Detachments (PEDs)

Case 6.2: ICSC with PEDs

Case Summary

A 30-year-old woman was seen with the diagnosis of pigment epithelial detachment right eye for which laser photocoagulation was done elsewhere. Her best corrected visual acuity was 20/70. Fundus right eye showed the presence of serous fluid in the center with a linear, hypopigmented band suggestive of fibrinous exudation (A). Fluorescein angiography showed multiple areas of hyperfluorescence with hypofluorescence corresponding to fibrin (B-D).

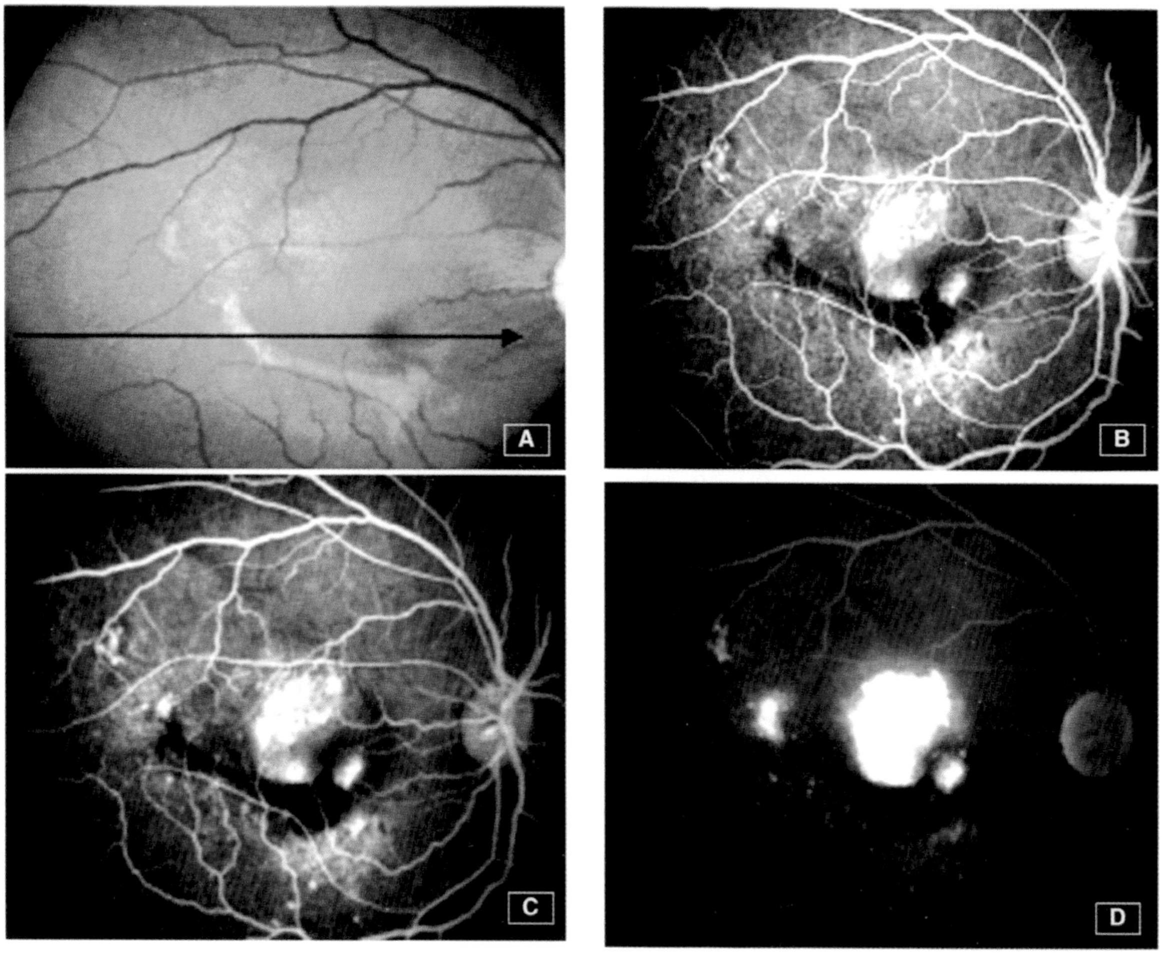

A

B

C

D

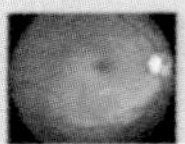

Optical Coherence Tomography

OCT right eye through the foveal center showed the presence of PED under the fovea measuring 410 microns in height with surrounding serous fluid (E). The fibrinous band was seen as hyper-reflective band on OCT (not shown in the picture).

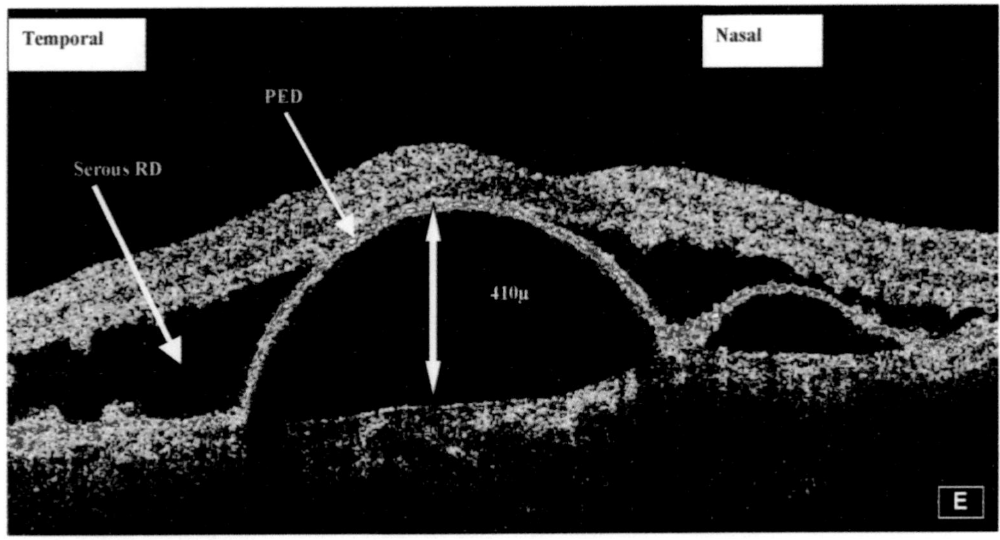

Follow-up

Repeat OCT scan 6 months later (F) showed resolution of serous fluid with persistent PED. However, there was a hyper-reflective area temporal to the fovea corresponding clinically to the area of laser scars. The RPE at the sites of PED was a bit irregular.

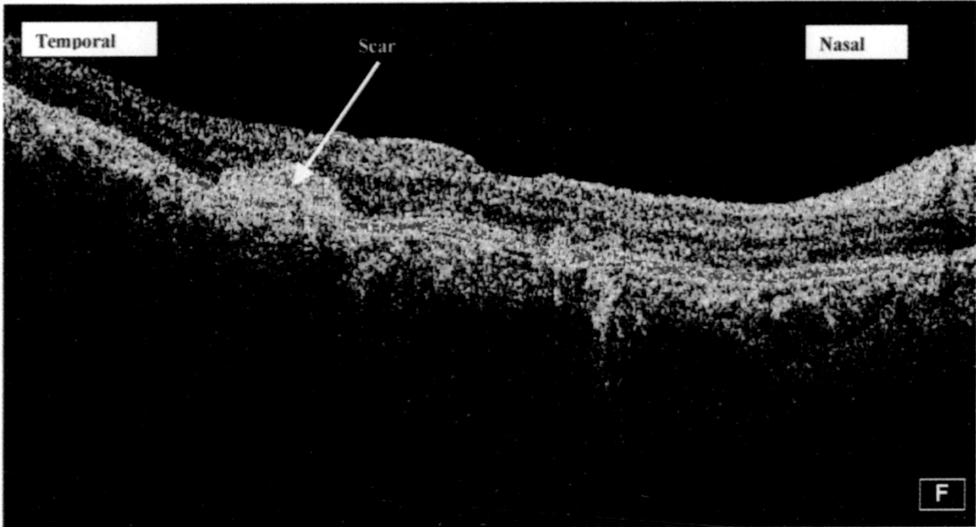

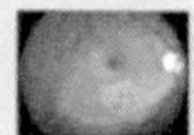

OCT IN DIAGNOSING COMPLICATIONS OF ICSC

Case 6.3: ICSC with Serous RD and PEDs in One Eye and Fibrinous Exudation in the Opposite Eye

Case Summary

A 32-year-old man presented with decreased vision of 10 days duration in the right eye. His best corrected visual acuity was 20/40 in this eye. Based on clinical picture and fluorescein angiography, a diagnosis of ICSC was established (A, B).

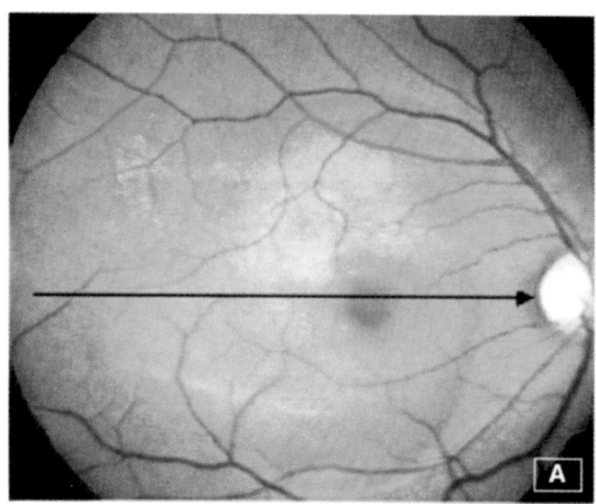

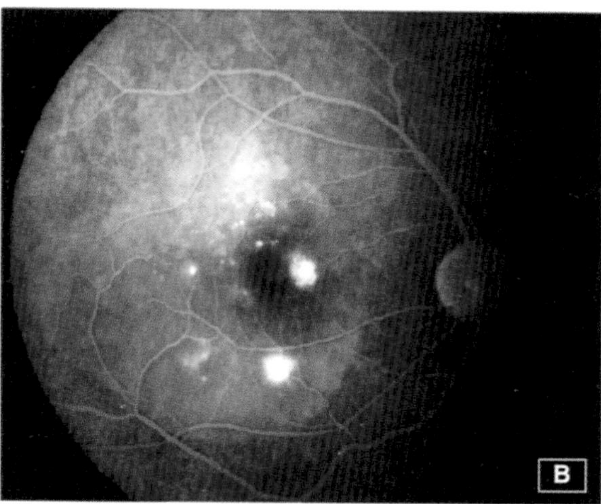

Optical Coherence Tomography

Horizontal OCT scan through foveal center in the right eye (C) showed the presence of hyporeflective area under the fovea suggestive of serous fluid accumulation measuring 270 microns in height with PED corresponding to the hyper-reflective spot nasal to the fovea on fluorescein angiography.

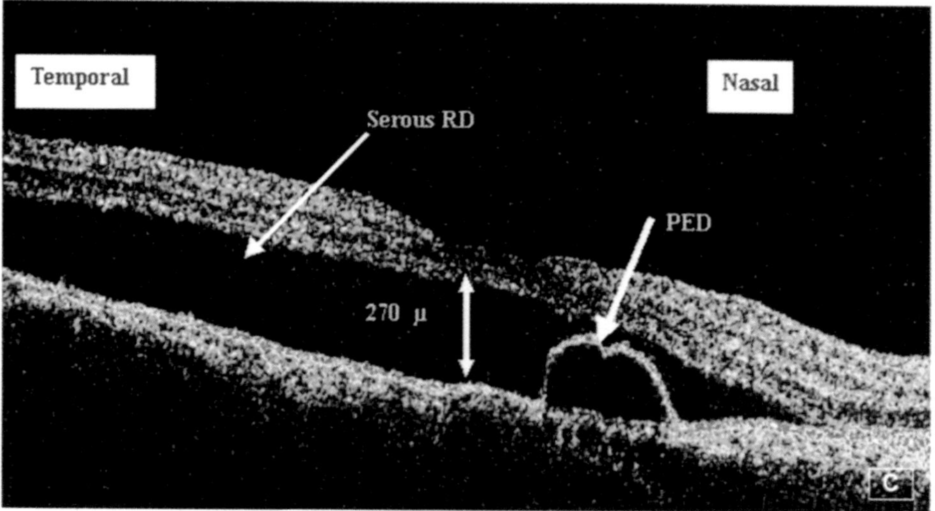

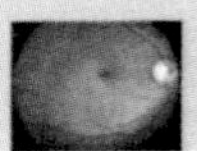

Follow-up

Eight weeks later, his visual acuity in this eye had improved to 20/25; the serous detachment and fibrinous exudation had resolved clinically (D). Repeat fluorescein angiography showed multiple hyperfluorescent spots suggestive of pigment epithelial detachments (E)

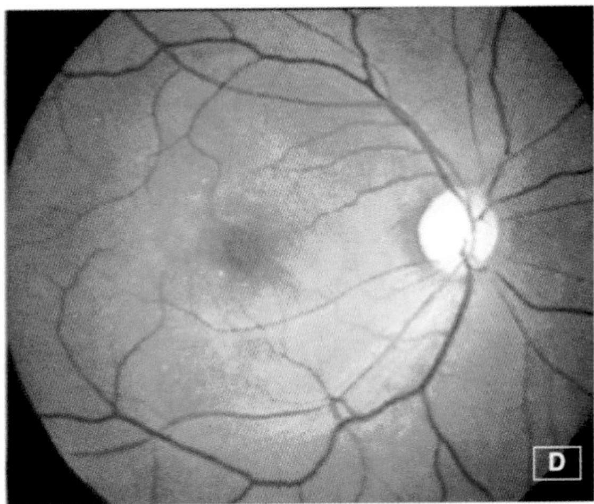
D

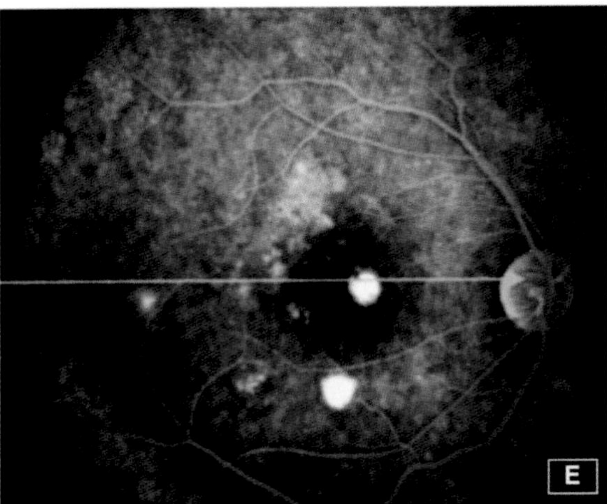
E

Repeat OCT at this stage through one such hyperfluorescent spot showed resolution of serous fluid with persistent PED, the height of which was reduced to 150 microns (F). The PED persisted at 6 months follow-up, though the height was reduced to 120 microns (G).

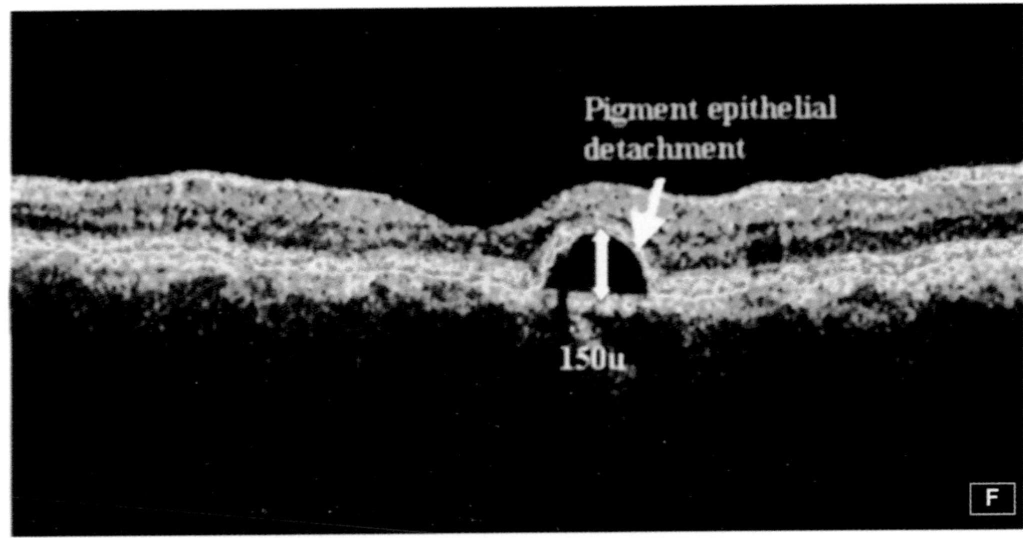

F

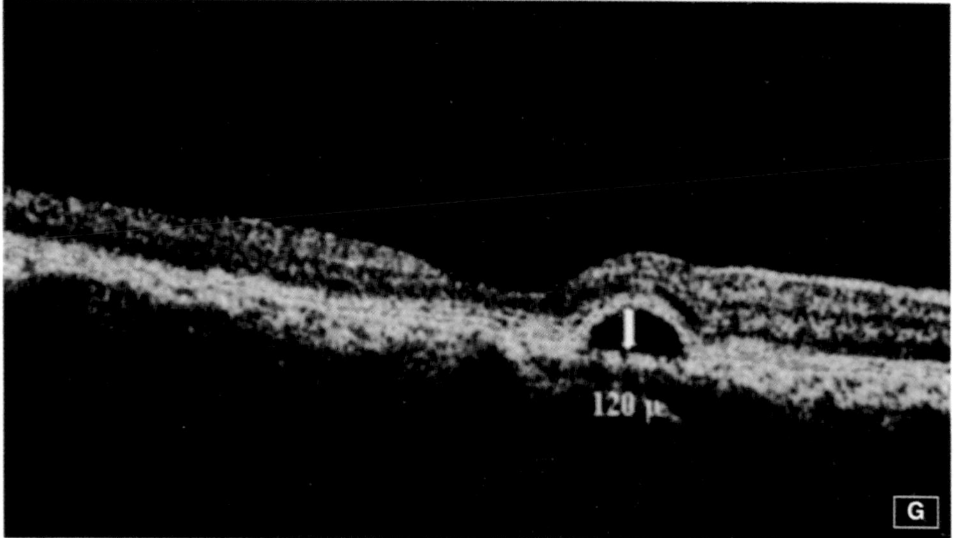

The patient also complained of decreased vision in his left eye of 3 months duration. His best corrected visual acuity in the left eye was 20/200. Based on clinical picture and fluorescein angiography (H, I), a diagnosis of ICSC with fibrinous exudation was established.

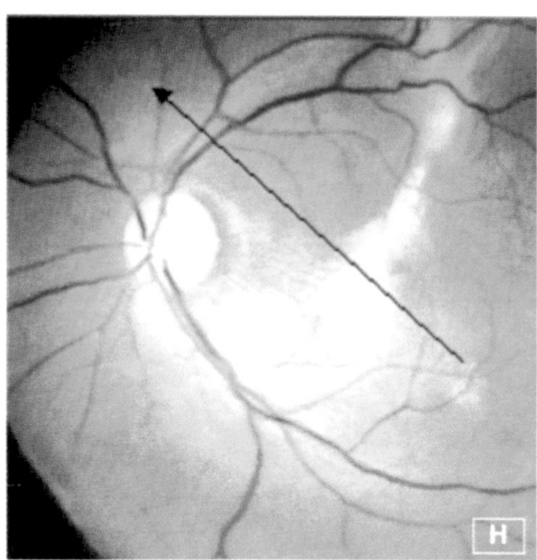

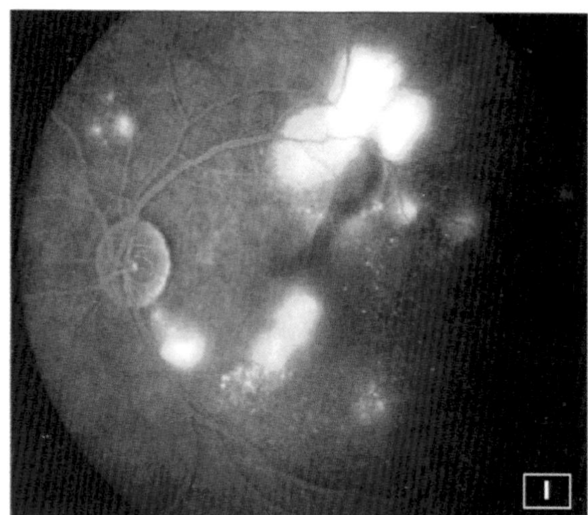

Optical Coherence Tomography

OCT scan at 45 degrees showed the presence of serous retinal detachment with a hyper-reflective area in the center corresponding clinically to fibrinous exudation (J).

A diagnosis of bilateral ICSC with left fibrinous exudation was made and patient was kept under follow-up. Eight weeks later, his visual acuity in the left eye was 20/200. The fibrin had partially resolved (K) and repeat fluorescein angiography (L) showed few areas of hyperfluorescence.

Repeat OCT scan through the center of fovea (M) showed normal foveal contour with a thin hyporeflective streak under the fovea suggestive of underlying serous fluid while a vertical scan passing through the fibrin (N) showed hyper-reflectivity (arrow) with underlying area of hyporeflectivity suggestive of underlying serous fluid.

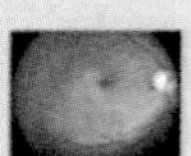

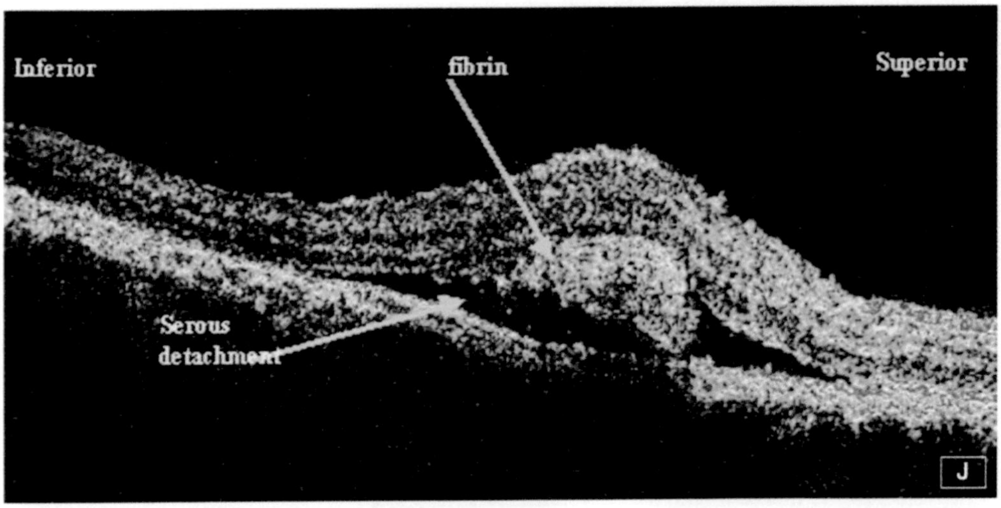

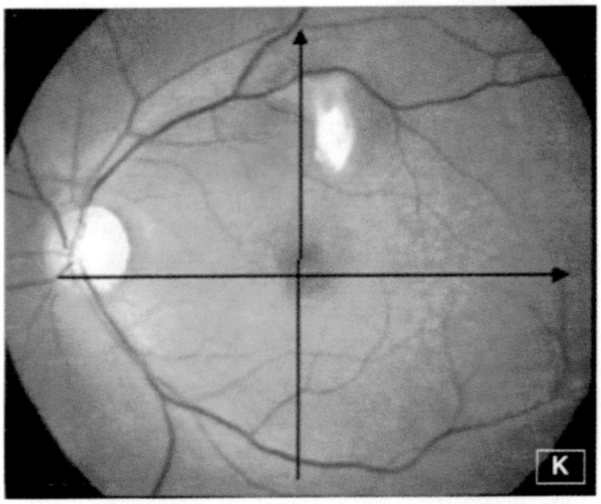

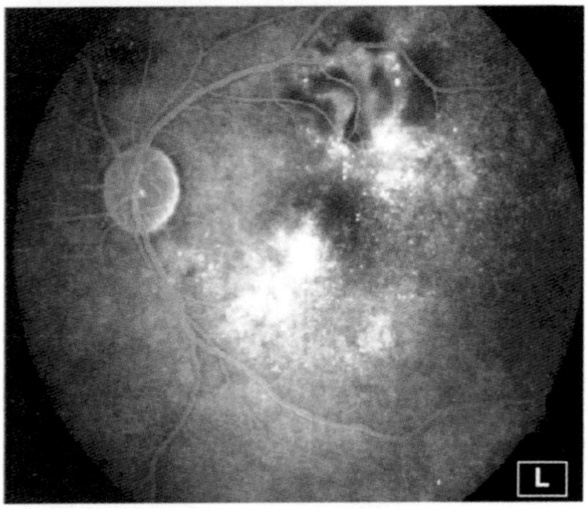

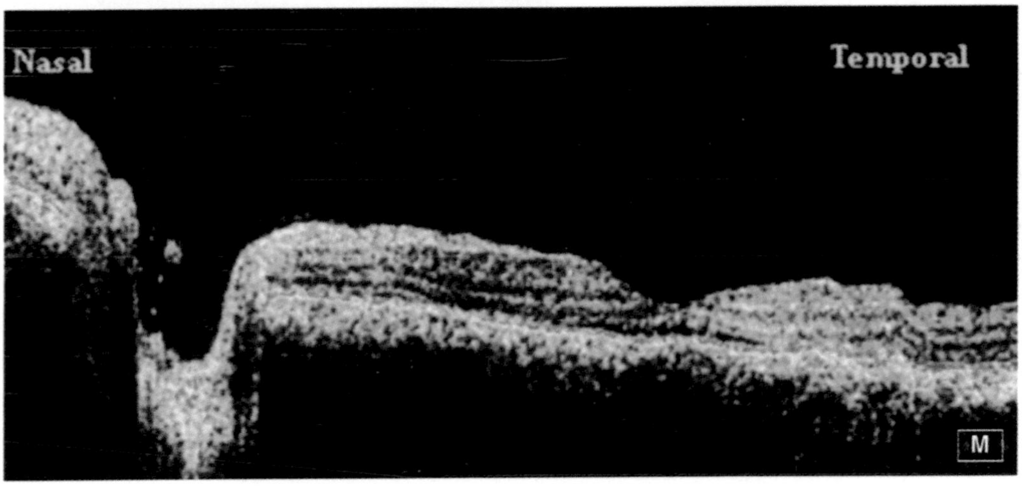

Focal laser photocoagulation was applied to the hyperfluorescent spot along the upper temporal vessel.

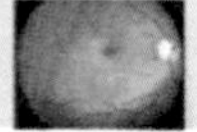

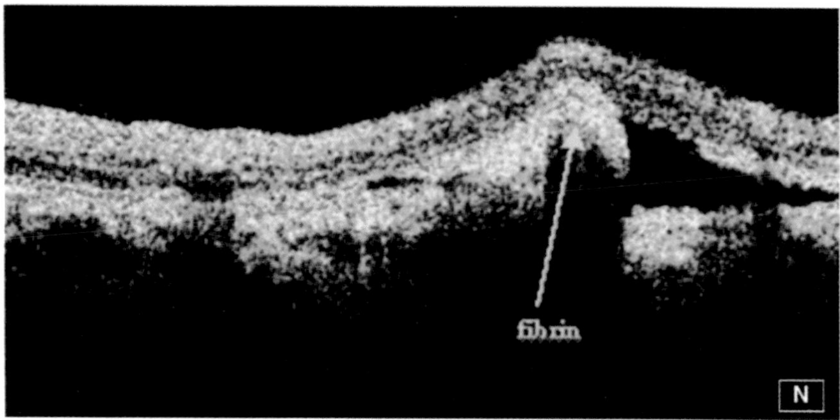

Six weeks later, his visual acuity was still 20/200 (O) with angiogram showing hypofluorescence corresponding to laser photocoagulation (P) and no serous detachment under fovea (Q).

More laser was applied to the residual hyperfluorescent spots. Six months later, his visual acuity had improved to 20/50 with normal looking fovea and organized fibrin along the upper temporal vessel (R). Horizontal line scan (S) through the foveal center showed normal looking fovea. Repeat vertical scan showed only fibrin, no serous fluid (not shown).

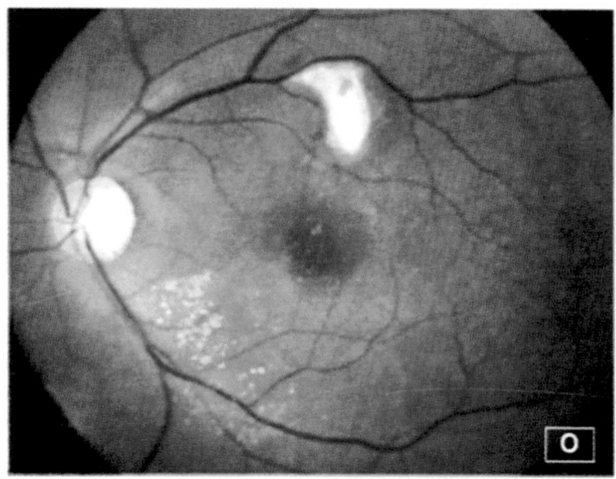

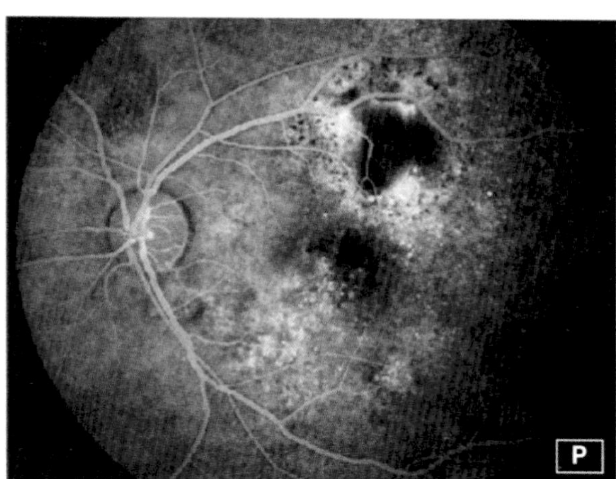

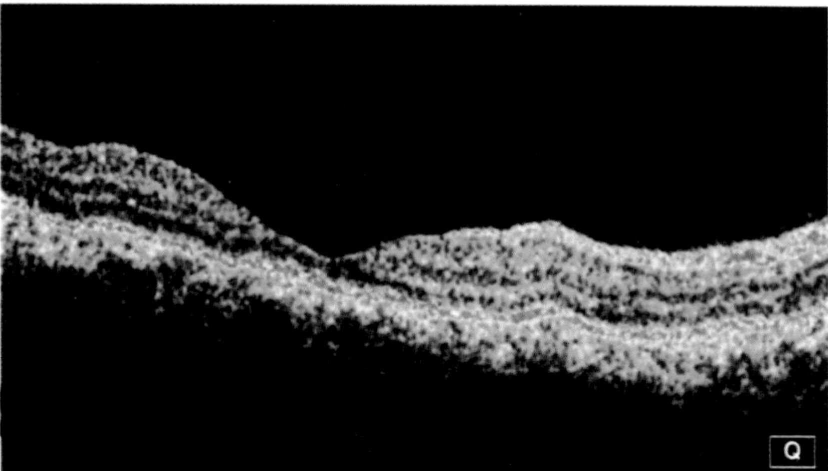

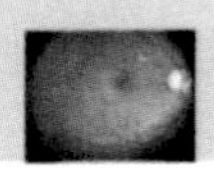

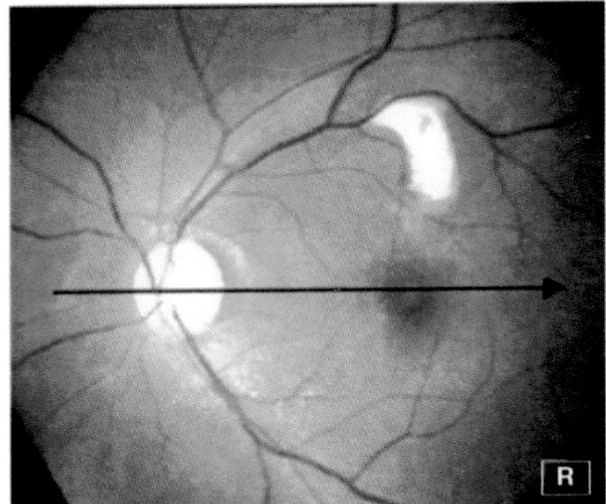
R

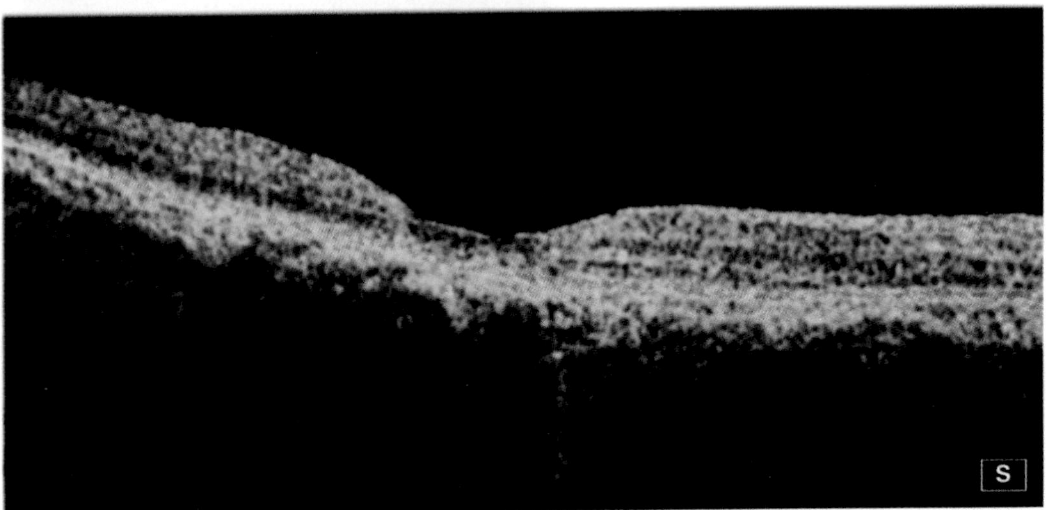
S

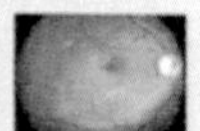

Case 6.4 : Chronic ICSC with Cystoid Macular Edema (CME)

Case Summary: ICSC with CME

A 56-year-old man presented with complaints of diminished vision in both his eyes of 6 months duration. His best corrected visual acuity was 20/200 in the right eye. Fundus right eye showed depigmentation temporal to fovea with few areas of hyperpigmentation (A) that showed hyperfluorescence on fluorescein angiography (B).

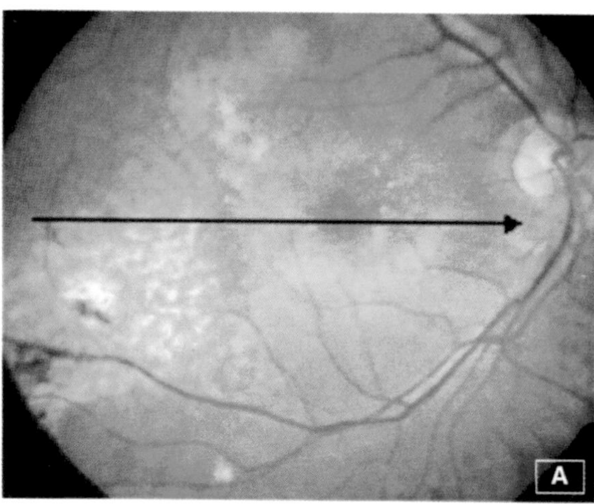

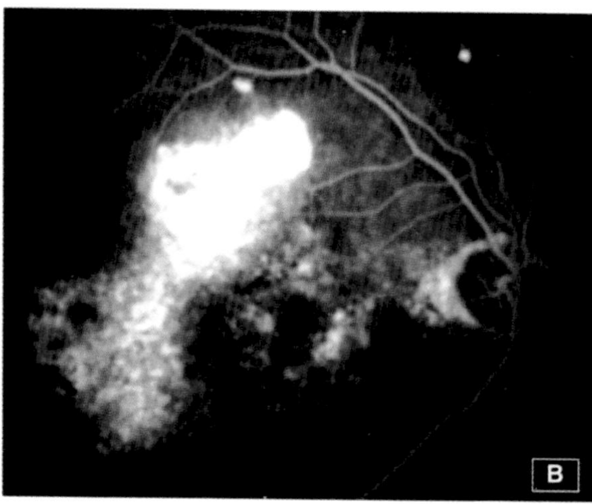

Optical Coherence Tomography

Optical coherence tomography showed hypo-reflective area under the fovea suggestive of serous retinal detachment measuring 450 microns in height. There were few hypo-reflective areas arranged in cyst-like pattern in the outer layers of the nasal retina (C).

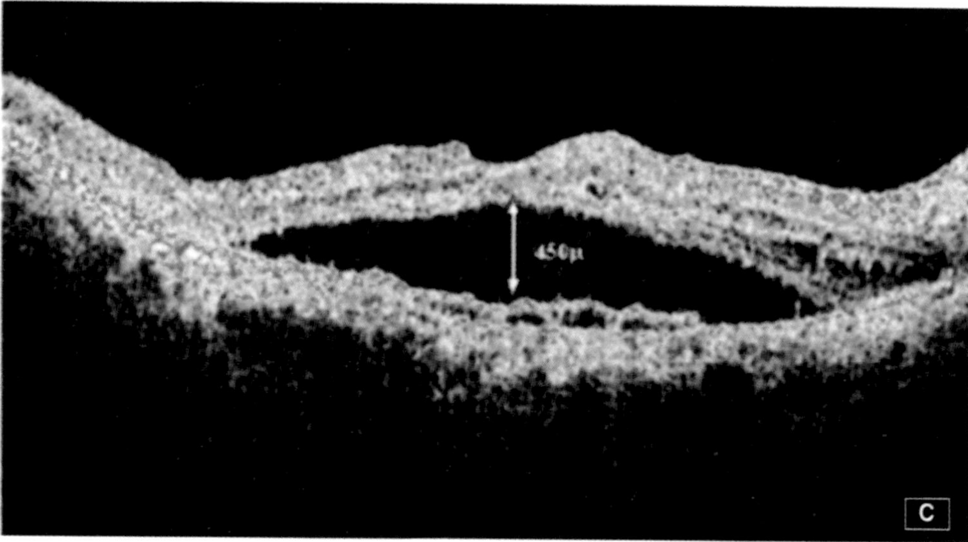

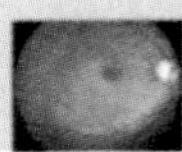

In view of chronicity of the disease, patient elected to receive focal laser photocoagulation of the leak. Four weeks later, his visual acuity was 20/125 (D). Repeat fluorescein angiography (E) showed hyperfluorescence that was less compared to the previous one (B).

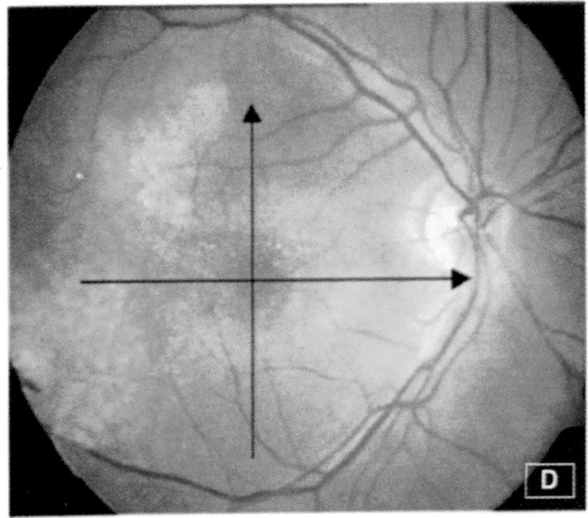

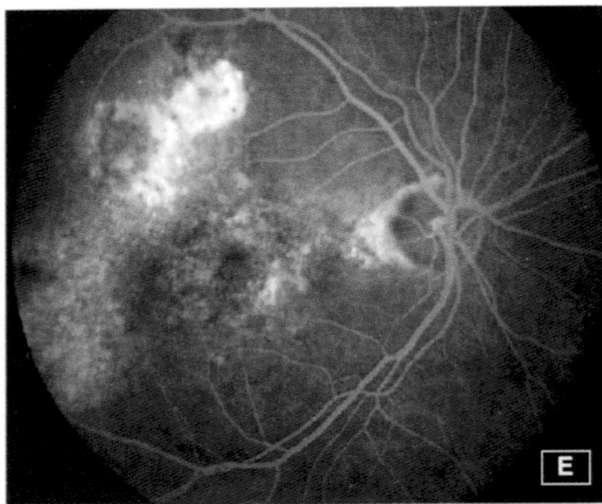

Repeat OCT scans (F and G) showed resolution of serous retinal detachment under the fovea, though a small area of detachment seen as hyporeflective area was seen nasal to the fovea and few cystoid spaces were seen as hyporeflective areas in the outer retina temporal to the fovea.

The left eye also had chronic ICSC (H) that showed hyperfluorescence on fluorescein angiography (I).

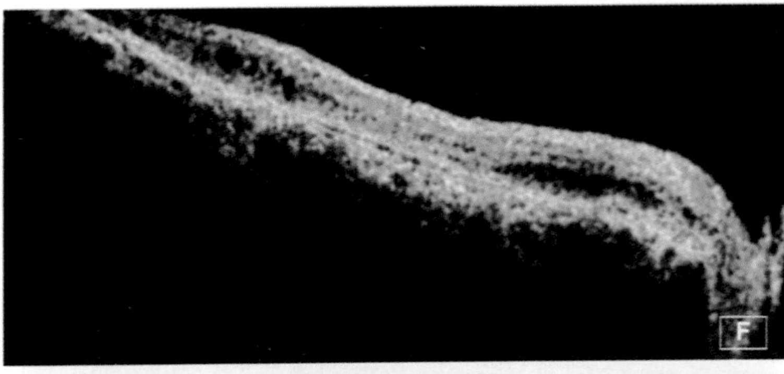

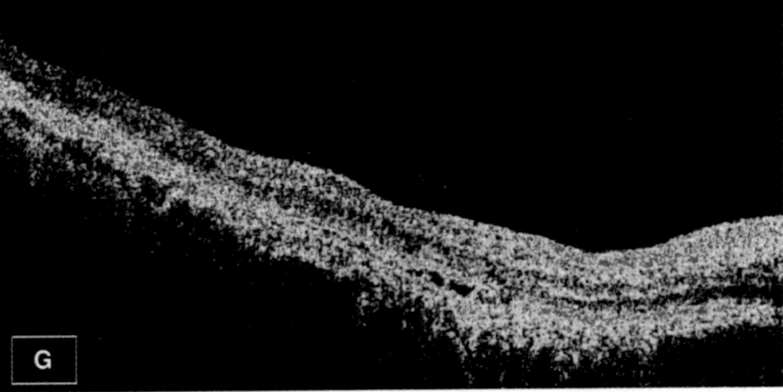

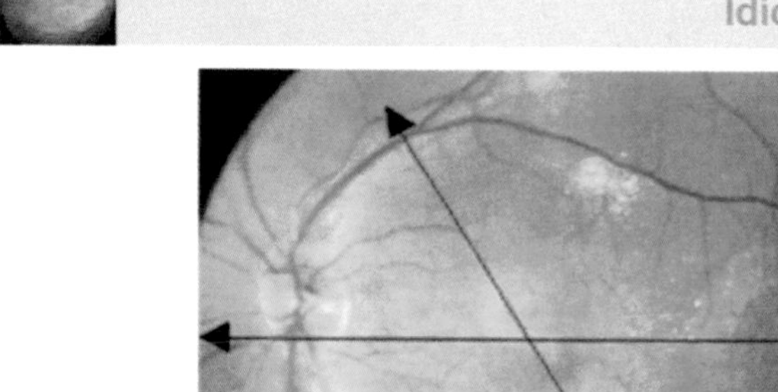

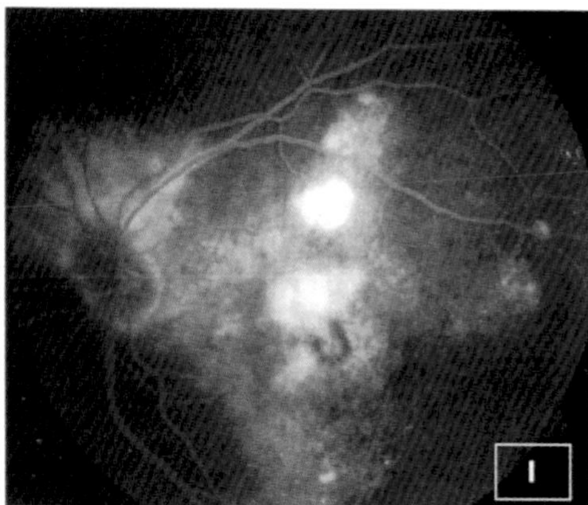

Optical coherence tomography scan (J) showed the loss of foveal contour, presence of small pigment epithelial detachments with an overlying hyporeflective band suggestive of small serous retinal detachment. Overlying this detachment were seen various hypo-reflective areas with intervening hyper-reflective walls conforming to the pattern of intraretinal cysts at different levels.

Four weeks later, following laser photocoagulation of the hyperfluorescent spot, the repeat OCT showed resolution of cysts with persistent PED and some serous fluid in the neurosensory retina (K).

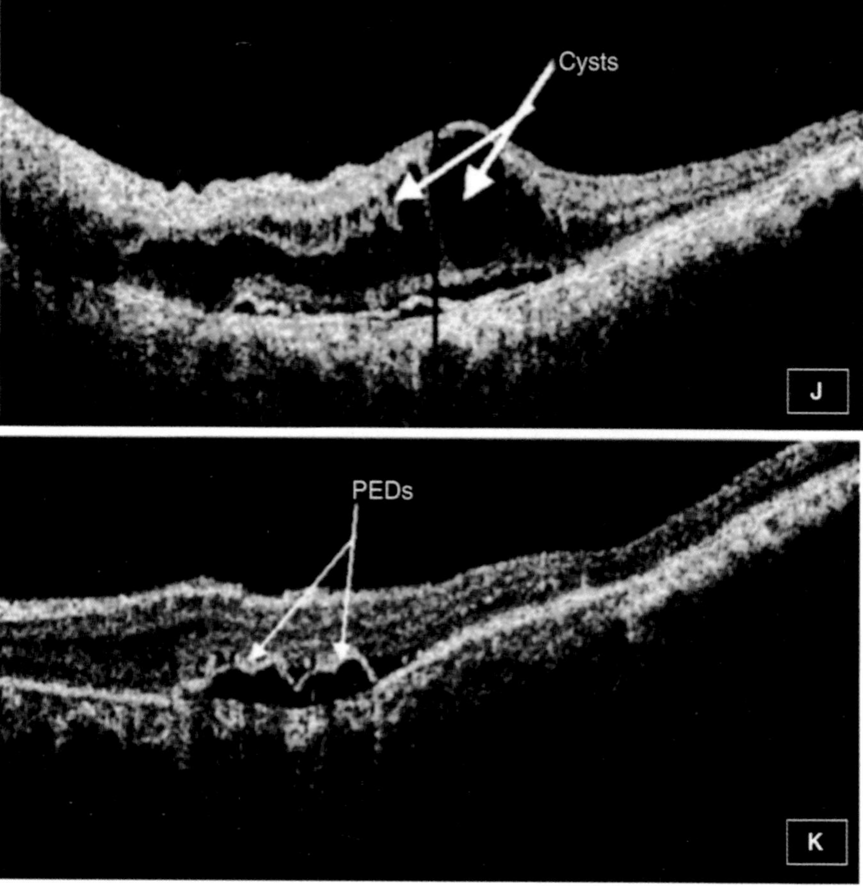

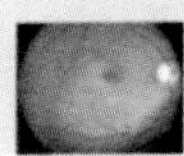

Case 6.5: ICSC with Idiopathic Polypoidal Choroidal Vasculopathy

Case Summary

A 45-year-old man was seen in 1991 with complaints of decreased vision in the right eye of one month duration. His best corrected visual acuity was 20/60. Fundus showed ICSC with PED (A) that was confirmed on fluorescein angiography. The ICSC showed spontaneous resolution in 6 weeks and patient regained a visual acuity of 20/20. Ten years later, he presented again with complaints of blurred vision in the same eye of 10 days duration. His visual acuity in this eye was 20/40 and fundus (B) showed the presence of subfoveal hemorrahage suggesting choroidal neovascular membrane (CNVM).

The patient received intravitreal TPA injection to clear the hemorrahage following which a fluorescein angiogram was done (not shown) that showed a juxtafoveal CNVM which was lasered and patient regained a vision of 20/20 (C).

Follow-up

Seven months later, the patient came back with metamorphopsia and a visual acuity of 20/30. Fundus examination showed the recurrence of CNVM nasal to the fovea (D).

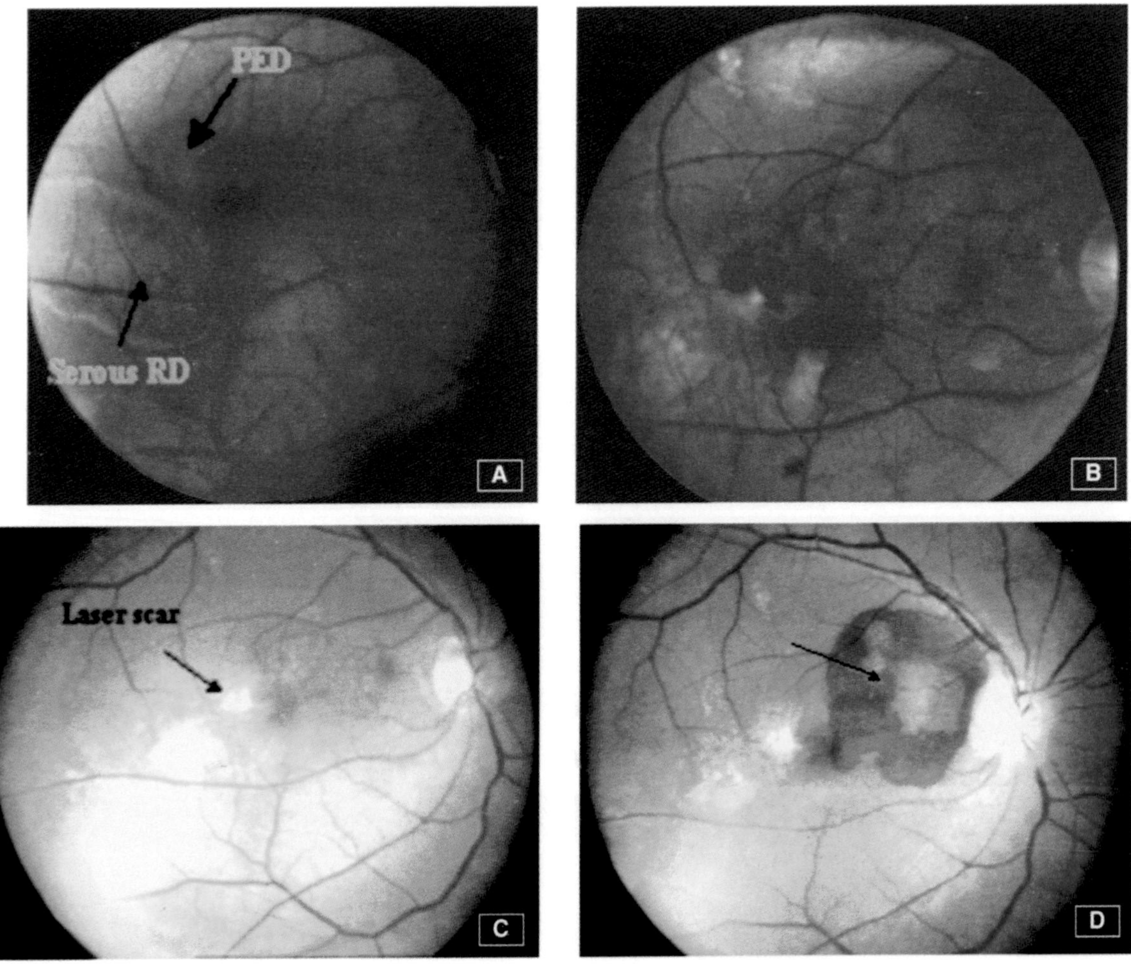

Fluorescein angiography showed the presence of a hyperfluorescent spot in the center of blocked fluorescence corresponding to subretinal hemorrahage (E). Indocyanine green angiography (F, G) showed multiple, rounded, saccular, hyperfluorescent spots (arrows) arranged in a bunch suggestive of idiopathic polypoidal choroidal vasculopathy (IPCV).

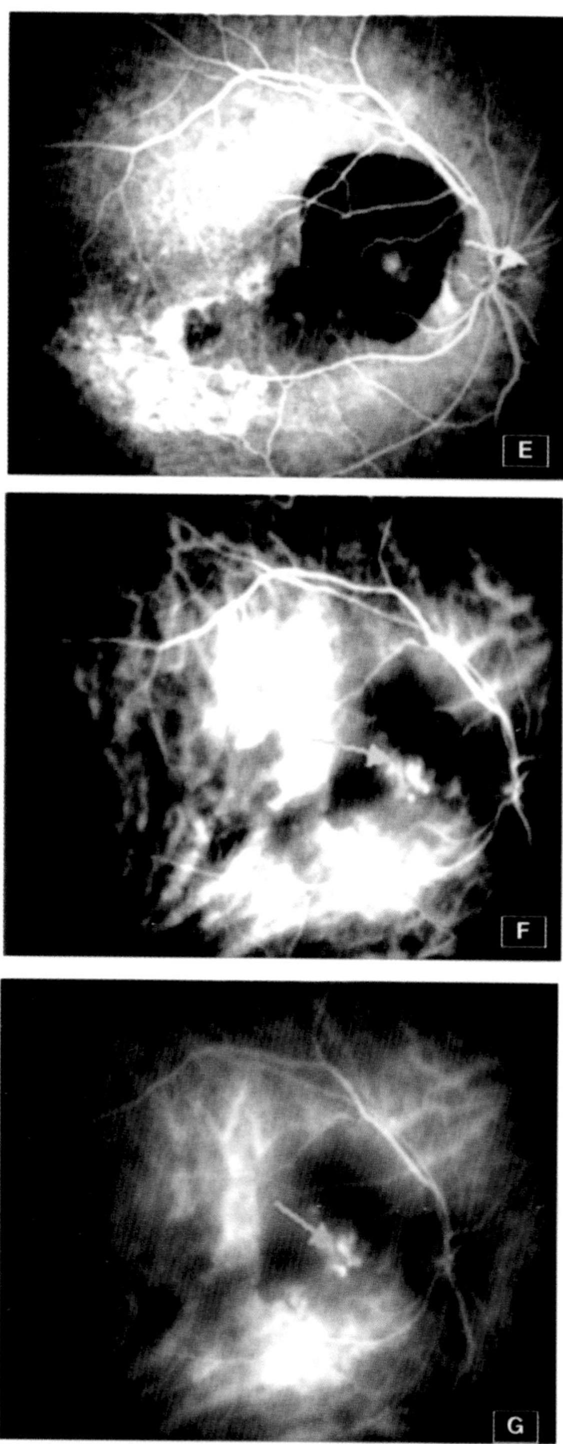

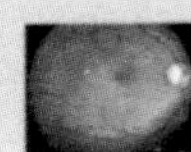

OCT scan (H) through these polyps showed multiple irregular, hyper-reflective areas at the level of choriocapillaries-RPE complex corresponding to polyps clinically with an overlying hyporeflective area corresponding to the area of bleed seen clinically.

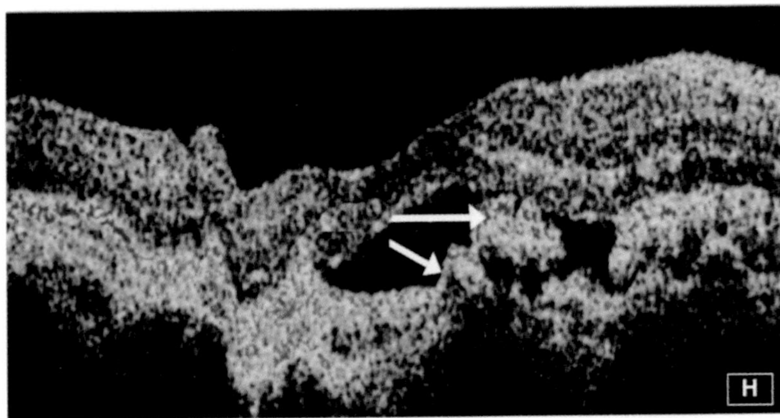

An overlay was prepared to delineate these areas (I) and thermal laser photocoagulation of these was done. Eight weeks later, following laser photocoagulation, repeat OCT scan showed resolution of the hyporeflective area with flattening of the hyper-reflective areas (J)

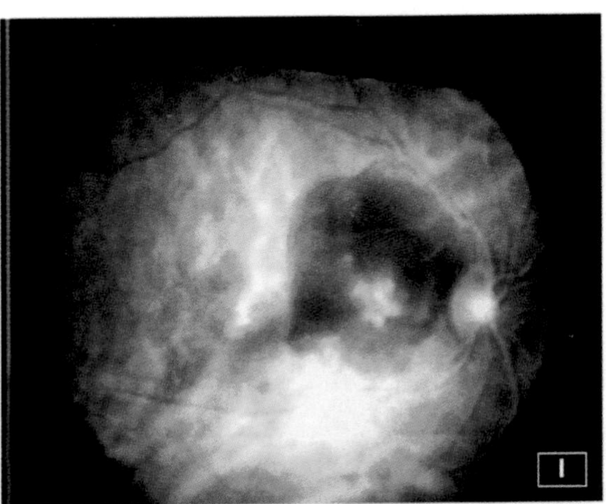

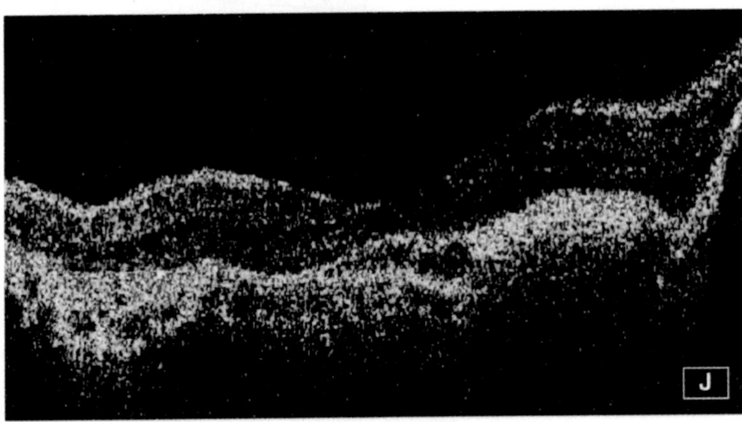

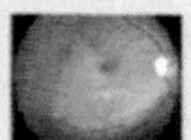

Follow-up

Over a follow-up of one year, the patient maintained a visual acuity of 20/20. The fundus showed a laser scar corresponding to the area of IPCV (K).

Repeat vertical OCT line scan (L) showed normal fovea with no serous fluid or saccular dilatations.

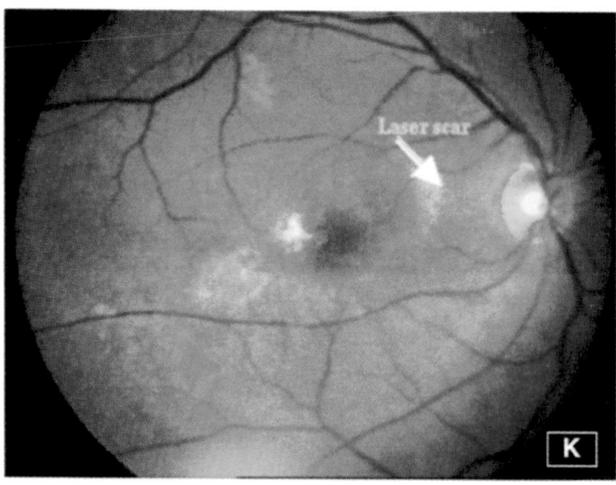

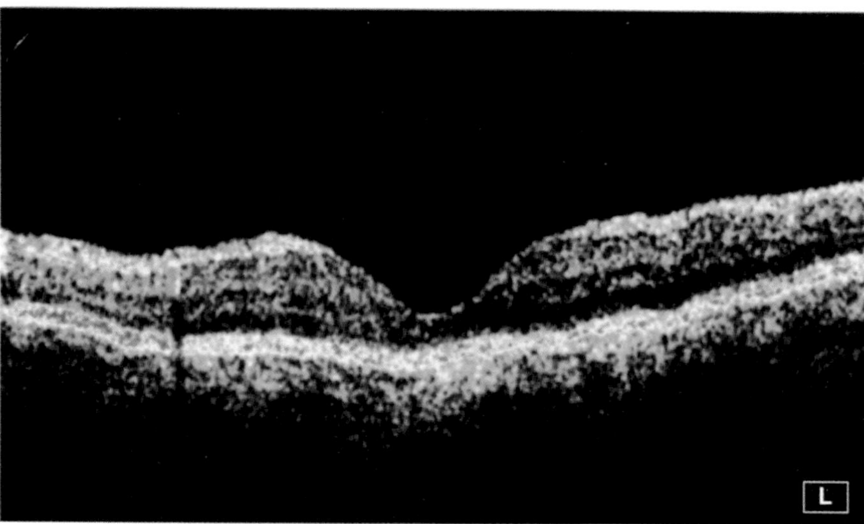

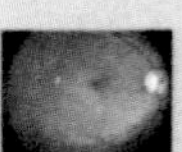

Case 6.6: ICSC with RPE Rip

Case Summary

A 30-year-old man presented with bilateral Idiopathic Central Serous Chorioretinopathy (ICSC) with subretinal fibrin and right eye RPE tear with inferior exudative retinal detachment (A, B). His best corrected visual acuity was 20/100 in the right eye. On fluorescein angiography RPE rip shows transmission hyperfluorescence and a few areas of focal leak (C)

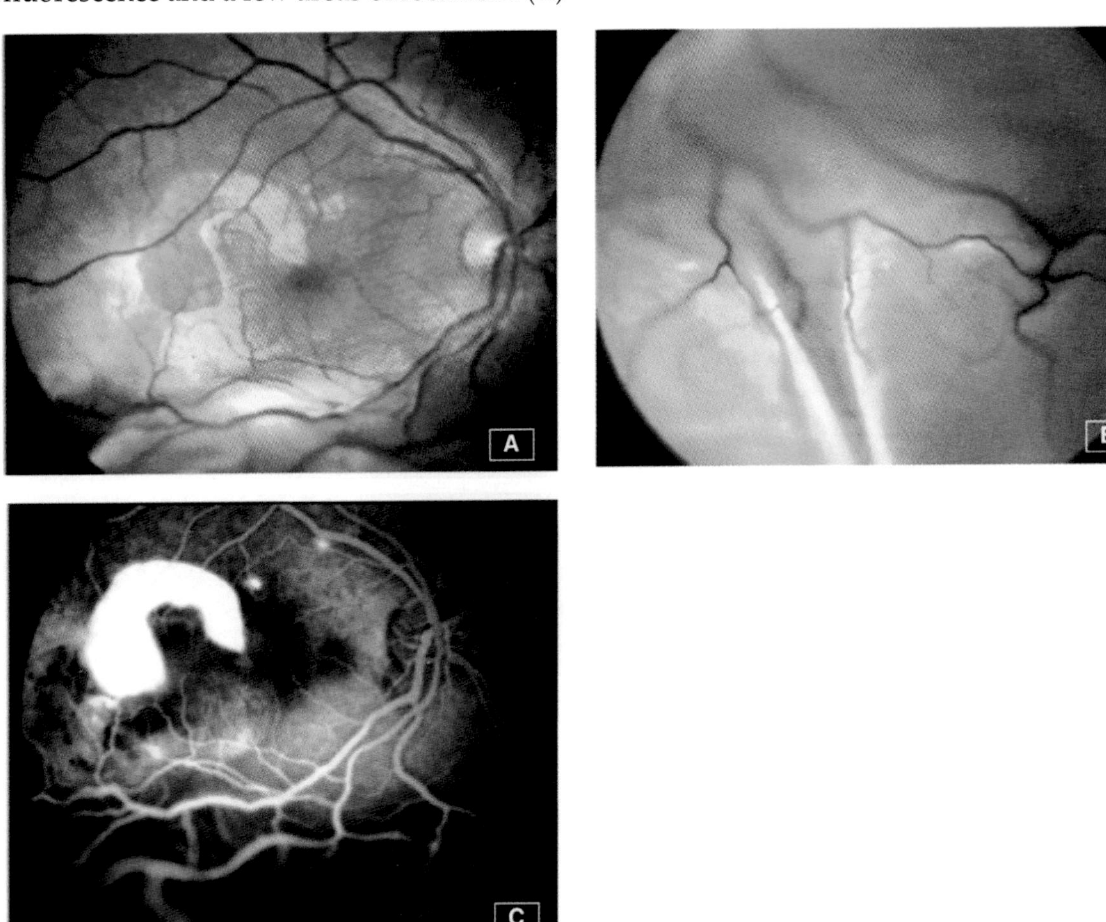

Optical Coherence Tomography

Vertical OCT line Scan (D) shows PED, serous RD and RPE disruption just above the foveal center (arrows). Horizontal OCT line Scan passing through the area of rip (E) shows adherence of fibrin to the margin of the RPE rip (arrow).

Four days later the rip progressed and retinal striations were directed towards contracting fibrin (F). Indocyanine green angiography showed hyperfluorescent areas between the rip and optic disc and hypofluorescence corresponding to RPE rip (G-I).

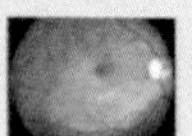

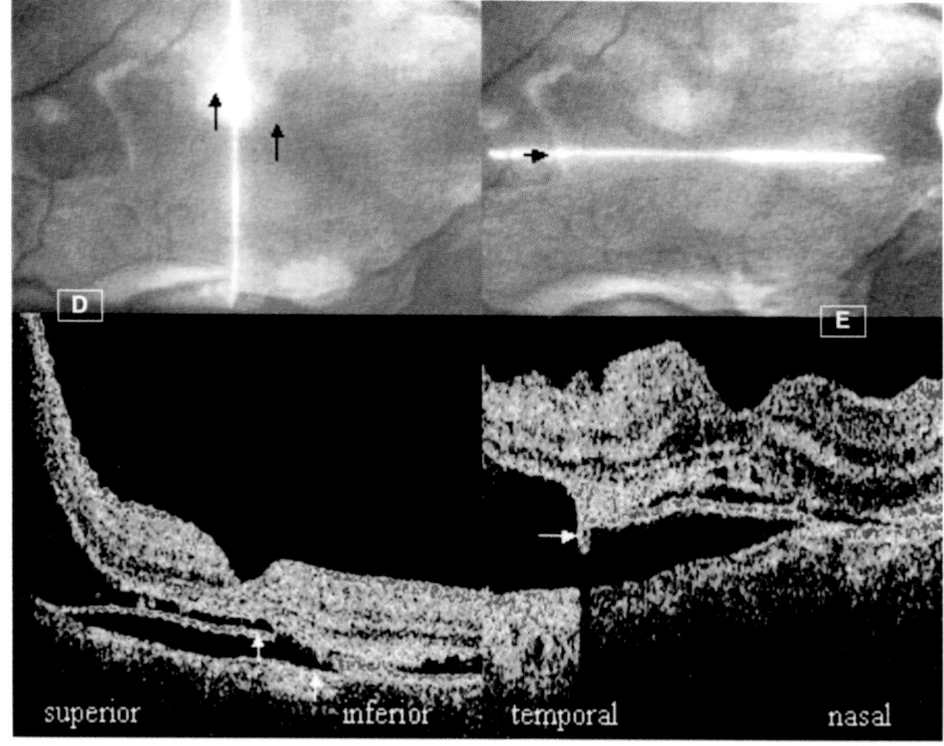
D
E
superior
inferior
temporal
nasal

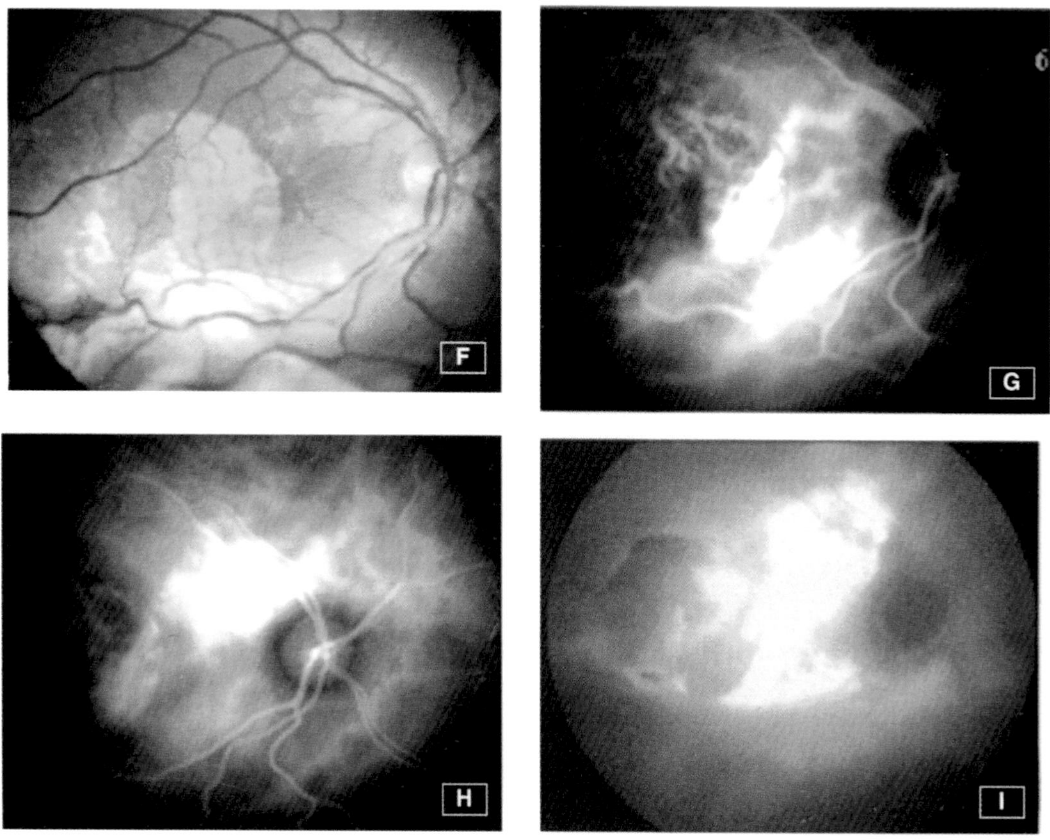
F
G
H
I

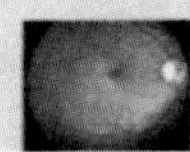

Repeat OCT at this stage was done (J) Solid arrows enclose area of RPE rip with subretinal fluid (arrow head). Note rolled over RPE. The rip continued to progress over next two weeks to become 360 degrees (K and L). Repeat OCT scan done two weeks later (M) showed detached RPE just nasal to the foveal center with exuberant fibrin and minimal subretinal fluid in the area of RPE rip temporal to foveal center. Patient was treated with anti-tuberculosis chemotherapy for pulmonary tuberculosis.

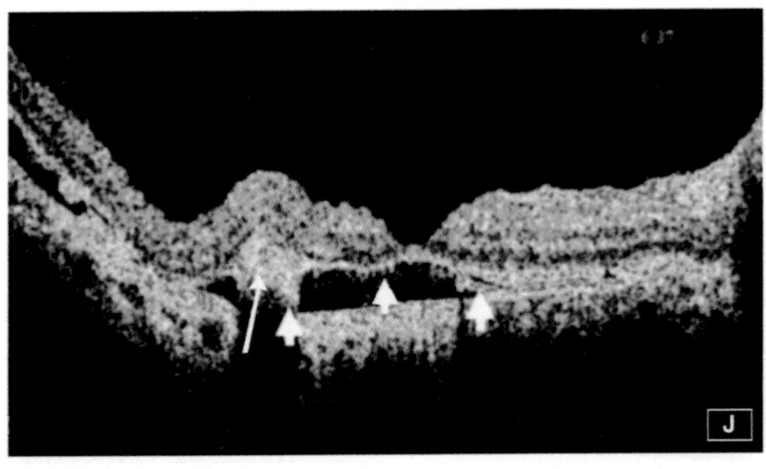

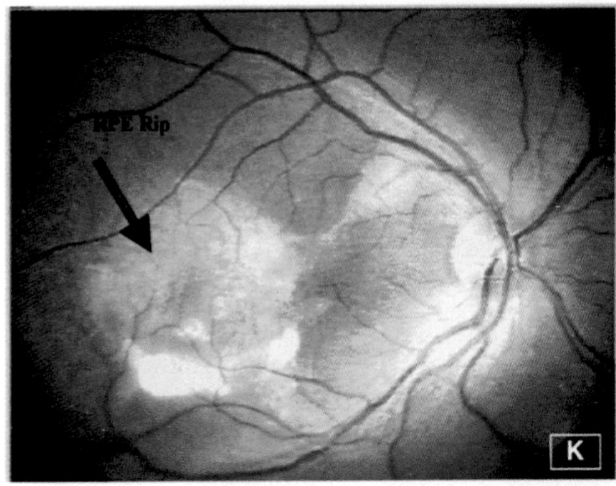

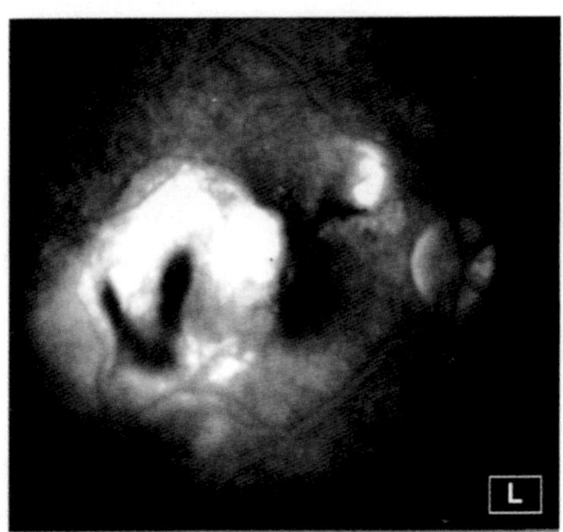

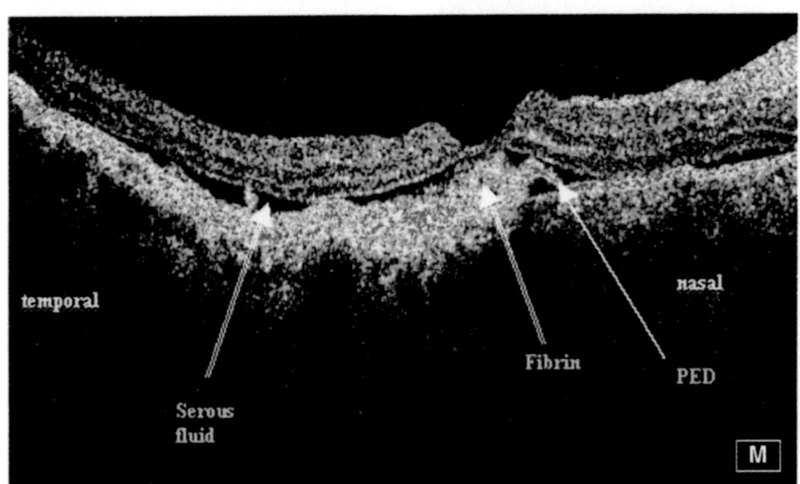

Four months later, his best-corrected visual acuity was 20/160 in the right eye and fundus showed healed scar in the right eye (N, O) that showed hyperfluorescence on fluorescein angiography (P, Q).

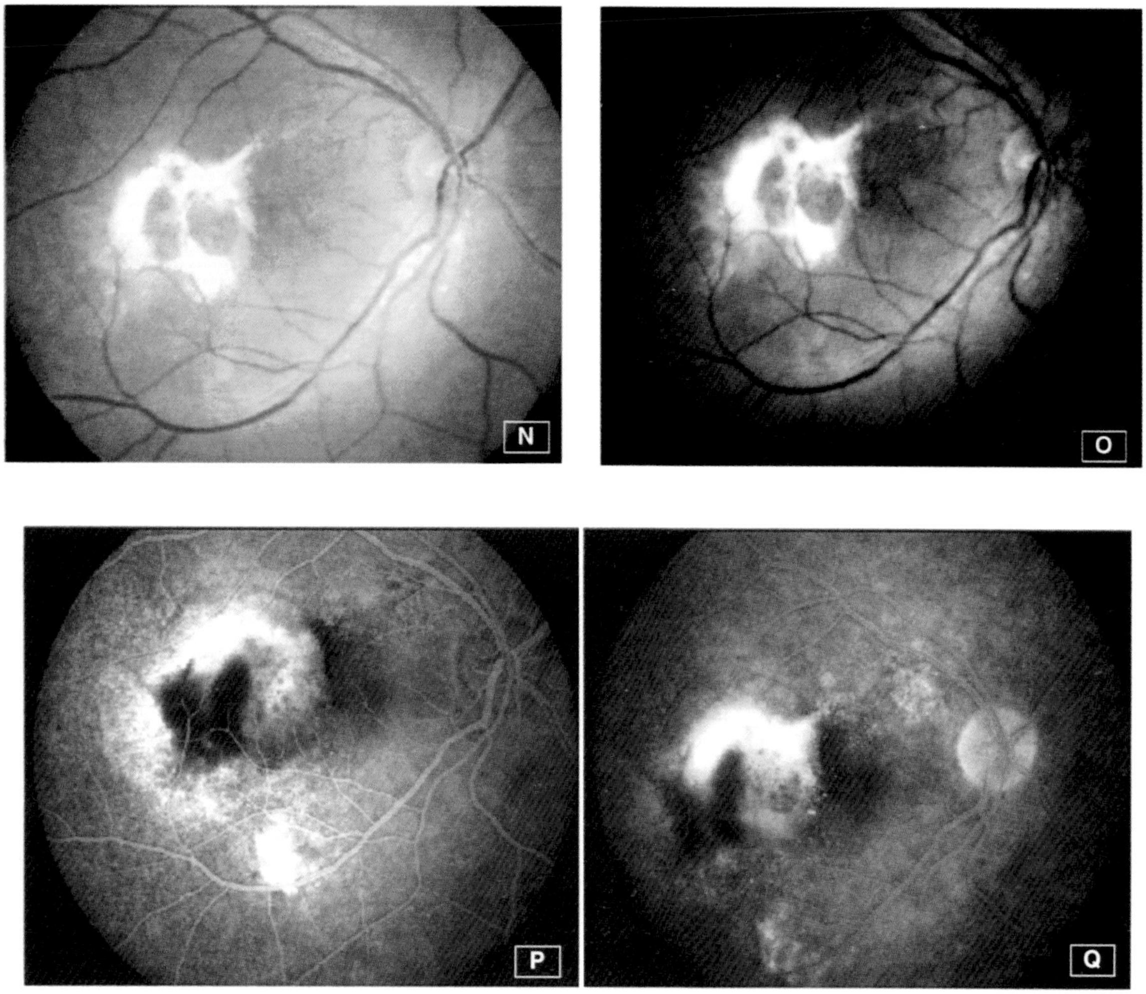

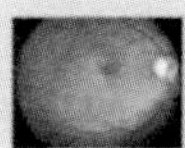

Repeat OCT showed normal foveal contour with rolled up RPE and minimal subretinal fluid as was indicated by the presence of hyporeflective band (R).

Over next eight months, he maintained a best corrected visual acuity of 20/30 with a healed scar in the fundus (S). The corresponding OCT showed normal foveal contour, no serous fluid or PED and hyper-reflective choroid corresponding to scars (T).

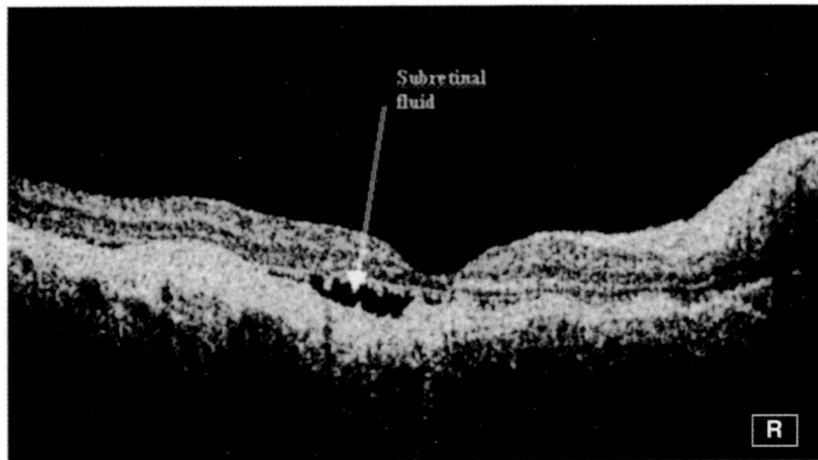

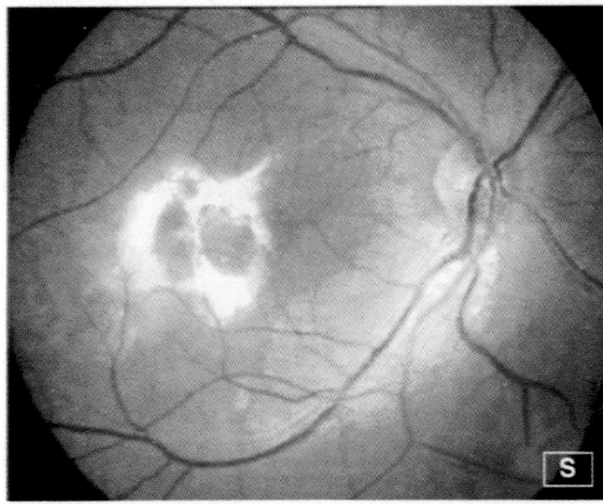

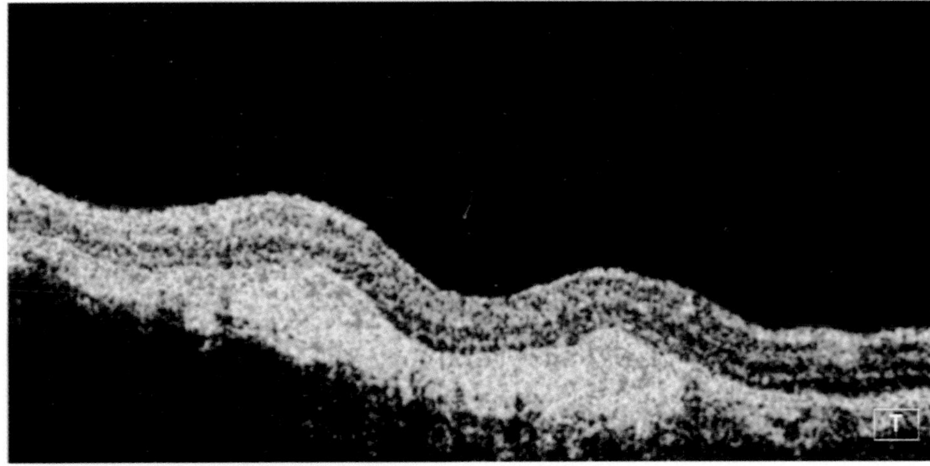

Case 6.7: Foveal Atrophy in ICSC

Case Summary

A 26-year-old man was seen with right eye chronic ICSC with visual acuity of 20/200 (A). Fluorescein angiography of the right eye (B) showed an area of mottled hyperfluorescence (arrow).

The OCT line scan (C) through the fovea showed foveal atrophy with central foveal thickness measuring 78 microns suggesting foveal atrophy following chronic ICSC.

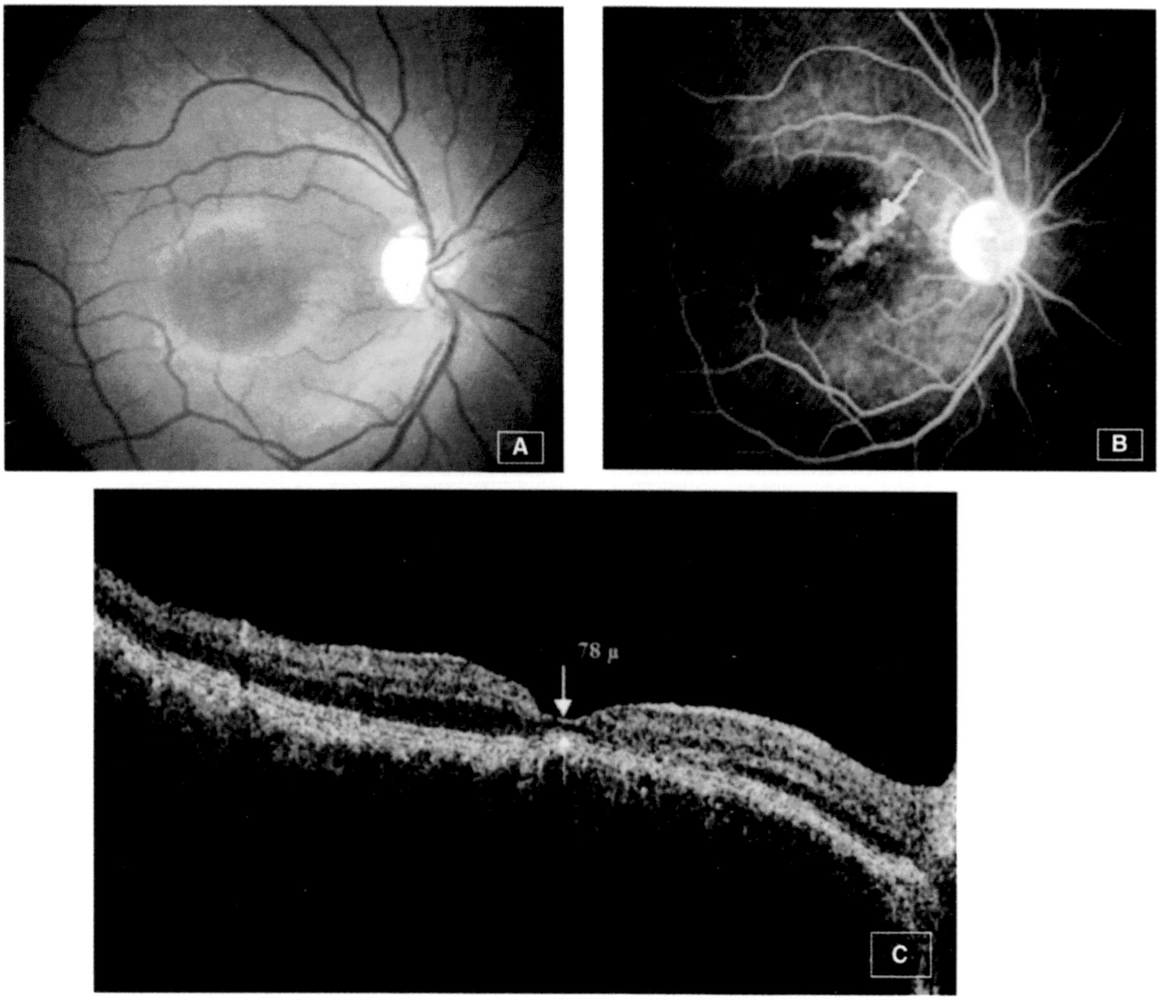

A

B

78 μ

C

C. OCT IN ATYPICAL ICSC

Case 6.8: Atypical ICSC in Elderly

Case Summary

A 64-year-old man was seen with decreased vision in both his eyes for one year duration. His best-corrected visual acuity was 20/60 in the right eye. Fundus in this eye showed the presence of multiple hard exudates (A) that showed hyperfluorescence on fluorescein angiography (B).

OCT scan through various angles (C-H) showed the hyporeflective area under the fovea that was suggestive of serous fluid with a small PED nasal to the fovea that corresponded to the hyperfluorescent spot seen on fluorescein angiography. The moderate backscatter seen within the PED was suggestive of possibly an occult CNVM.

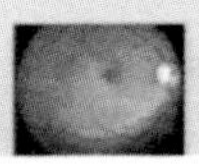

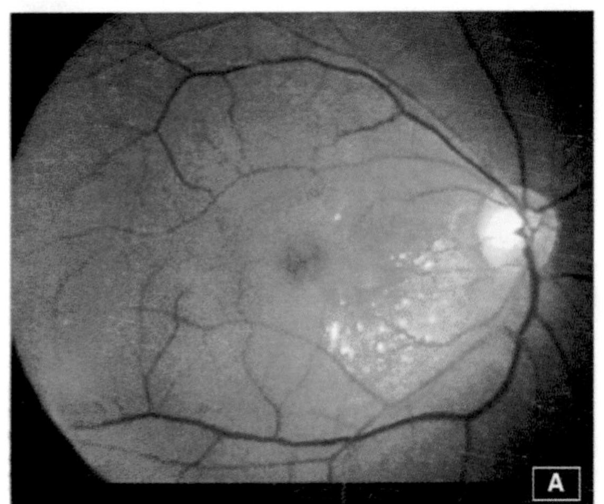
A

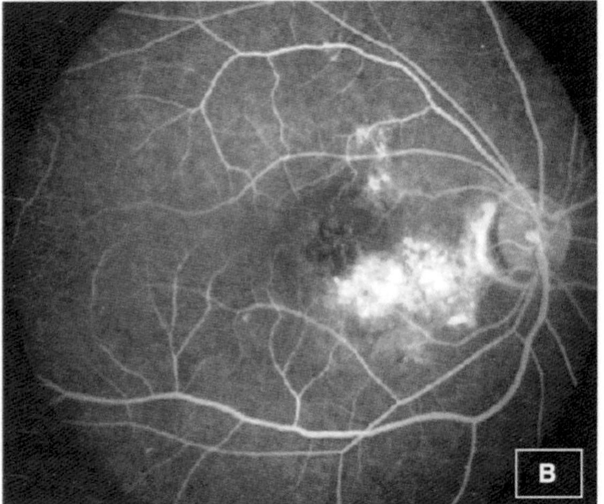
B

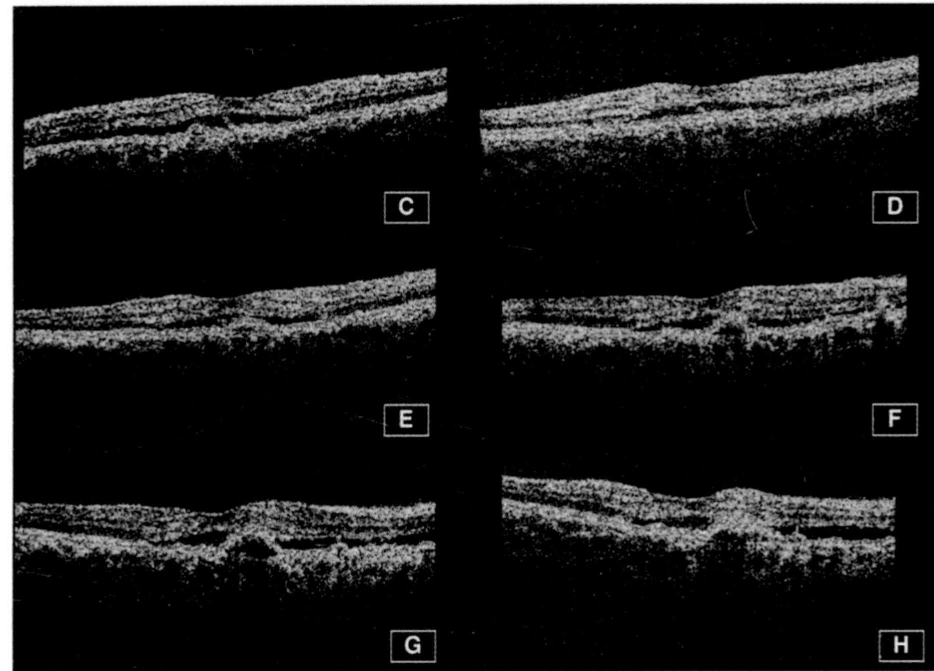
C
D
E
F
G
H

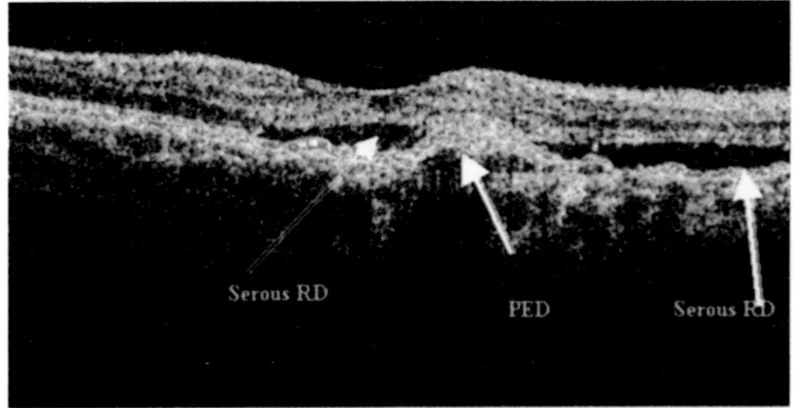
Serous RD
PED
Serous RD

Case 6.9: Atypical ICSC in Diabetes

Case Summary

A 46-year-old Type II diabetic was seen with the clinical diagnosis of clinically significant macular edema (A). On fluorescein angiography, besides microaneurysms, there were three discrete areas of hyperfluorescence that showed pooling of the dye in the later phases that was unlike leak from the microaneurysms or dilated capillary bed (B-D).

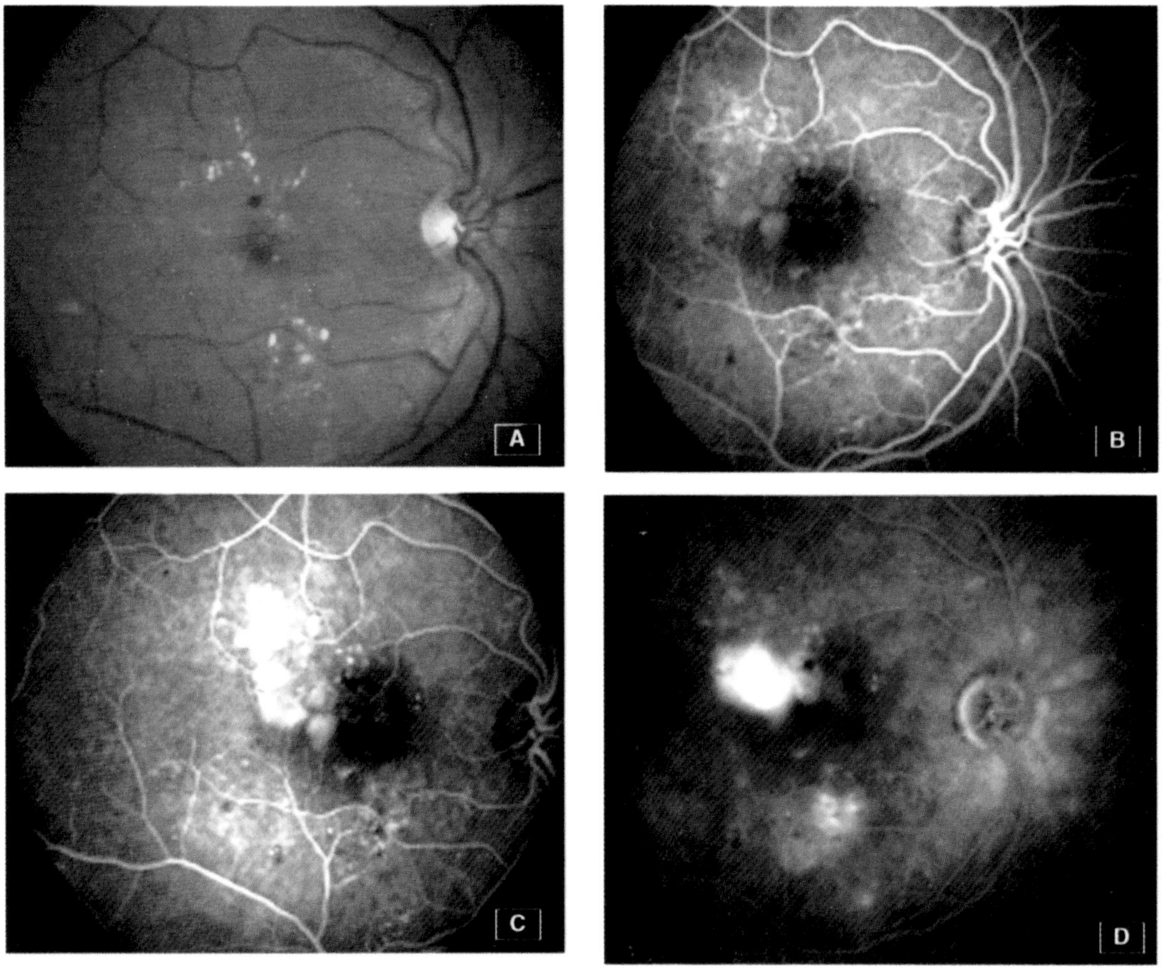

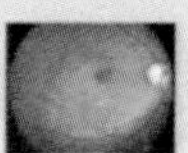

Optical Coherence Tomography

OCT line scan through the areas of dye pooling (E) showed mild elevation of the hyper-reflective layer corresponding to RPE with underlying hyporeflective band suggesting shallow PED. In addition, there was a hyporeflective band just anterior to it suggesting the presence of a probable fluid pocket of ICSC.

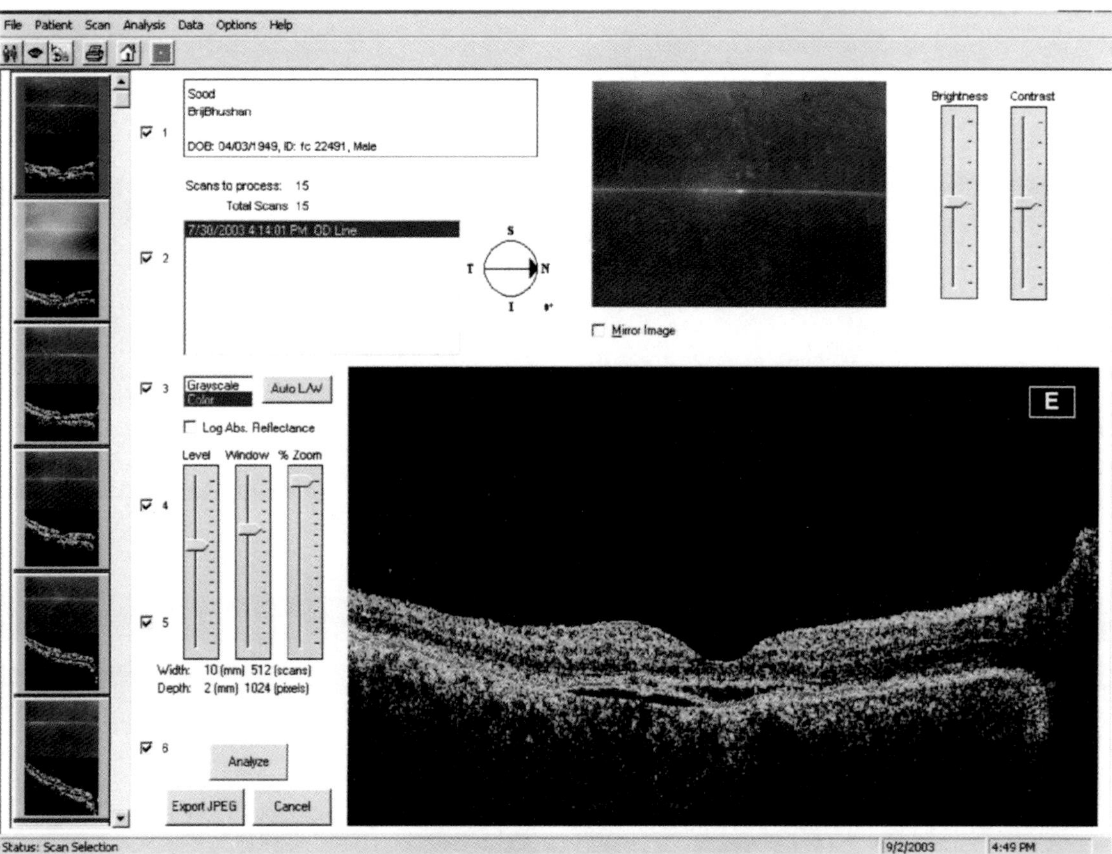

CONCLUSIONS

From these cases, it becomes clear that OCT is a very useful tool in monitoring the structural changes in the underlying retina. Since it is a noninvasive tool, it can be repeated easily and the repeat mode ensures reproducibility of the scan from the same area. This reduces the need for repeat fluorescein angiography in these patients. In short, we found that (A) PED is a very common feature of both typical as well as atypical ICSC (B). OCT is helpful in diagnosis the complications of ICSC (C) OCT is helpful in diagnosing Atypical cases.

SUGGESTED READINGS

1. Wang M,Sander B, Larsen M. Retinal Atrophy in Idiopathic Central Serous Chorioretinopathy. Am J Ophthalmol 2002,133 : 787-93.
2. Hee MR, Puliafito CA, Wong C et al. Optical coherence tomography of central serous chorioretinopathy. Am J Ophthalmol 1995; 120:65-74.
3. Wang M, Larsen M, Sander R, Lund-Andersen H. Central serous chorioretinopathy with foveal detachment demonstrated by optical coherence tomography. Acta Ophthalmol Scand 1999; 77:402-05.

Chapter 7

Macular Hole

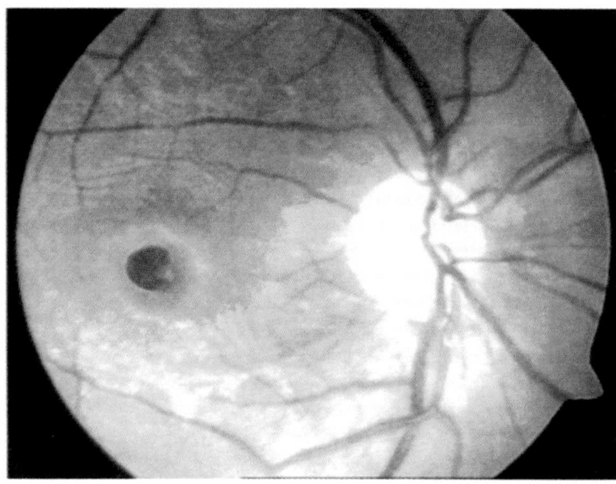

OCT is a very useful tool in the diagnosis and management of macular holes. It helps by providing a cross-section of retina that helps in many ways.

1. It helps in differentiating various retinal lesions that cannot be clinically distinguished, i.e. lamellar or full thickness macular holes, macular cysts, foveal detachments of retinal pigment epithelium or neurosensory retina and epiretinal membrane with pseudo-hole. Full thickness macular holes show a breach in all the layers of retina while lamellar macular hole shows only partial loss of tissue with steep foveal contour. Retinal pigment epithelium (RPE) detachments and macular cysts are characterized by the presence of a well-defined, round, localized area of hypo-reflectivity in the outer retinal layers/subretinally.
2. OCT helps in staging of macular holes that helps in evaluating surgical intervention. It has clarified the pathoanatomy of the macular holes. It has provided new evidence that the presence of a localized perifoveal vitreous detachment is a rule in the earliest stages of macular hole formation. It has been shown experimentally that the discrete linear signal (DLS) seen on OCT is the signal from posterior vitreous face. OCT has led to a new classification of macular holes as follows:
   Stage 1A: Foveal pseudocyst
   Stage 1B: Impending macular hole characterized by disruption of outer retina
   Stage 2: Full thickness retinal dehiscence.
   In a recently proposed 'hydration theory 'of the macular hole genesis, it has been suggested that following the posterior hyaloid traction, there is a tear in the inner fovea that allows seepage of fluid vitreous into the spongy layer of the macula, thus creating a cavity in the inner retina. The fluid

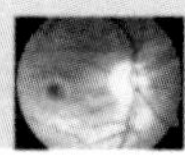

dissects and spreads into the outer retinal layers, which causes enlargement of the macular hole. Since RPE and Bruchs membrane are rigid, the swollen retina extends inwards. The swollen retina then elevates and retracts. If there is posterior vitreous detachment, the separated vitreous pulls a tag of inner retina along with.

3. OCT helps in diagnosing vitreofoveal traction in the fellow eyes of the patients with macular holes.
4. OCT is an excellent modality for studying vitreoretinal interface and is helpful in studying the progression of the macular hole in the fellow eyes.
5. OCT gives quantitative information regarding the diameter of macular hole that helps in prognosticating response to surgical intervention.
6. OCT helps in providing other information like the presence of cystic changes in the adjacent retina, presence of surrounding subretinal fluid etc.
7. Following PPV, two patterns of hole closure have been described on OCT :
   Type 1 closure: Close without neurosensory deficit.
   Type 2 closure: Close with neurosensory deficit.
   The smaller sized holes have better prognosis because they tend to show type 1 closure pattern.
   In clinical practice, OCT has 4 major roles:
   A In disease staging
   B. Understanding disease pathogenesis
   C. Follow-up following surgery
   D. Prognosticating the surgical outcome.

A. OCT IN STAGING OF MACULAR HOLES BASED ON PERIFOVEAL VITREOUS DETACHMENTTHEORY

Case 7.1: Stage 1 A Macular Hole: Foveal Pseudocyst

Case Summary

A-70-year-old-woman underwent routine check-up of her left eye. Her best-corrected visual acuity was 20/30 in this eye and she had posterior subcapscular cataract. Fundus was unremarkable (A). She had a stage 2 macular hole in the opposite eye.

Optical Coherence Tomography

OCT line scan of the fovea showed a perifoveal detachment of the posterior hyloid that was still attached to the center of the foveola. An intraretinal pseudocyst was seen in the inner part of the foveola (B). **OCT helped in diagnosing the foveal pseudocyst in this patient, which is the first step in the formation of macular hole.**

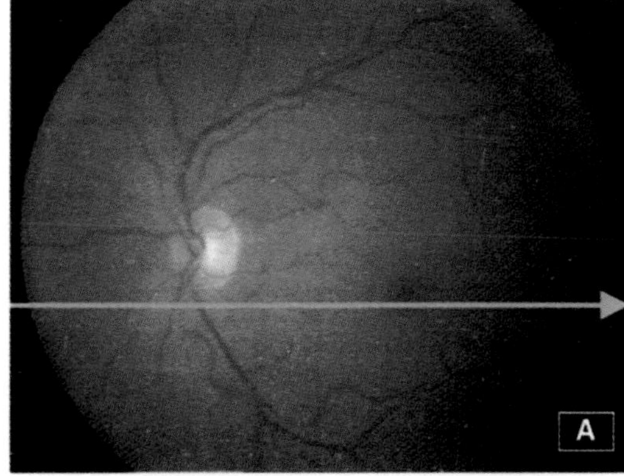

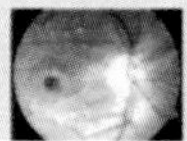

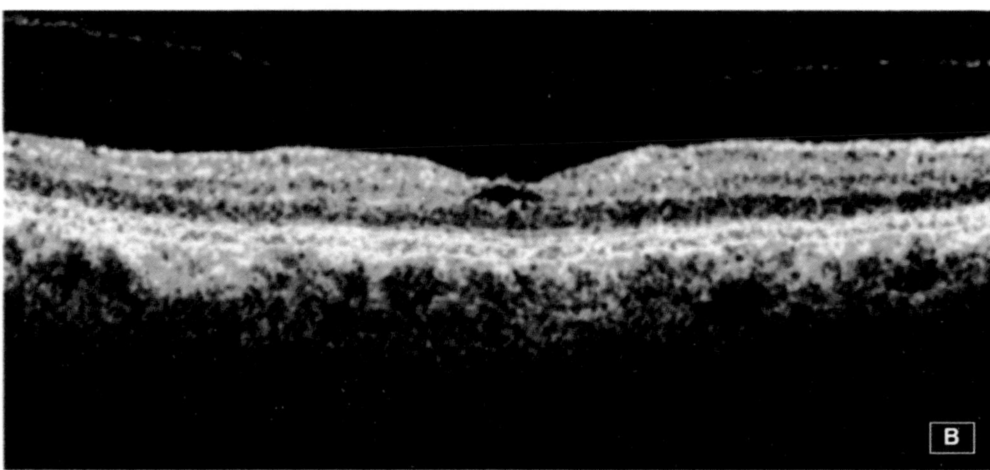

Case 7.2: Stage 1 B Impending Macular Hole

Case Summary

A 76-year-old man complained of metamorphopsia of one month duration. His best corrected visual acuity in the right eye was 20/30. He also gave history of undergoing pars plana vitrectomy in the opposite eye 6 years back for macular hole. Fundus showed a slight alteration in the macular color (arrows) (A). Fluorescein angiography revealed an area of punctate hyperfluorescence (B).

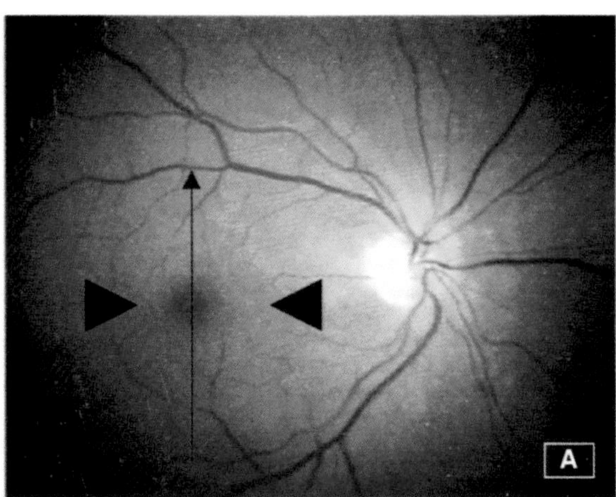

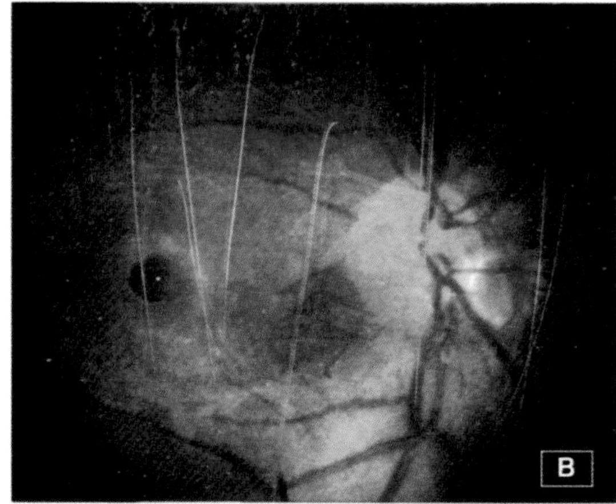

Optical Coherence Tomography

A vertical OCT image through the fixation showed loss of foveal contour. There was perifoveal detachment of posterior hyaloid membrane that remained attached to the center of the foveola. The foveal traction has resulted in disruption of foveal pit and hyporeflectivity in the inner retinal layers suggesting an intraretinal cyst, i.e. stage IB macular hole (C). **In this patient, the macula looked apparently normal on biomicrocsopy except mild discoloration of the fovea. OCT was able to detect the significant changes occurring in the retina suggesting that the foveal pseudocyst had expanded posteriorly causing partial disruption of the outer retinal layer at the umbo. The continued traction from perifoveal vitreous causes opening of the roof of pseudocyst, thus resulting in stage 2 macular hole.**

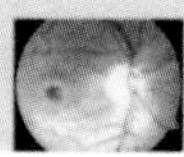

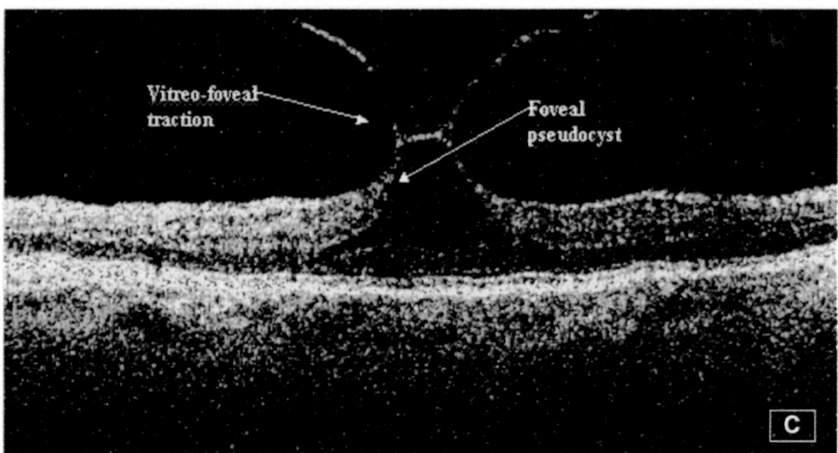

Case 7.3 : Stage 2 Lamellar Macular Hole

Case Summary

A 52-year-old woman presented with floaters in the right eye of 5 months duration. She had macular hole and her best-corrected visual acuity was 20/100 (A). OCT (B) showed retinal dehiscence confined to the inner retinal layers suggestive of lamellar macular hole. **The avulsion of the roof of foveal pseudocyst has resulted in the development of Stage 2 macular hole.**

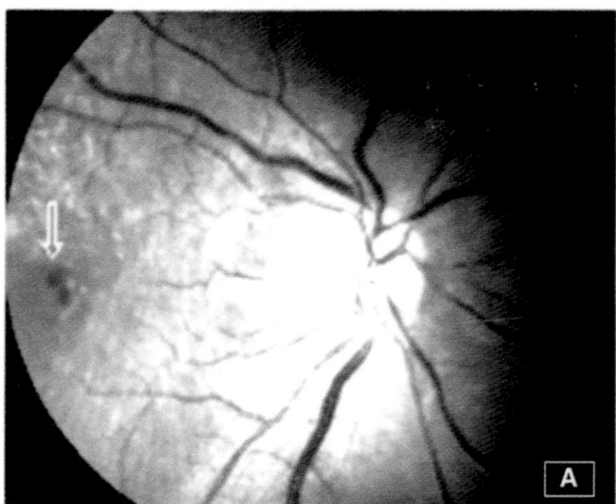

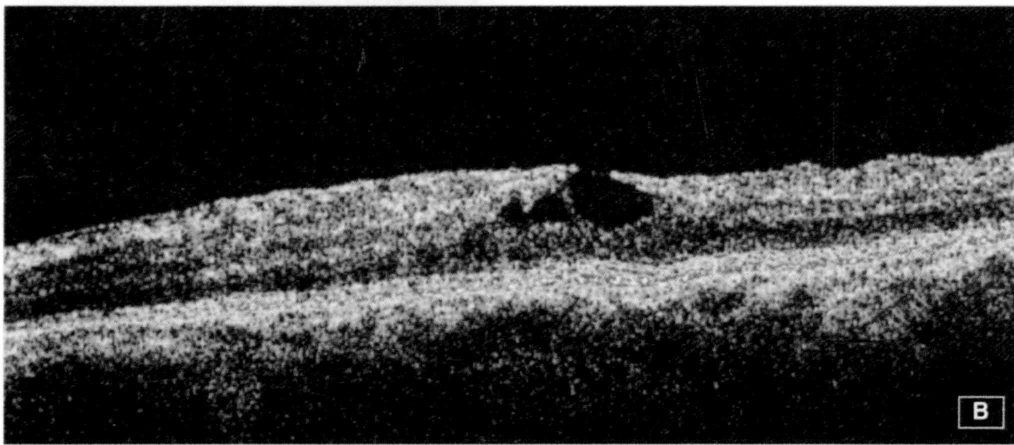

The patient underwent R/E pars plana vitrectomy with internal limiting membrane peeling and SF6 internal tamponade. Three weeks later, her vision had improved to 20/50 (C) and OCT showed closure of macular hole with return of foveal contour (D).

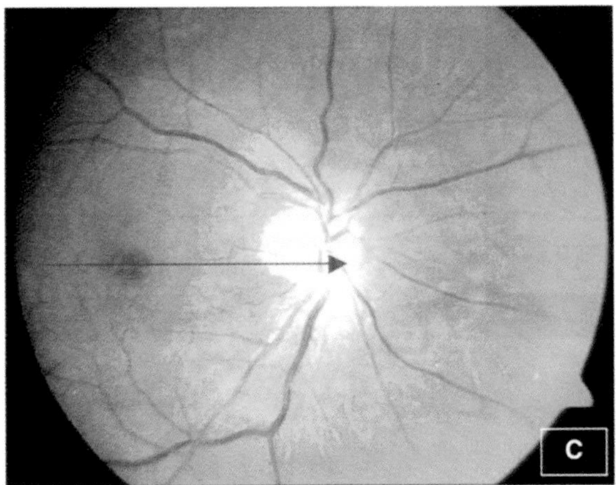

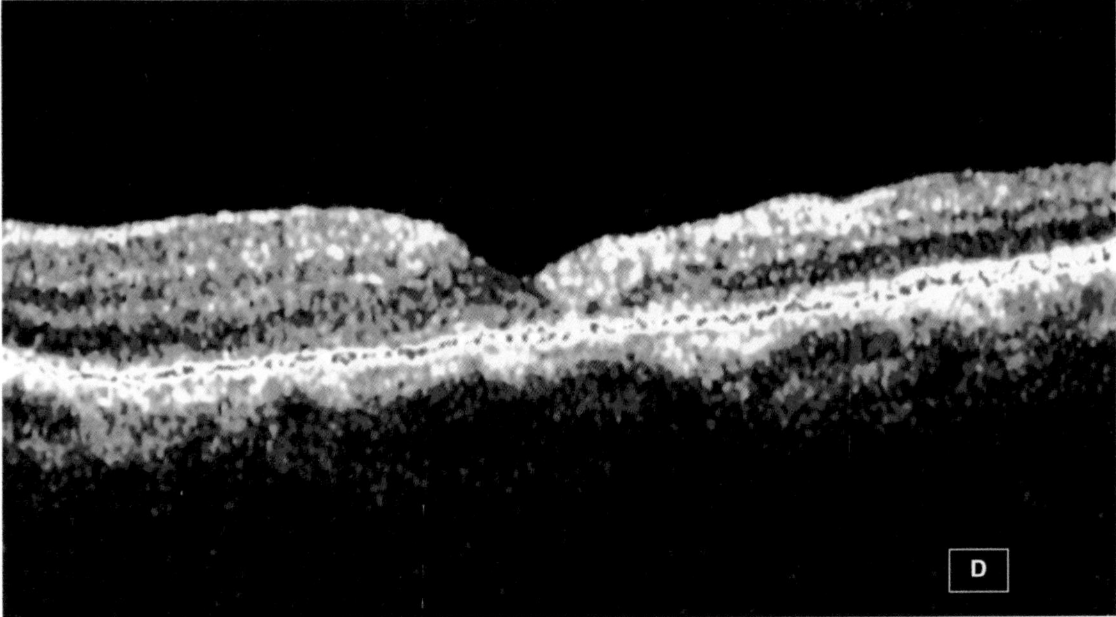

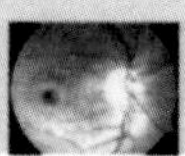

Case 7.4: Stage 2 Macular Hole

Case Summary

A 56-year-old woman complained of decreased vision of three months duration. Her best-corrected visual acuity in the right eye was 20/200. Fundus showed stage II macular hole (A). Watzke Allen sign was positive.

Optical Coherence Tomography

Horizontal OCT scan through the fovea (B) showed full thickness retinal dehiscence consistent with stage II macular hole. Surrounding retina showed thickening measuring 390 microns from the bottom of the hole along with cystic changes characterized by hyporeflective spaces in the neurosensory retina. The diameter of hole as measured on OCT was 390 microns.

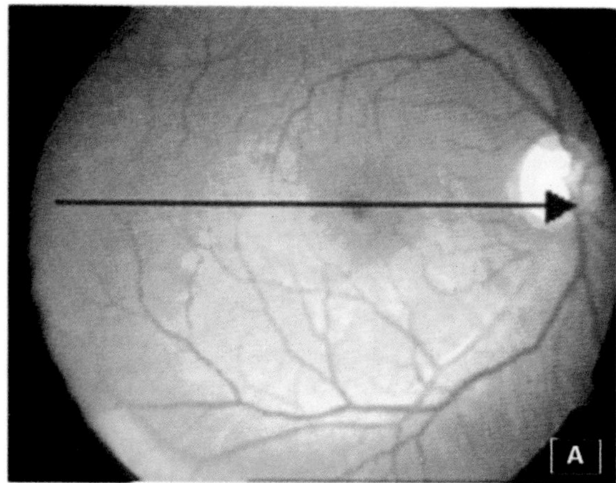

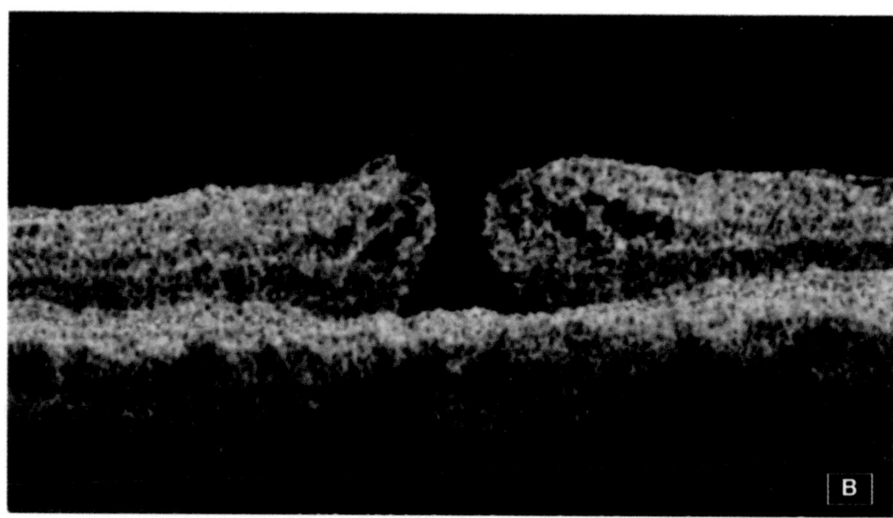

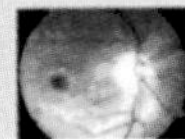

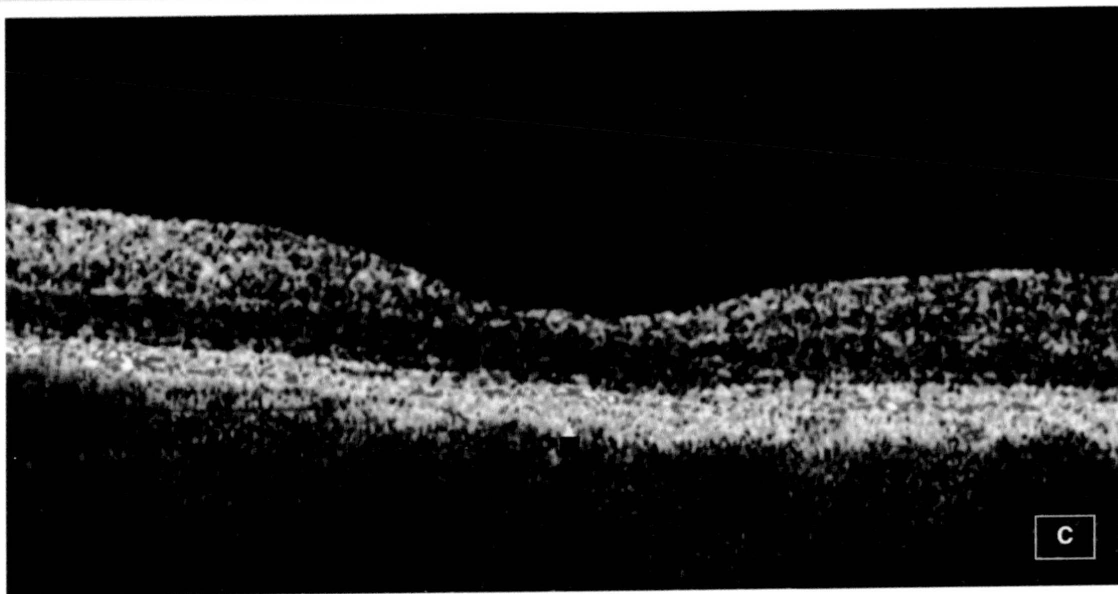

The patient underwent right eye pars plana vitrectomy with internal limiting membrane peeling. Repeat OCT (C) done 3 weeks later showed closure of hole with restoration of photoreceptor layer. The perifoveal retinal thickening and cystic changes showed resolution. The visual acuity improved to 20/30.

Case 7.5: Idiopathic Macular Hole with Retinal Detachment

Case Summary

A-72-year-old woman was seen with left eye macular hole with surrounding cuff of fluid (A).

Optical Coherence Tomography

OCT scan of the left eye (B) showed macular hole with hyporeflective space underneath suggesting the presence of retinal detachment.

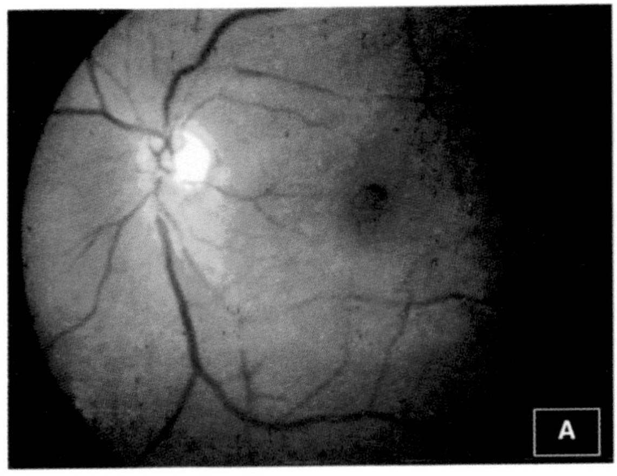

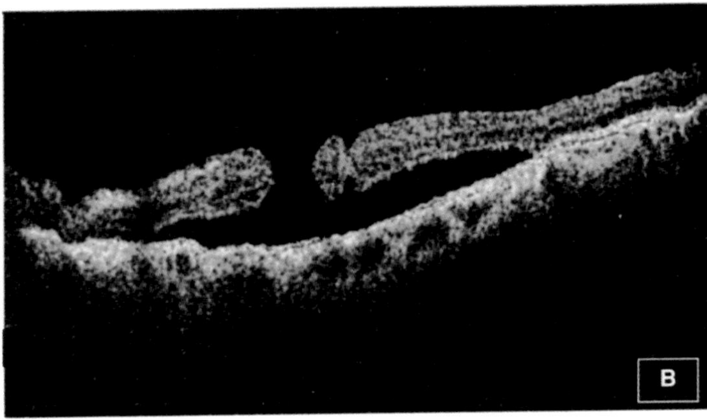

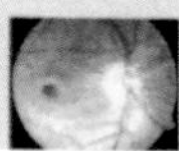

Case 7.6: Macular Hole with Retinal Detachment

Case Summary

A-62-year-old diabetic woman was seen with tractional macular hole and retinal detachment (A).

OCT line scan (B) through the foveal center shows full thickness macular hole with underlying retinal detachment.

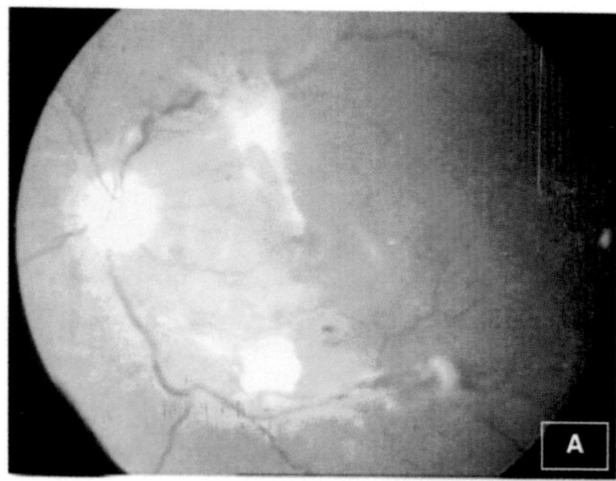

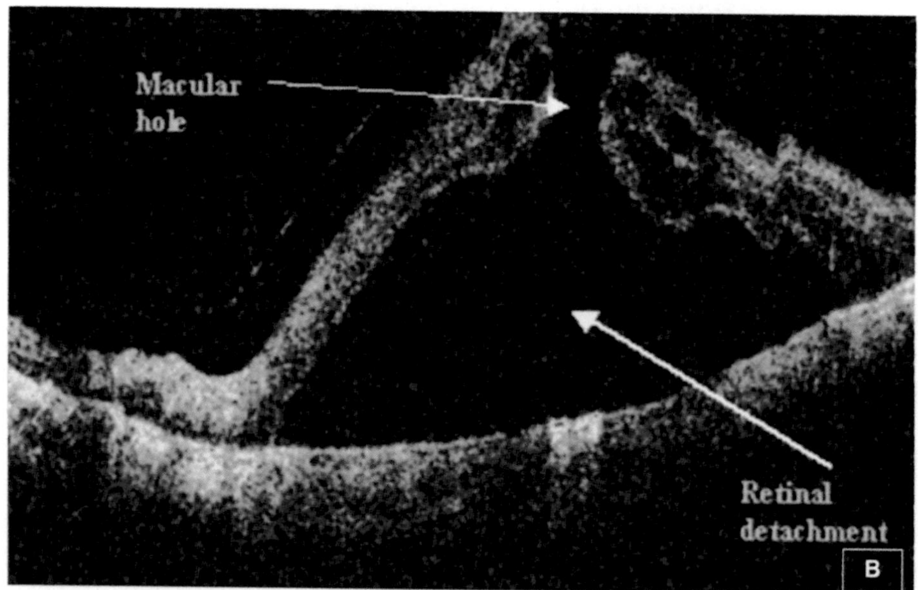

B. OCT IN DISEASE PATHOGENESIS

The two most prevalent current theories in the pathogenesis of macular hole are : 1, Perifoveal vitreous detachment theory that has been shown in the preceding cases and 2. The hydration theory.

Case 7.7: The Hydration Theory

Case Summary

A 60-year-old man was seen with right eye small macular hole with prefoveolar opacity suggesting operculum (A).

The OCT shows accumulation of the fluid within the retinal layers with partially detached posterior hyaloid membrane that was attached to the optic disc and foveal edge (B) (arrows).

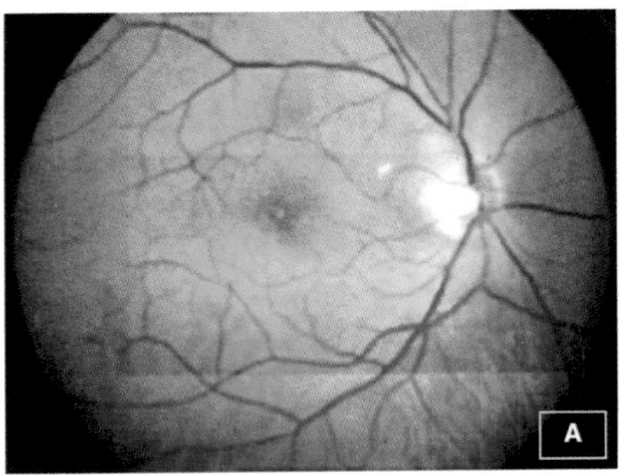

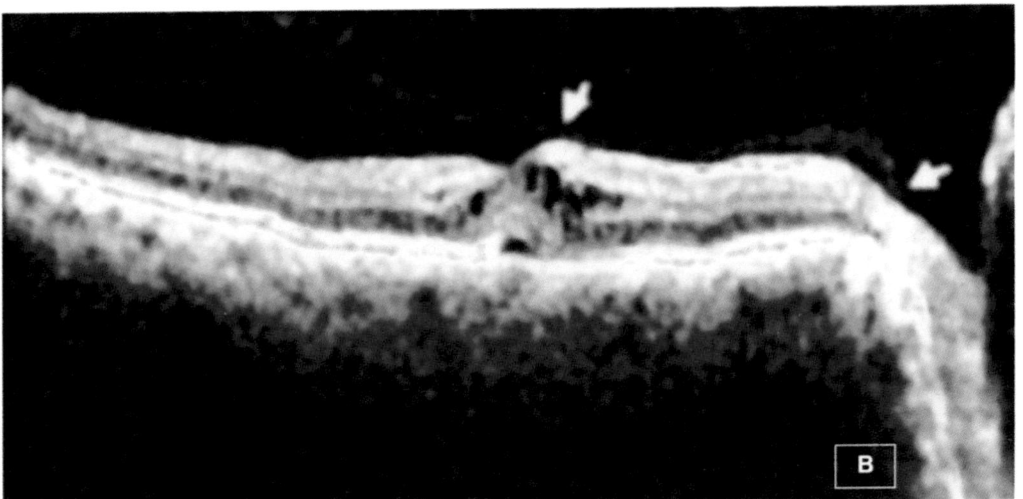

The fluid migrates into the outer plexiform layer. The rigidity of Bruchs membrane-RPE complex causes the inward movement of the swollen retina that elevates and retracts the overlying internal limiting membrane and inner retina complex (C). The posterior hyloid separation might pull a tag of inner retinal tissue seen as the avulsed operculum suspended in the detached posterior hyloid (D).

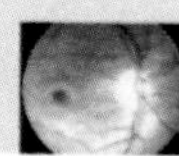

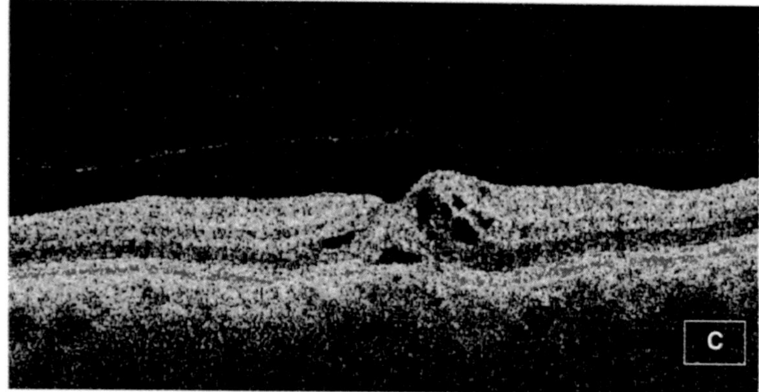

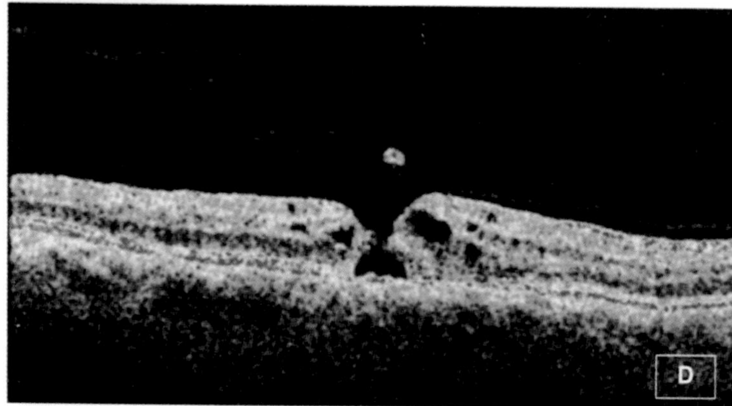

C. FOLLOW-UP FOLLOWING SURGERY

Case 7.8: Stage 2 Macular Hole with Operculum

Case Summary

A 72-year-old woman presented with complaints of difficulty in reading from the right eye for the last one month. Her best-corrected visual acuity was 20/80. Fundus showed a macular hole with positive Watzke's sign (A).

OCT (B) showed the presence of full thickness retinal dehiscence with an overlying operculum (thin arrow). The posterior hyloid membrane was seen lying 240 microns anterior to the retina (thick arrow) that seemed to cause traction on the fovea, presumably resulting in the formation of the hole.

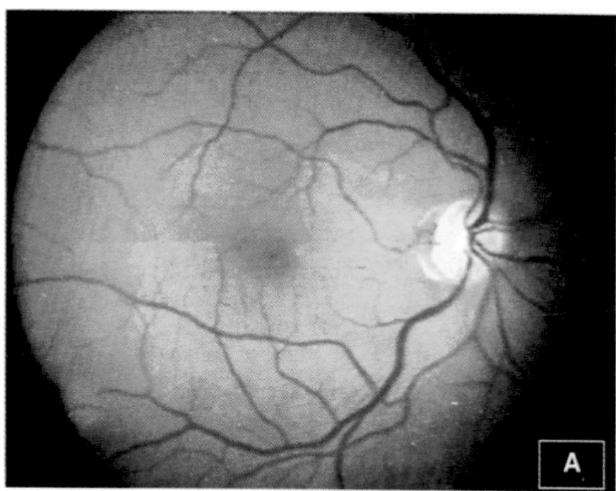

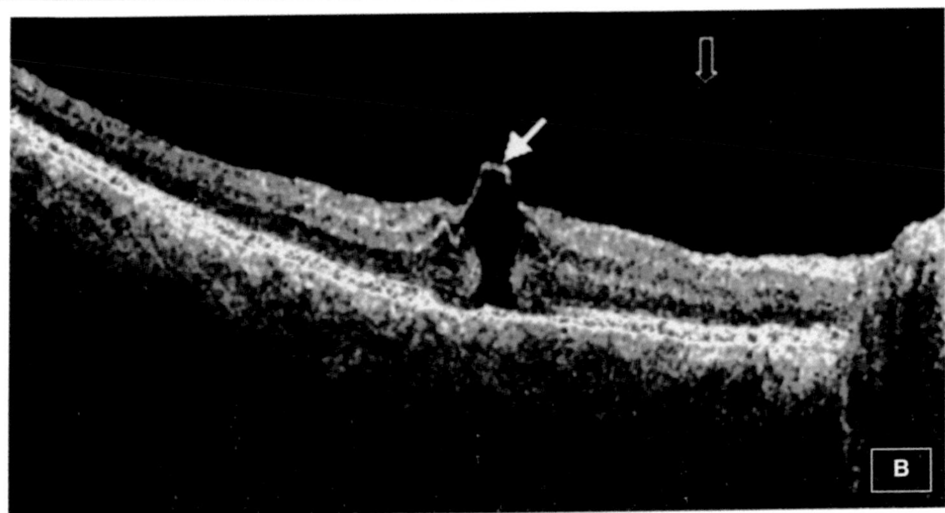
B

The patient underwent right eye pars plana vitrectomy with internal limiting membrane peeling and C_3F_8 temponade. Three weeks later, her visual acuity had improved to 20/40 and repeat OCT showed closure of the hole (C, D).

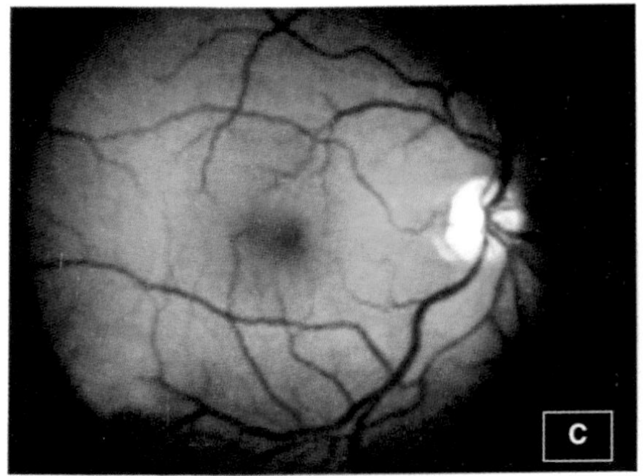
C

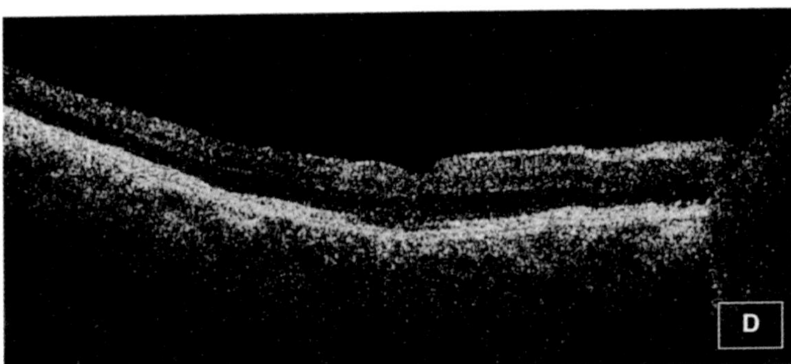
D

PATTERNS OF CLOSURE OF MACULAR HOLES

Case 7.9: Pattern 1 Closure

Case Summary

Pattern 1 closure : normal foveal contour with restoration of photoreceptor layer indicating closure without neurosensory deficit.

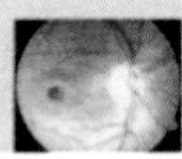

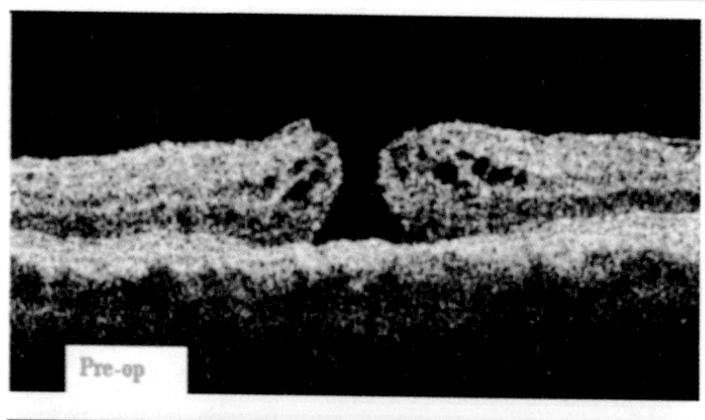

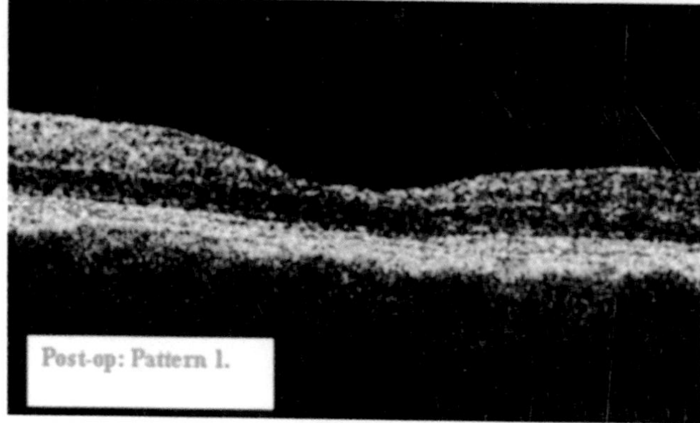

Case 7.10: Pattern 1 Closure with Restoration of Photoreceptor Layer (A and B)

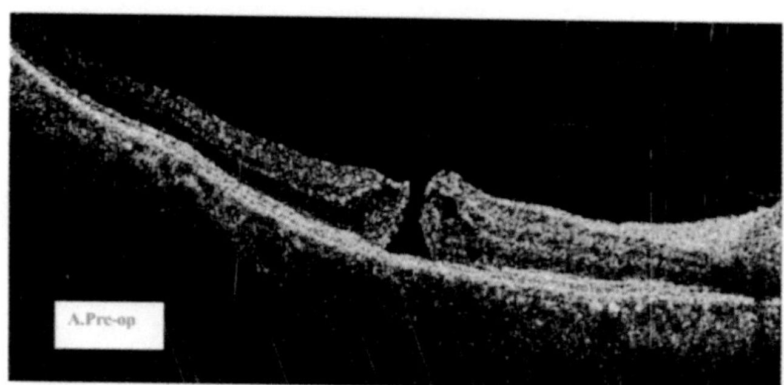

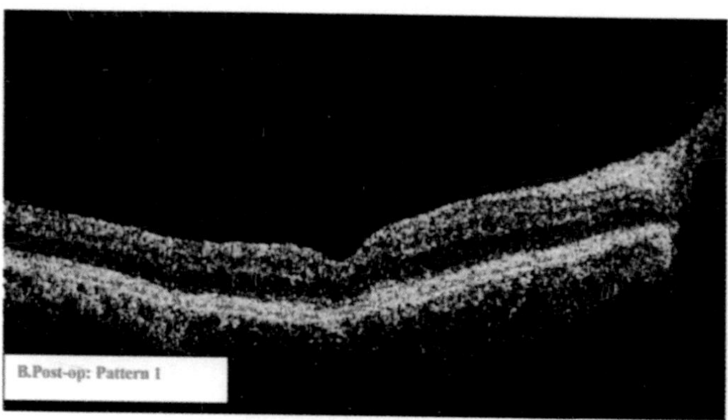

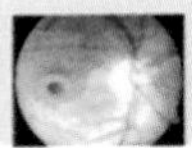

Case 7.11: Pattern 2

Case Summary

Closure of macular hole without restoration of photoreceptor layer (A, B).

Note the pre-op large size of the hole; large sized holes commonly close without restoration of photoreceptor layer.

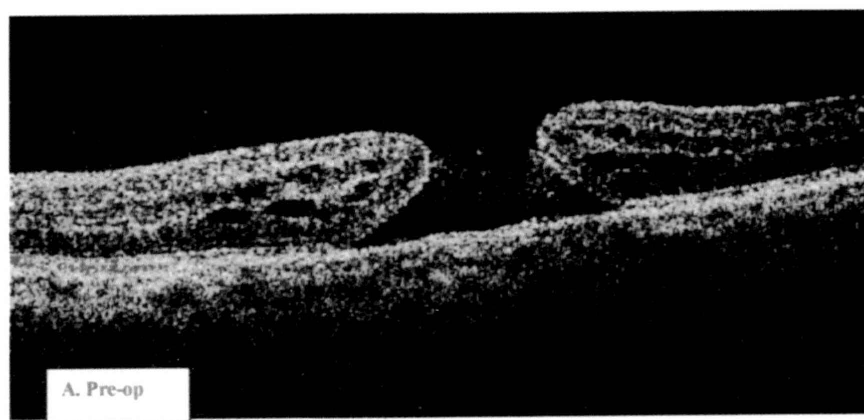

A. Pre-op

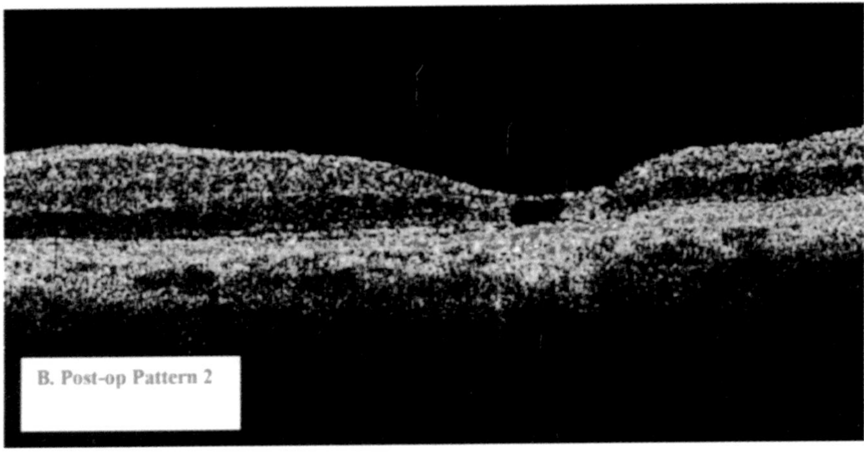

B. Post-op Pattern 2

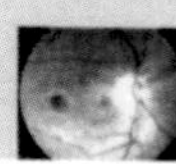

Case 7.12: Pattern 2

Case Summary

Closure of macular hole without restoration of photoreceptor layer (A, B). Note the V-shaped foveal contour with absent photoreceptor layer under the fovea.

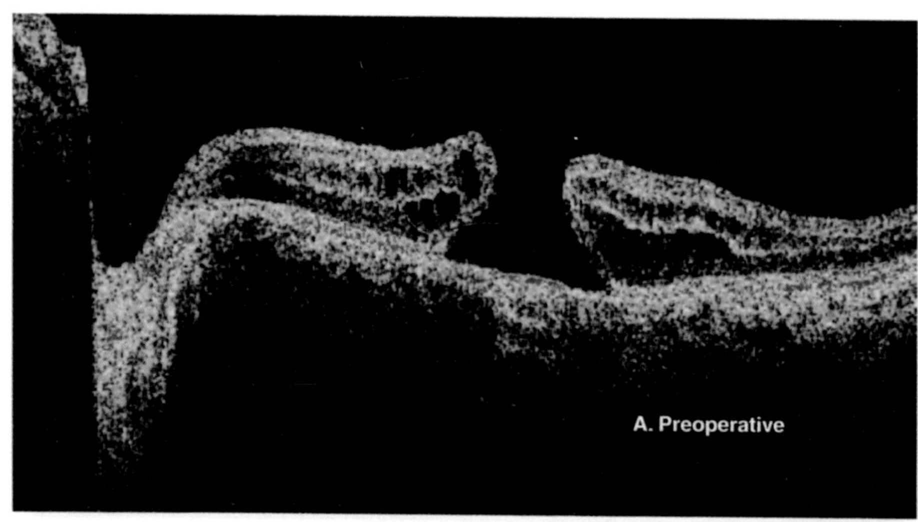

A. Preoperative

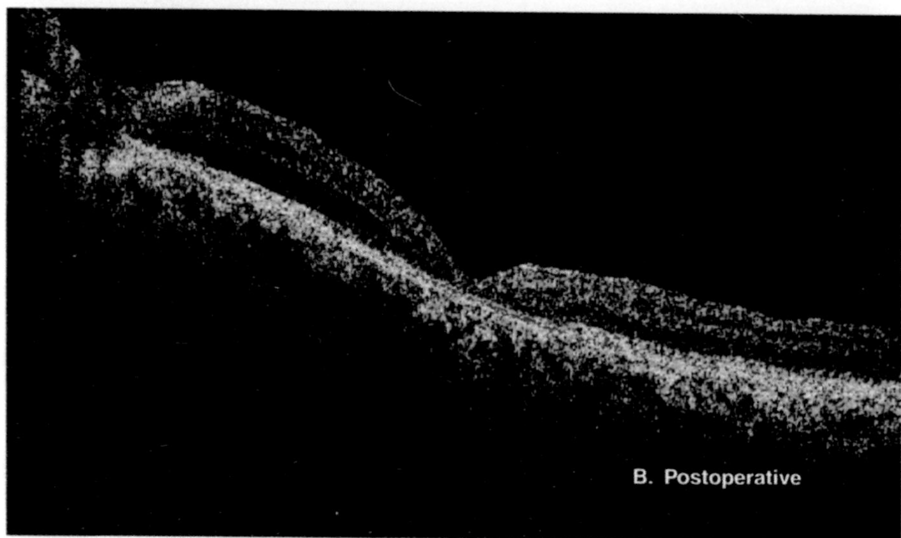

B. Postoperative

D. PROGNOSTICATING SUCCESS OF MACULAR HOLE SURGERY

Calculation of Hole Form Factor

The diameter of macular hole is a predictor of surgical success. The larger holes are associated with poor visual outcome and closure without restoration of neurosensory retina. Hole form factor (HFF) of less than 0.5 is reported to be associated with poor surgical closure rates.

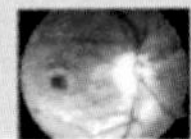

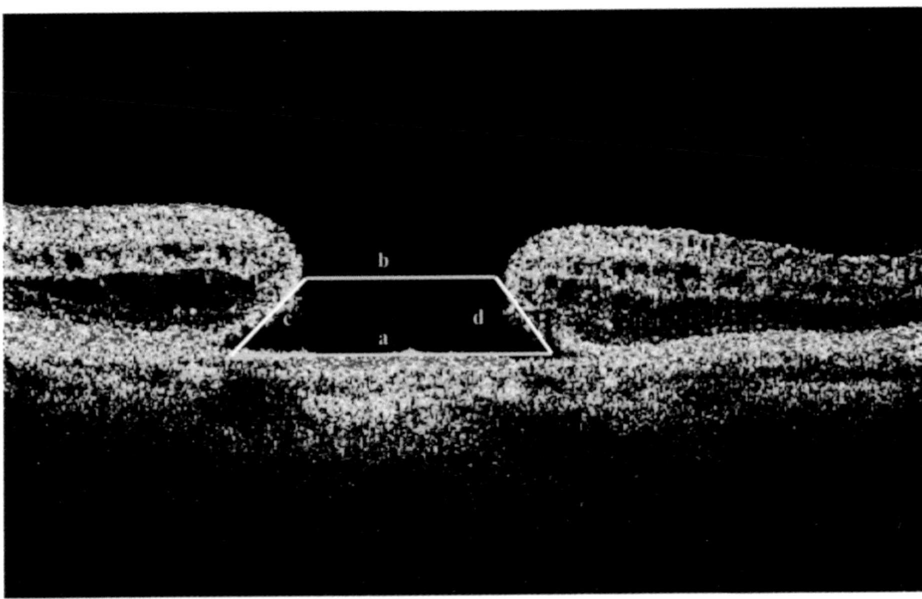

a= diameter at the base of hole.
b=minimum diameter of the hole.
c= length of left arm.
d=length of right arm.

Hole form factor = $\frac{c+d}{d}$

CONCLUSIONS

It is beyond doubt that OCT is contributory in almost every stage of macular hole management.

1. Starting from giving insight into the pathogenesis, various theories are being proposed as we are now able to study the vitreoretinal interface with the help of OCT. We have discussed the perifoveal vitreous traction and hydration theories and apparently the pathogenesis of macular hole may be multifactorial with number of factors playing a role.
2. OCT is a very useful tool in diagnosing the early stages of macular holes even when the biomicroscopic examination is normal.
3. OCT helps in monitoring the hole closure following pars plana vitrectomy.
4. Calculation of hole size preoperatively can help one predict the prognosis following surgery.

SUGGESTED READINGS

1. Hee MR, Puliafito CA, Carlton W et al. Optical coherence tomography of macular holes. Ophthalmol 1995; 102:748-56.
2. Ullrich S, Haritoglou C, Gass C et al. Macular hole size as a prognostic factor in macular hole surgery. Br J Ophthalmol 2002;86:390-93.
3. Johnson MW. Improvements in understanding and treatment of macular holes. Curr opin Ophthalmol 2002; 13:152-60.
4. Chauhan DS, Antcliff RJ, Rai PA ,et al. Papillofoveal traction in macular hole formation. Arch Ophthalmol 2000;118:32-38.
5. Tornambe PE Macular hole genesis: The Hydration Theory. Retina 2003; 23: 421-24.
6. Imani M, Iijima H, Gotoh T, Tsukahara S. Optical coherence tomography of successfully repired idiopathic macular holes. Am J Ophthalmol 1999;128:621-27.

Chapter 8

Retinal Vascular Occlusions

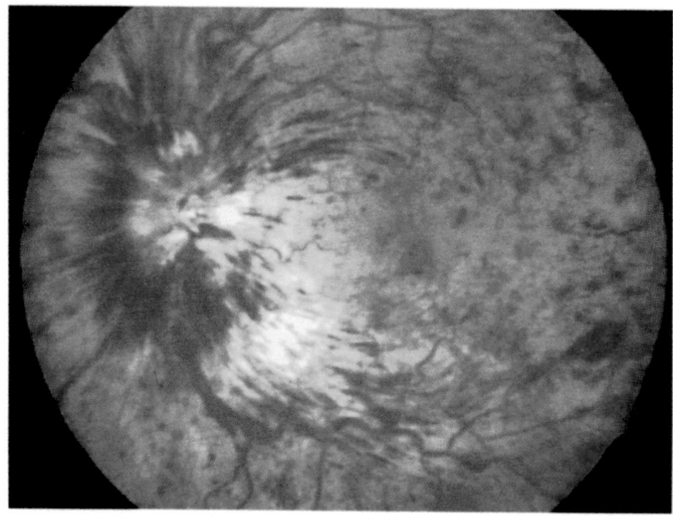

The vascular occlusions can be either arterial or venous.

OCT plays a major role in studying the macula in various venous occlusions. The quantification and tomography of macular edema as is demonstrated on OCT during the natural history helps one to decide the management strategies for these eyes. The macula in venous occlusions shows intraretinal fluid accumulation, serous retinal detachment, cystoid macular edema, state of vitreo-retinal interface including epiretinal membranes and lamellar macular hole formation. It is an excellent modality to study the response of the macula to any intervention namely, intravitreal triamcinolone acetonide injection, sheathotomy, etc.

In retinal arterial occlusions, OCT documents either macular edema or atrophy. The area of ischemic pale retina appears hyper-reflective during acute phase and regains its original reflectivity over a period of time.

Case 8.1: Branch Retinal Vein Occlusion

Case Summary

A 55-year-old woman was seen with visual loss in her right eye of 15 days onset. Her best corrected visual acuity was 20/90. Fundus showed R/E lower temporal BRVO (A). Fluorescein angiography showed late leakage of dye in the infero-temporal quadrant and in the fovea (B).

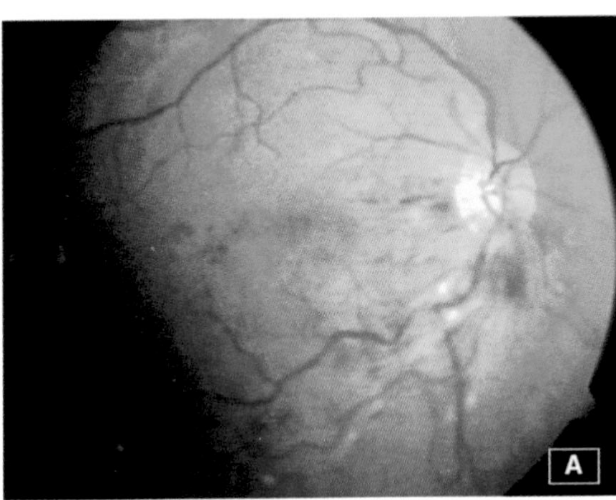

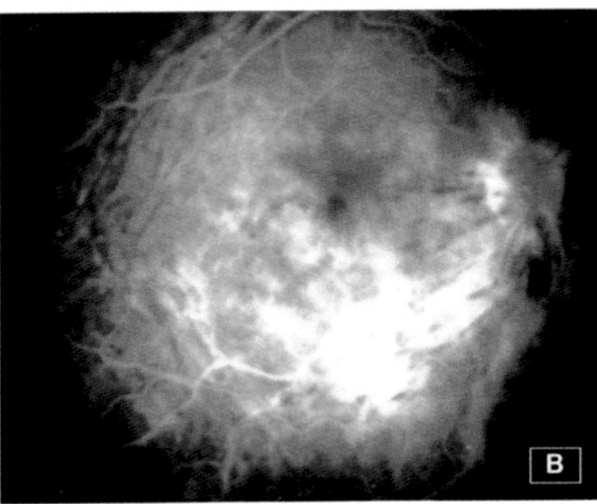

Optical Coherence Tomography

OCT showed loss of foveal contour with hyporeflective spaces corresponding probably to serous fluid in the neurosensory retina (C). The patient elected to receive intravitreal triamcinolone acetonide 4 mg. Four weeks later, her visual acuity improved to 20/40 and OCT showed reduction in macular edema (D). Three months later, macular photocoagulation was done to the leaking microaneurysms.

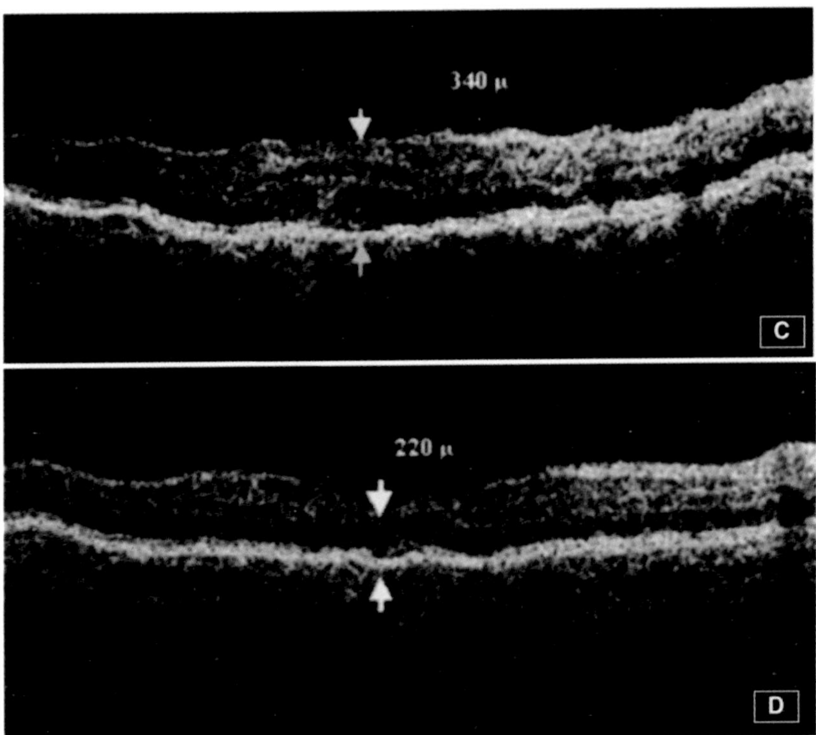

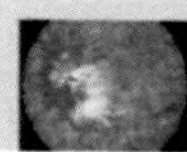

The macular edema started reappearing 4 months after intravitreal injection and repeat OCT done at 6 months showed reappearance of macular edema with hyporeflective spaces in the outer retina corresponding probably to cysts (E). **The OCT helped in monitoring response to the intervention in this patient. It showed the initial resolution following intravitreal triamcinolone acetonide. However, the effect of triamcinolone acetonide was only transient with reappearance of edema after 4 months.**

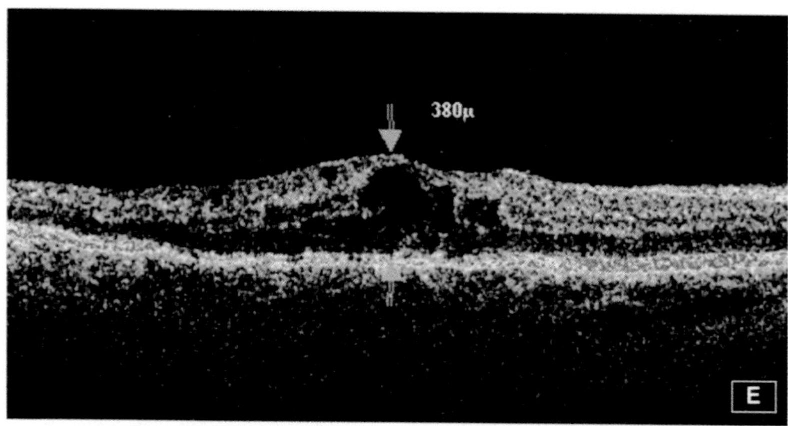

Case 8.2: OCT in Macular BRVO

Case Summary

A 65-years-old woman was seen with left eye macular BRVO with cuticular drusens (A). Her visual acuity in this eye was counting fingers. Fluorescein angiography showed hyperflurescence corresponding to the territory of macular vein (B-D).

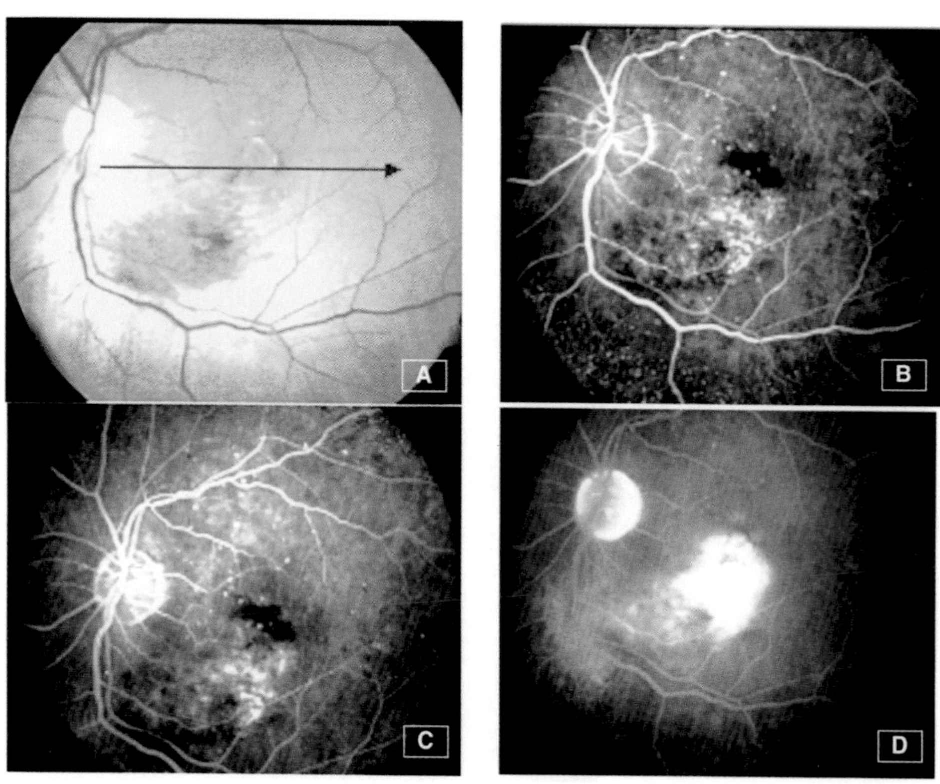

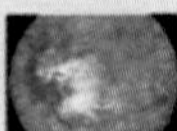

Optical Coherence Tomography

OCT scan through the fovea showed hyporeflective areas with intervening hyper-reflective walls consistent with cysts in the neurosensory retina (E). The retinal mapping showed increased retinal thickeness (F) in the central 6 mm retina.

The patient received intravitreal triamcinolone acetonide 4 mg. Two weeks later, her vistual acuity was counting fingers. She had pigmented scar in the center. Fluorescein still showed leakage, though it was less than before (G, H).

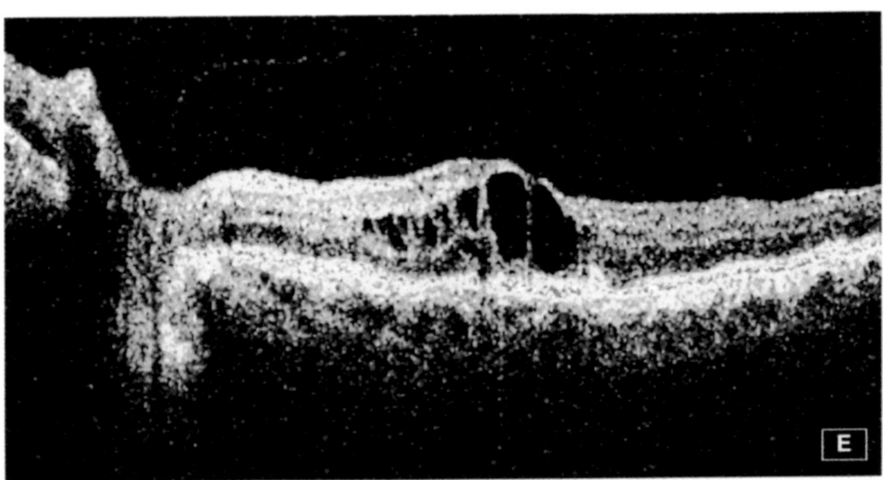

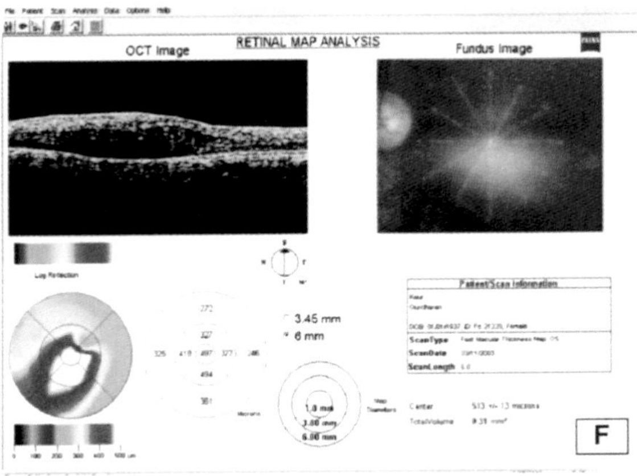

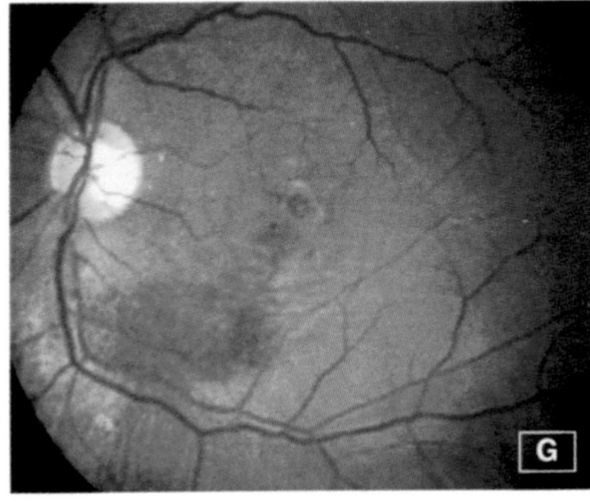

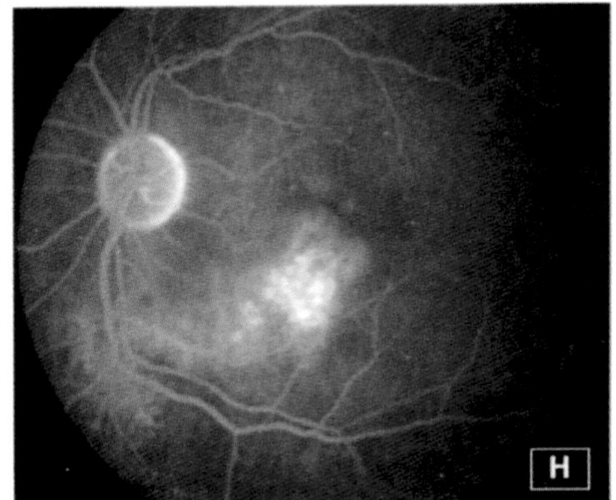

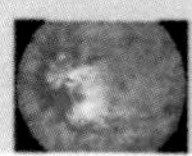

Repeat OCT scan showed normal foveal contour, reduction in retinal thickness with resolution of cystoid spaces (I, J). **The OCT helped in documenting precise improvement by quantifying the retinal thickness.**

Six months later, she showed resolved edema clinically (K). The vision, however, did not improve due to the presence of a macular scar. Optical coherence tomography done at this stage showed normal foveal contour, irregular RPE beneath the fovea corresponding to the scar and absence of cystoid spaces in the neurosensory retina (L). **OCT helped in monitoring response to therapy at the ultrastructural level.**

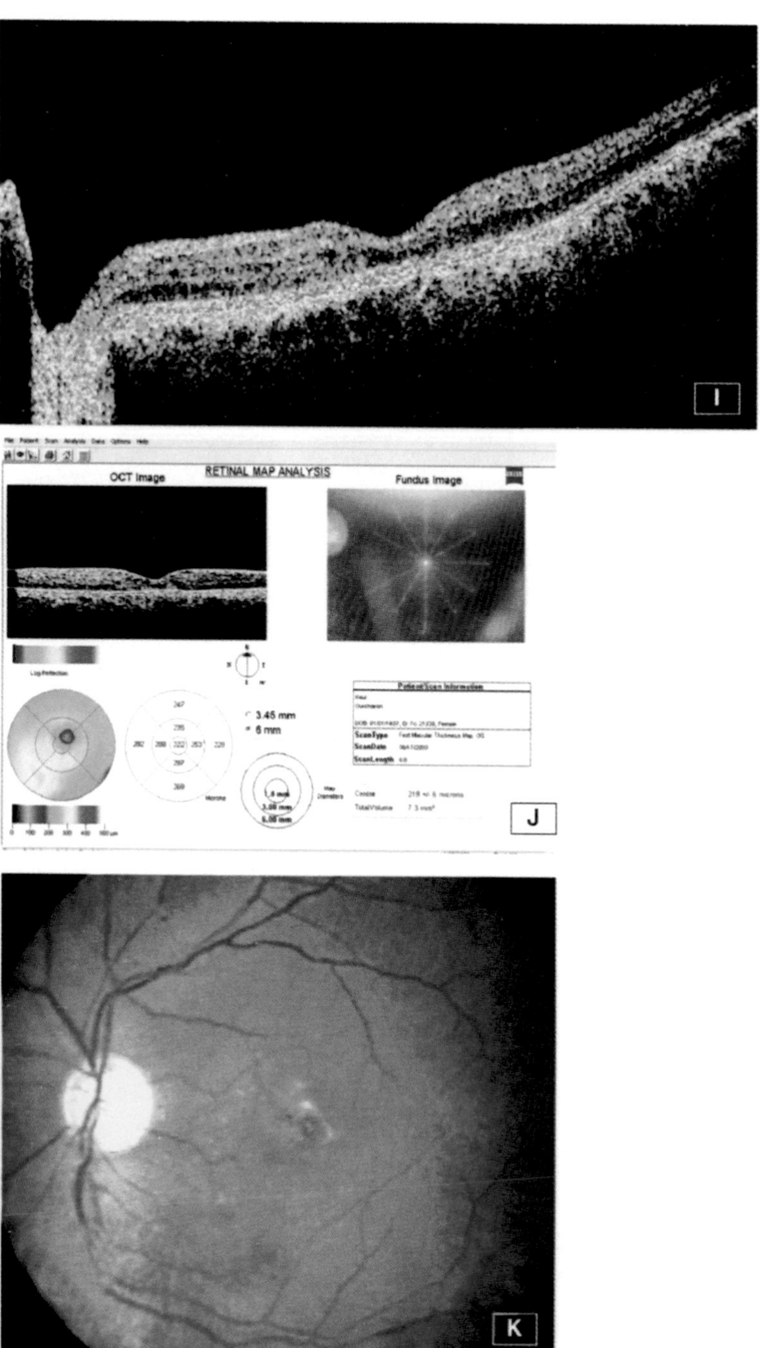

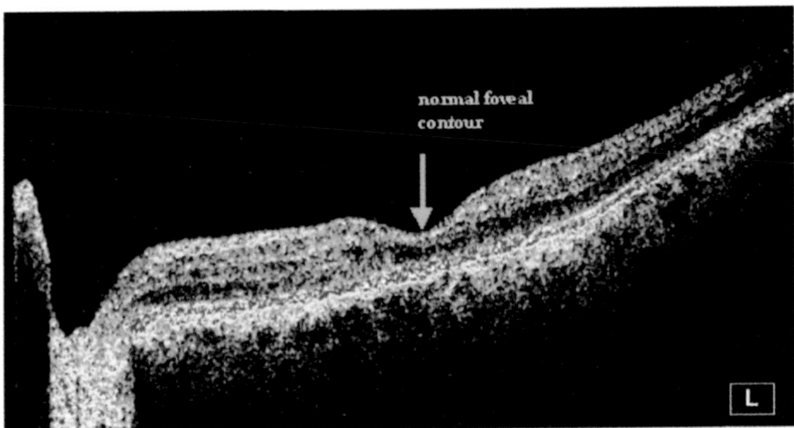

Case 8.3: OCT in Hemispheric CRVO

Case Summary

A 57-year-old type II diabetic patient with non-proliferative diabetic retinopathy developed hemispheric central retinal vein occlusion in the inferior half of right eye (A). His best corrected visual acuity was 20/200. Fluorescein angiography showed hyperfluorescence in the inferior half and in the macula (B-D).

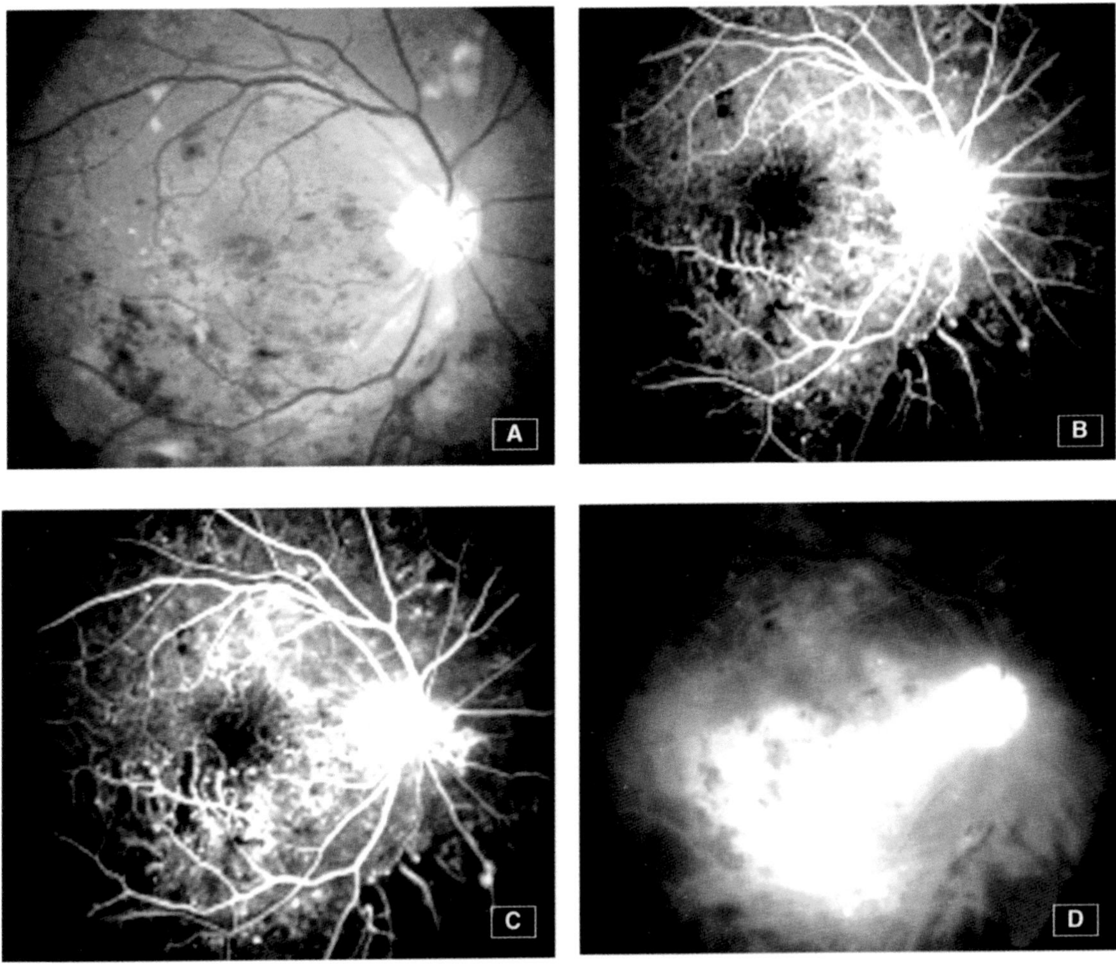

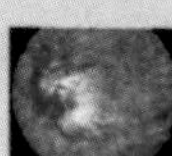

Optical Coherence Tomography

OCT through the fovea at different angles showed the presence of retinal thickening in the macula with hypo-reflective areas separated by hyper-reflective septae corresponding probably to intraretinal cysts (E, F).

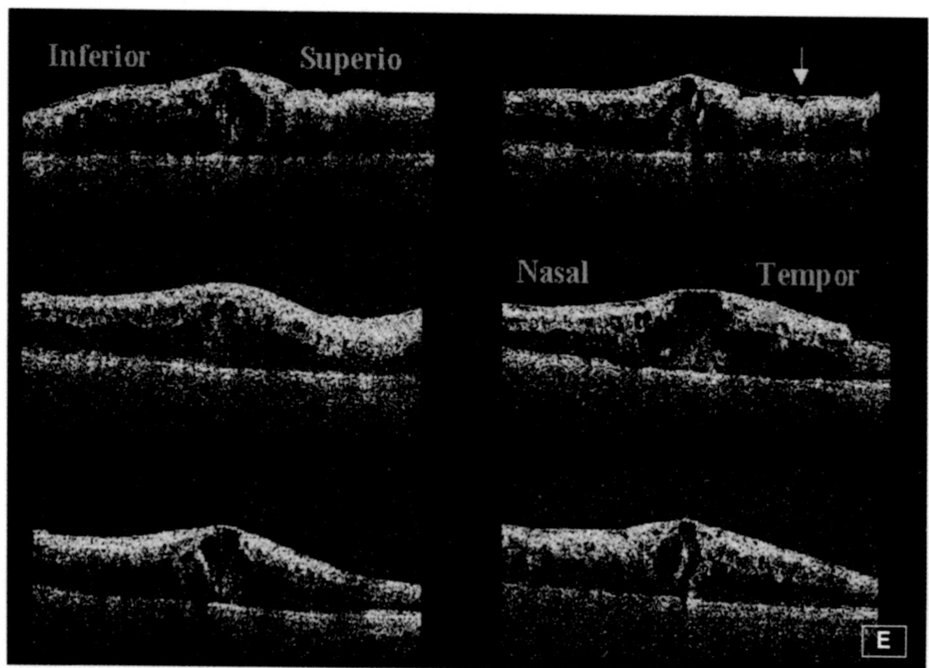

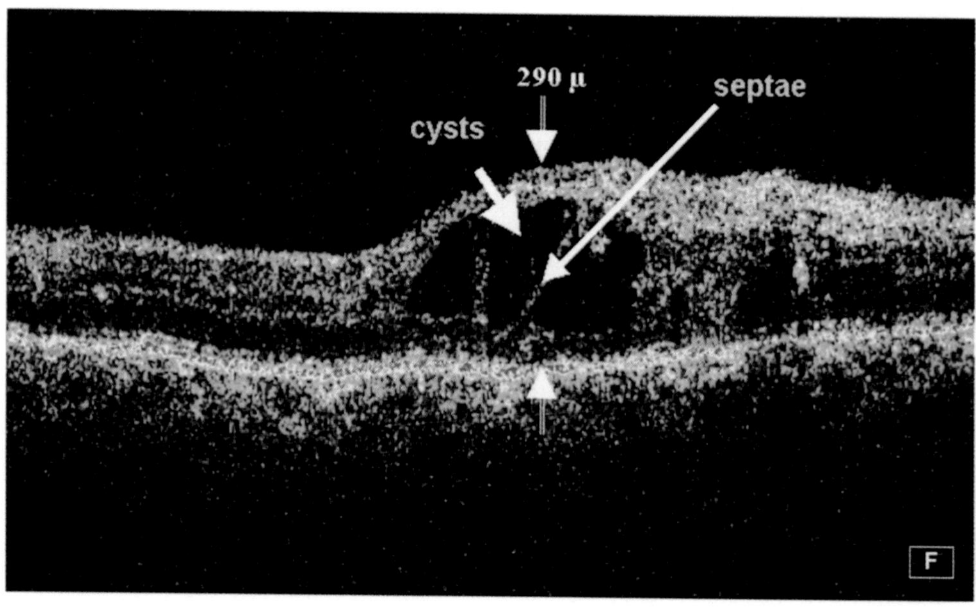

The patient received intravitreal triamcinolone acetonide 4 mg. Seventy two hours later, repeat OCT showed reduction in the retinal thickening with resolution of retinal cysts (G,H).

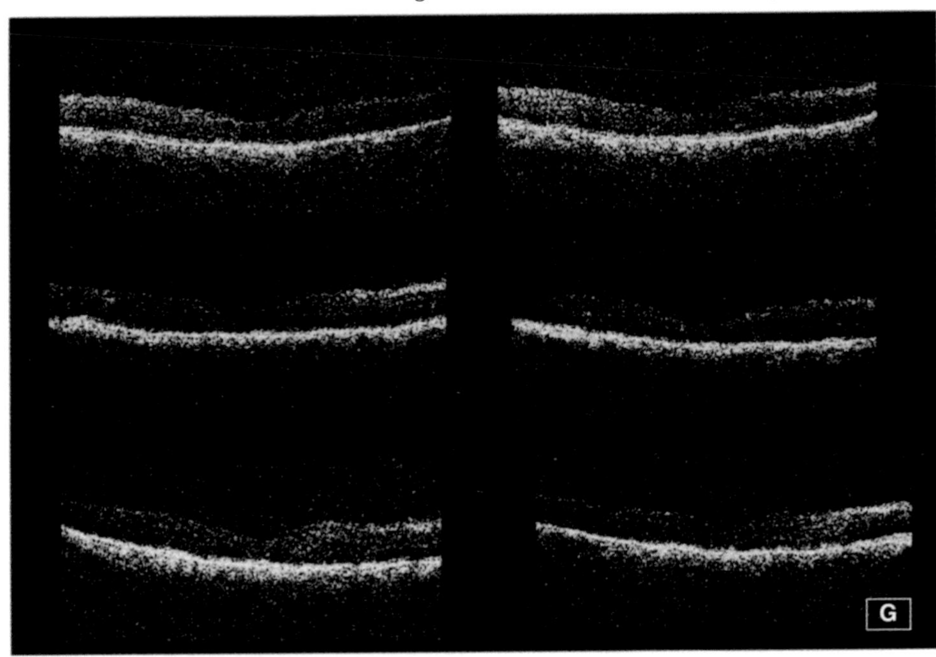

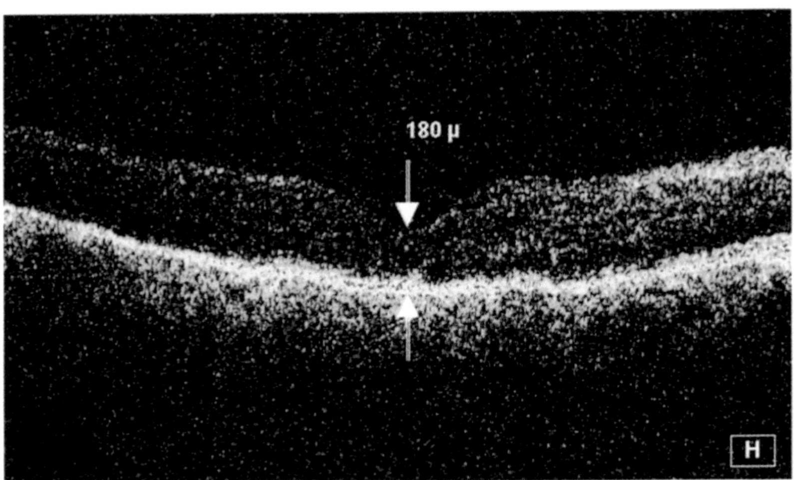

Six weeks following triamcinolone injection, grid laser photocoagulation of the macula was done. Three months later, he was subjected to panretinal photocoagulation for proliferative diabetic retinopathy. Over a follow up of four months, patient maintained a visual acuity of 20/30 and OCT shows no macular edema (I, J).

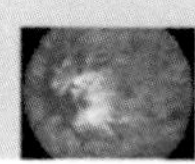

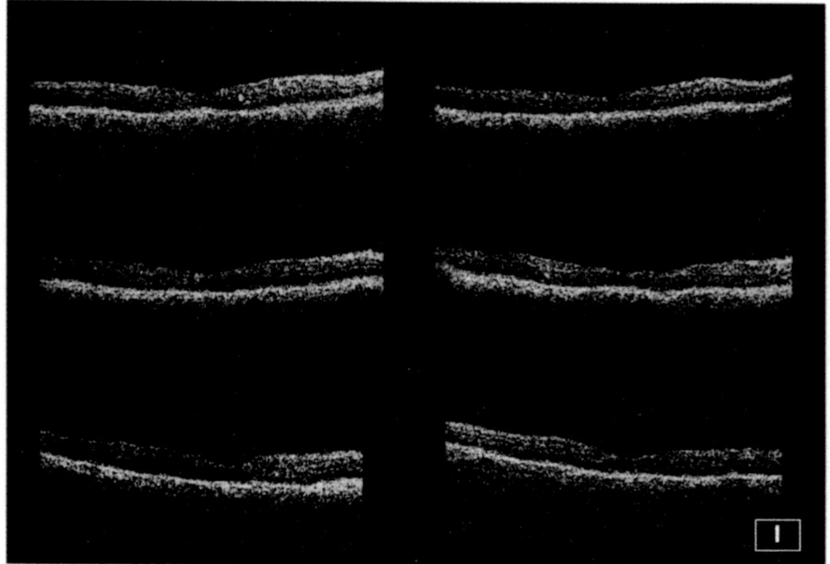

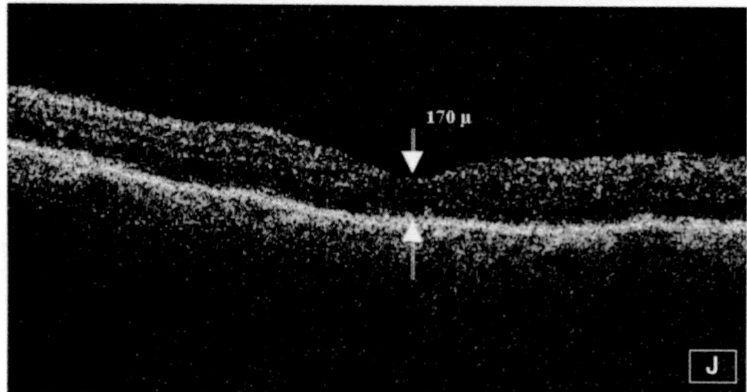

Six months, later, however he had decreased vision again and repeat OCT (K) showed reappearance of retinal thickening with full thickness hypo-reflective areas separated by hyper-reflective longitudinal lines suggestive of cystoid spaces with intervening septae. Also seen was posterior hyloid membrane 176 microns in front of retinal surface. The OCT was helpful in documenting the response to intervention, thus obviating the need for repeated fluorescein angiography.

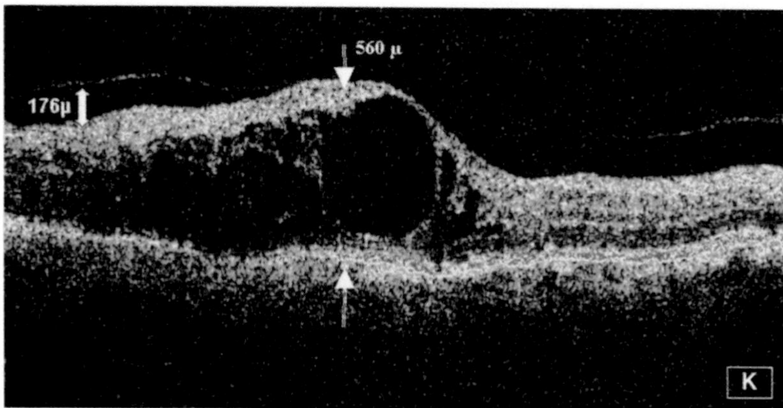

CENTRAL RETINAL VEIN OCCLUSION

Case 8.4: Intravitreal Triamcinolone Acetonide in Non-ischemic CRVO with Cystoid Macular Edema

Case Summary

A 35-year-old woman was seen with non-ischemic CRVO and cystoid macular edema (A). Her visual acuity was reduced to 20/70. Fluorescein angiography showed dye leak in the posterior pole with accumulation in the cystic spaces in the late phase (B).

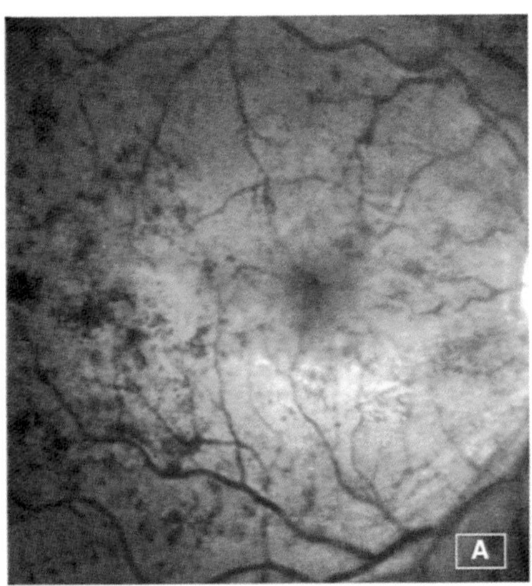
A

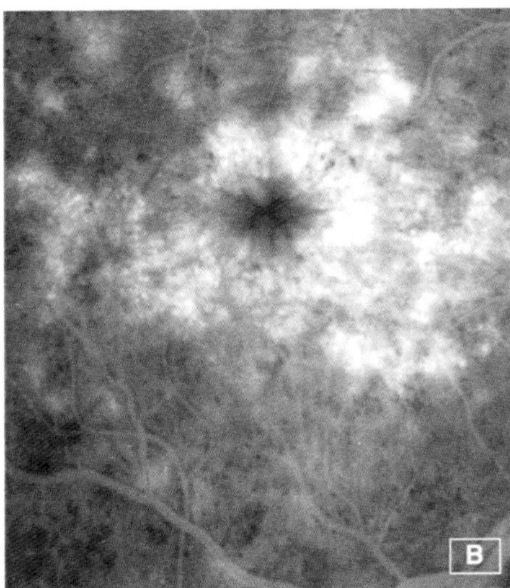
B

Optical Coherence Tomography

Horizontal OCT line scan through the foveal center (C) showed loss of foveal contour, central retinal thickening measuring 585 microns, multiple hypo-reflective areas consistent with cystic spaces at various levels in the neurosensory retina and another hyporeflective area beneath the cysts under the foveal center that was suggestive of serous retinal detachment under the fovea (thick arrow).

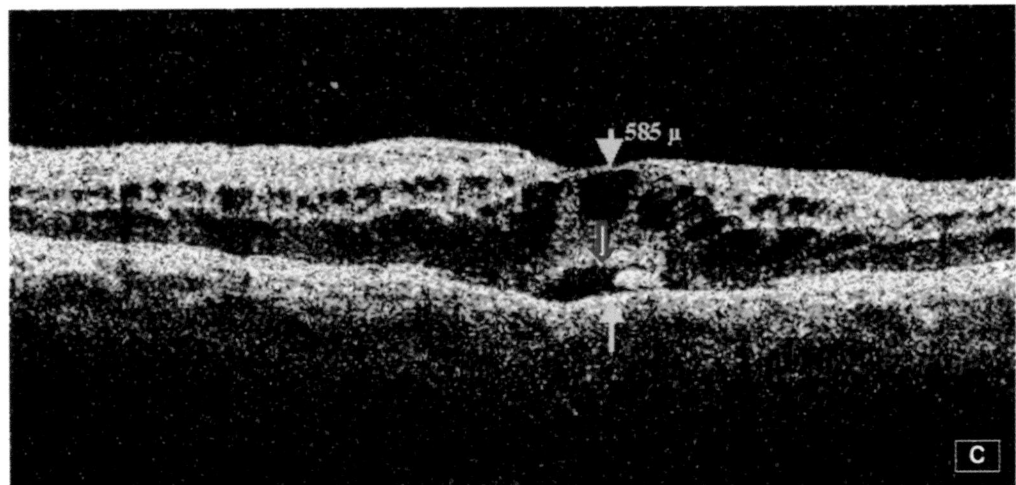

C

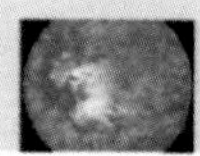

The patient received intravitreal triamcinolone acetonide 4 mg. Eighteen weeks later; her visual acuity had improved to 20/20 (D). No leakage was seen in repeat fluorescein angiography (E).

Repeat OCT (F) showed resolution of cystoid spaces as well as of foveal serous detachment. The central foveal thickness was reduced to 280 microns.

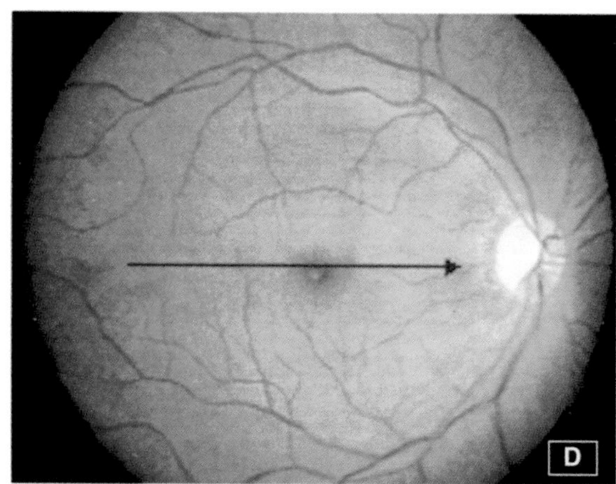

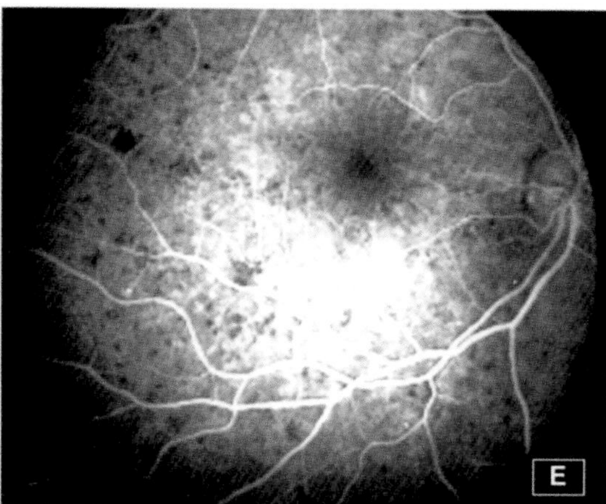

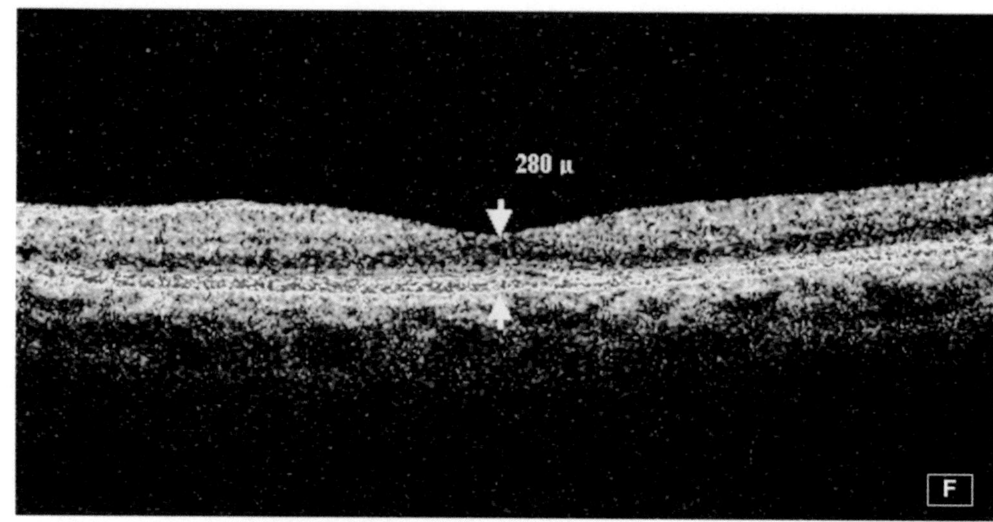

Case 8.5 : CRVO with Taut Posterior Hyloid Membrane

Case Summary

A 45-year-old woman was seen with visual acuity of counting fingers in her right eye of one year duration. The right eye showed old central retinal vein occlusion for which she had undergone grid laser elsewhere. Posterior pole showed taut posterior hyloid membrane causing an apparent traction on the retina (A). Fluorescein angiography (B) showed hyperfluorescence temporal to the fovea with hyperfluorescence in the posterior pole in late phase.

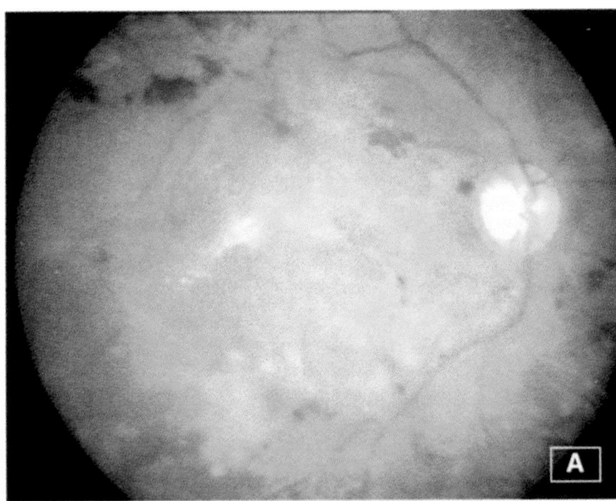

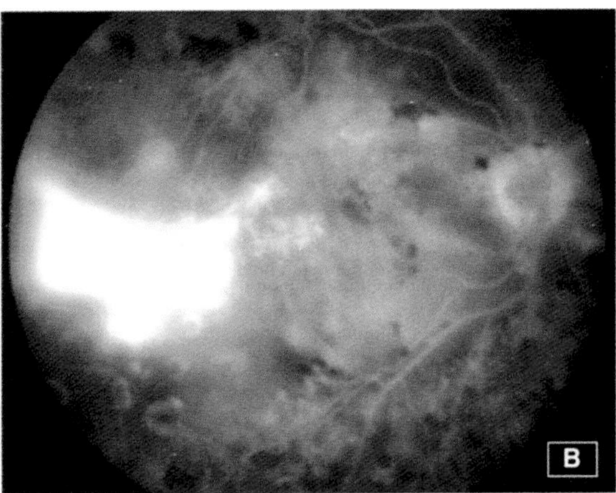

Optical Coherence Tomography

OCT scans through different angles passing through the foveal center (C) showed vitreoschisis of the posterior hyloid membrane (thick arrows) with posterior lamella causing traction between the disc and macula resulting in the development of internal limiting membrane folds seen as villi-like projections of the inner retinal layers (thin arrows).

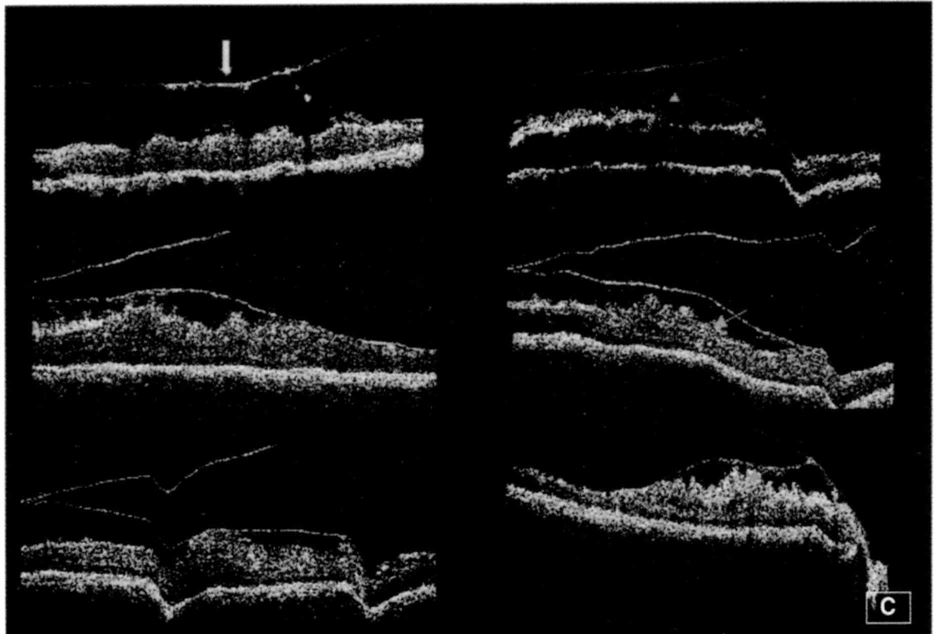

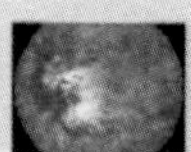

The patient underwent pars plana vitrectomy in this eye to remove the traction caused by the posterior hyloid. Eight weeks postoperatively, she had a visual acuity of 20/60. Fundus showed cystoid spaces in the center (D) that showed dye pooling in the late phase of angiogram (E).

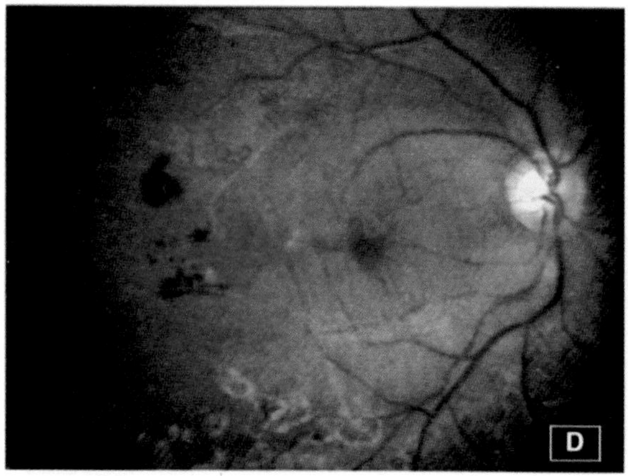
D

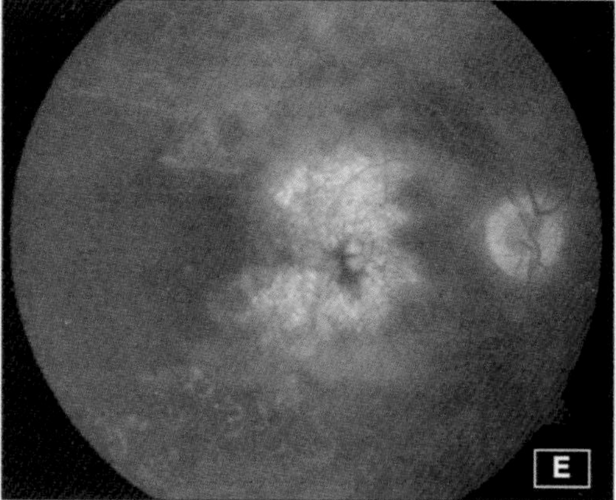
E

Repeat OCT done at 4 weeks showed foveal thickness measuring 460 microns with multiple hyporeflective areas seen at the level of both inner and outer retina, arranged in cystic pattern consistent with cystoid macular edema seen on fluorescein angiography. In addition, there was reduced backscattering from the outer retinal layers suggestive of intraretinal fluid accumulation. Note the absence of posterior hyloid membrane that was surgically removed (F). The patient was initiated on topical NSAID for the same.

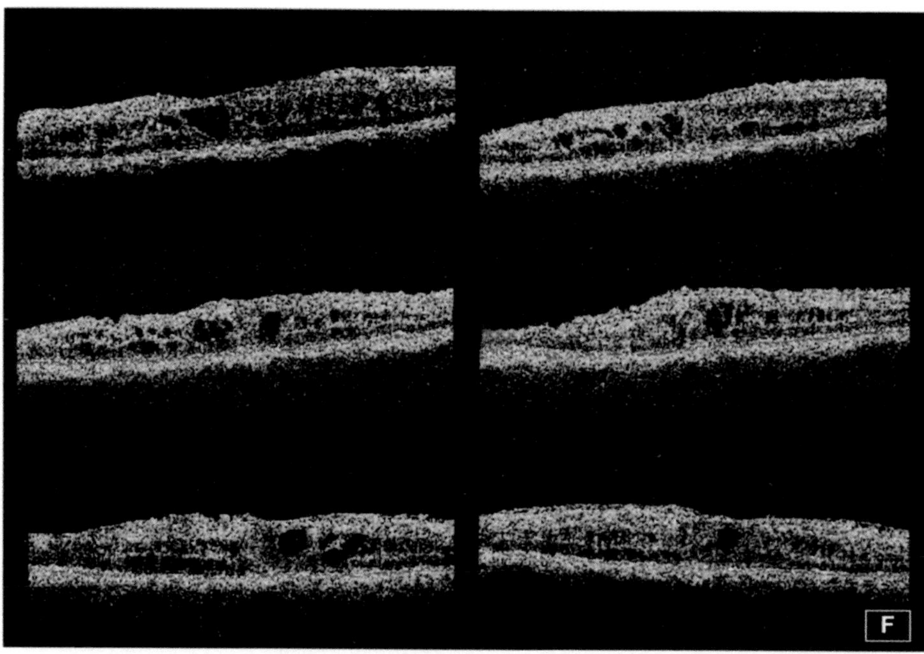
F

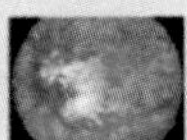

OCT IN BRANCH RETINAL ARTERY OCCLUSION (BRAO)

Case 8.6: BRAO

Case Summary

A 20-year-old girl presented with complaints of diminished vision in her left eye of two days duration. Her visual acuity was 20/40 in this eye. Fundus showed retinal opacification of inferior retina (A) with delayed arterial filling in the nasal as well as inferior retinal circulation on fluorescein angiography (B). However there was no evidence of macular edema even during late phase of angiography (C) .

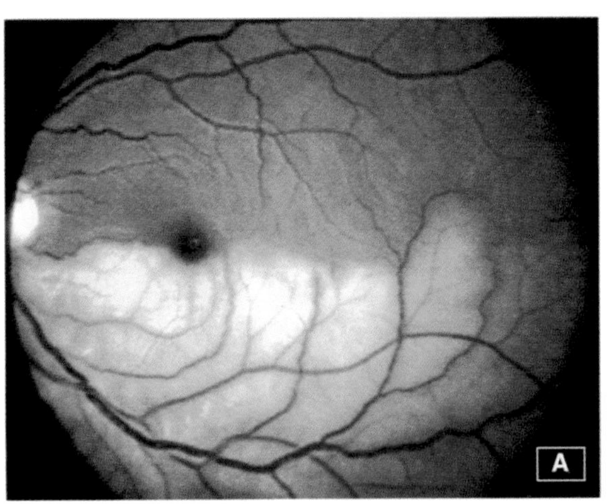

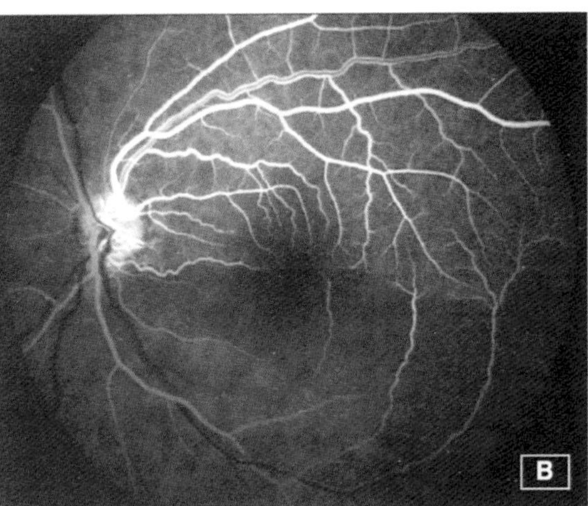

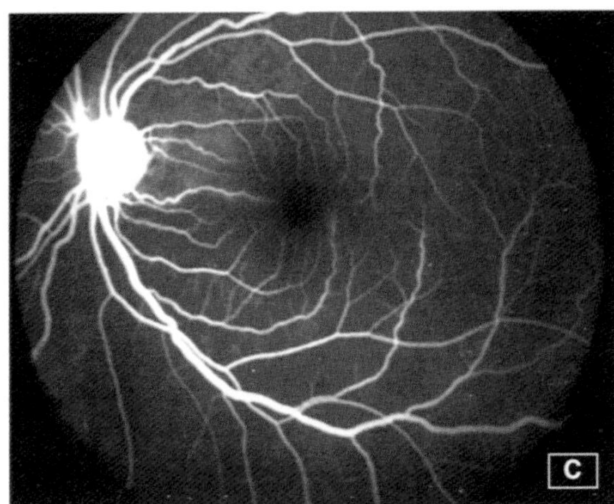

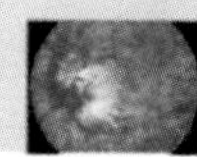

Optical Coherence Tomography

OCT done at this stage through various angles (D) showed hyper-reflectivity in the inner retinal layers of the inferior retina, corresponding to the opaque retina clinically.

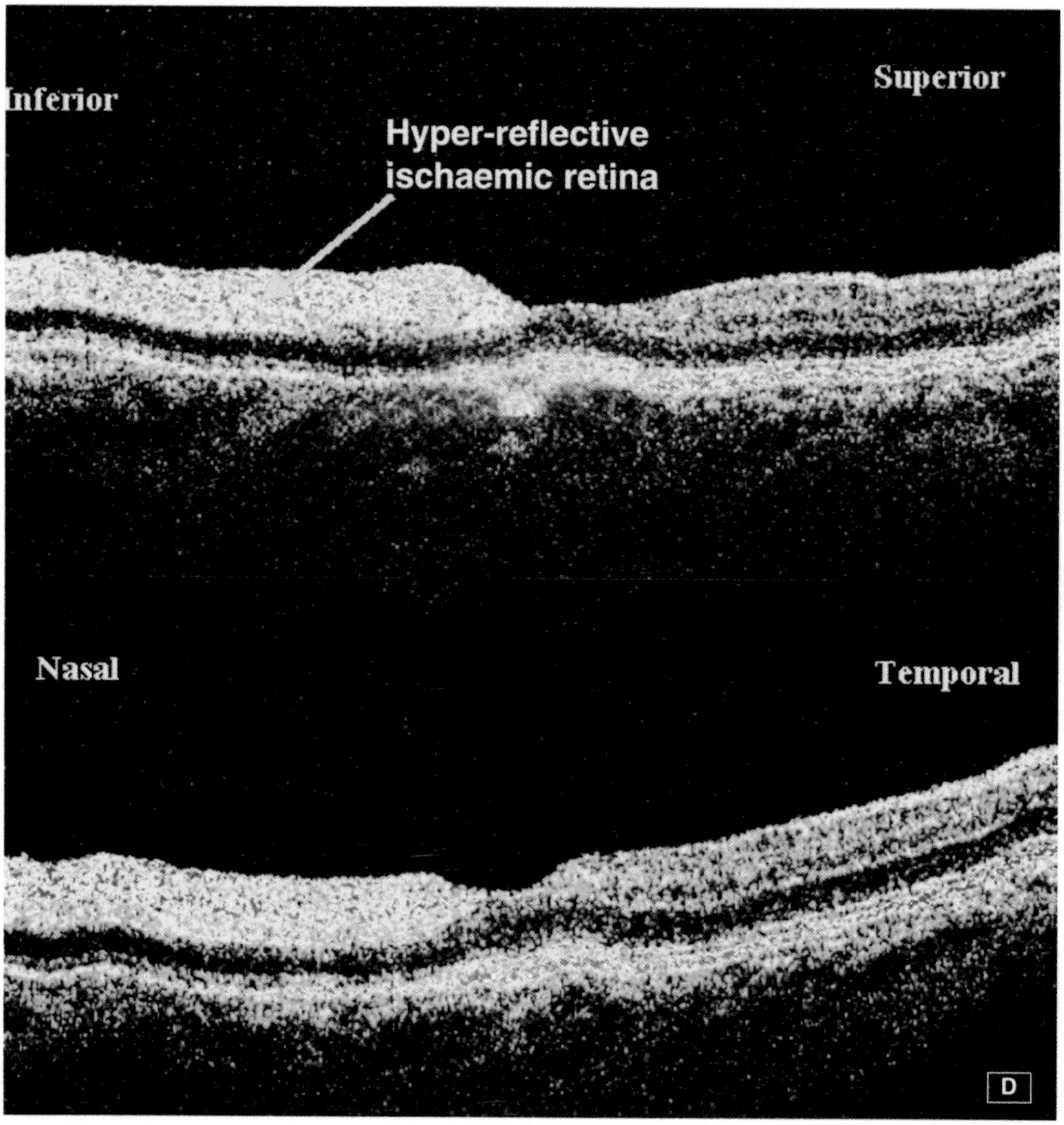

The areas of inner layer hyper-reflectivity were persistent at one week (E) whereas at 3 weeks follow-up, the inner retina did not show any hyper-reflectivity (F).

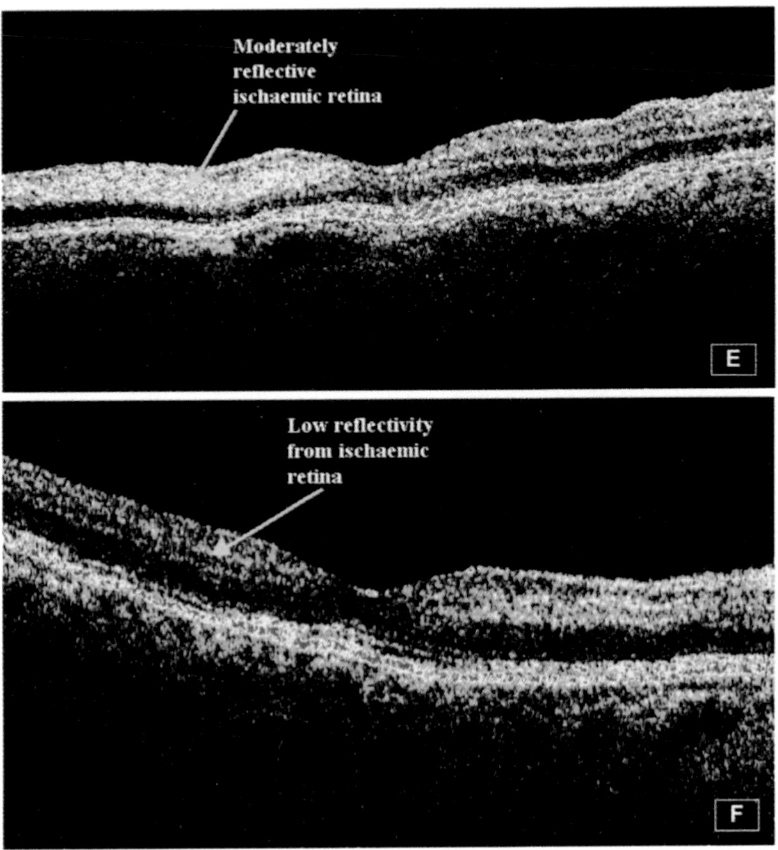

Follow-up

Two months later, the patient had regained a visual acuity of 20/20 with normal retinal perfusion on fluorescein angiography. There was no hyper-reflectivity in the inner retinal layers now (G).

The OCT in this patient documented that the ischemic retina becomes hyper-reflective compared to the non-ischemic retina.

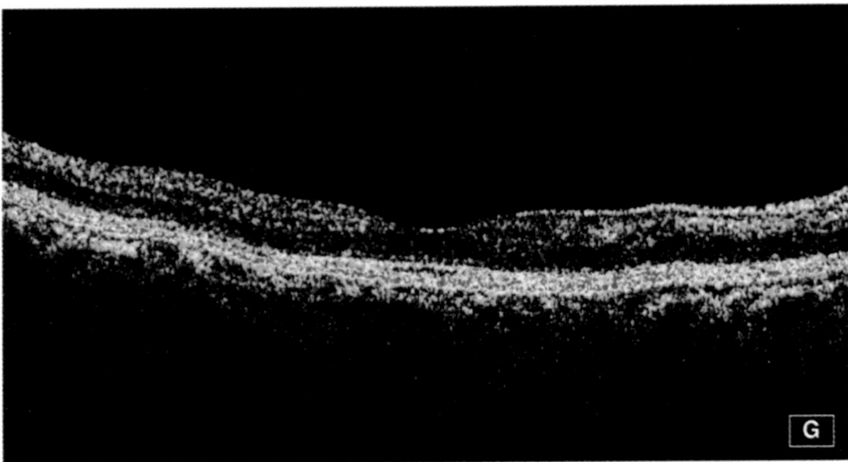

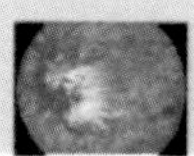

OCT IN CENTRAL RETINAL VEIN OCCLUSION (CRVO) WITH BRANCH RETINAL VEIN OCCLUSION (BRAO)

Case 8.7: CRVO with BRAO

Case Summary

A 65-year-old man was seen with retinal hemorrhages in the superior half of the retina in his left eye (A). He had lost vision in the opposite eye due to neovascular glaucoma following ischemic central retinal vein occlusion (CRVO). His visual acuity in the left eye at presentation was 20/90. Fluorescein angiography showed hypofluorescent areas in the superior retina corresponding to retinal hemorrahages with delayed hyperfluorescence in the macula suggestive of macular edema (B-D).

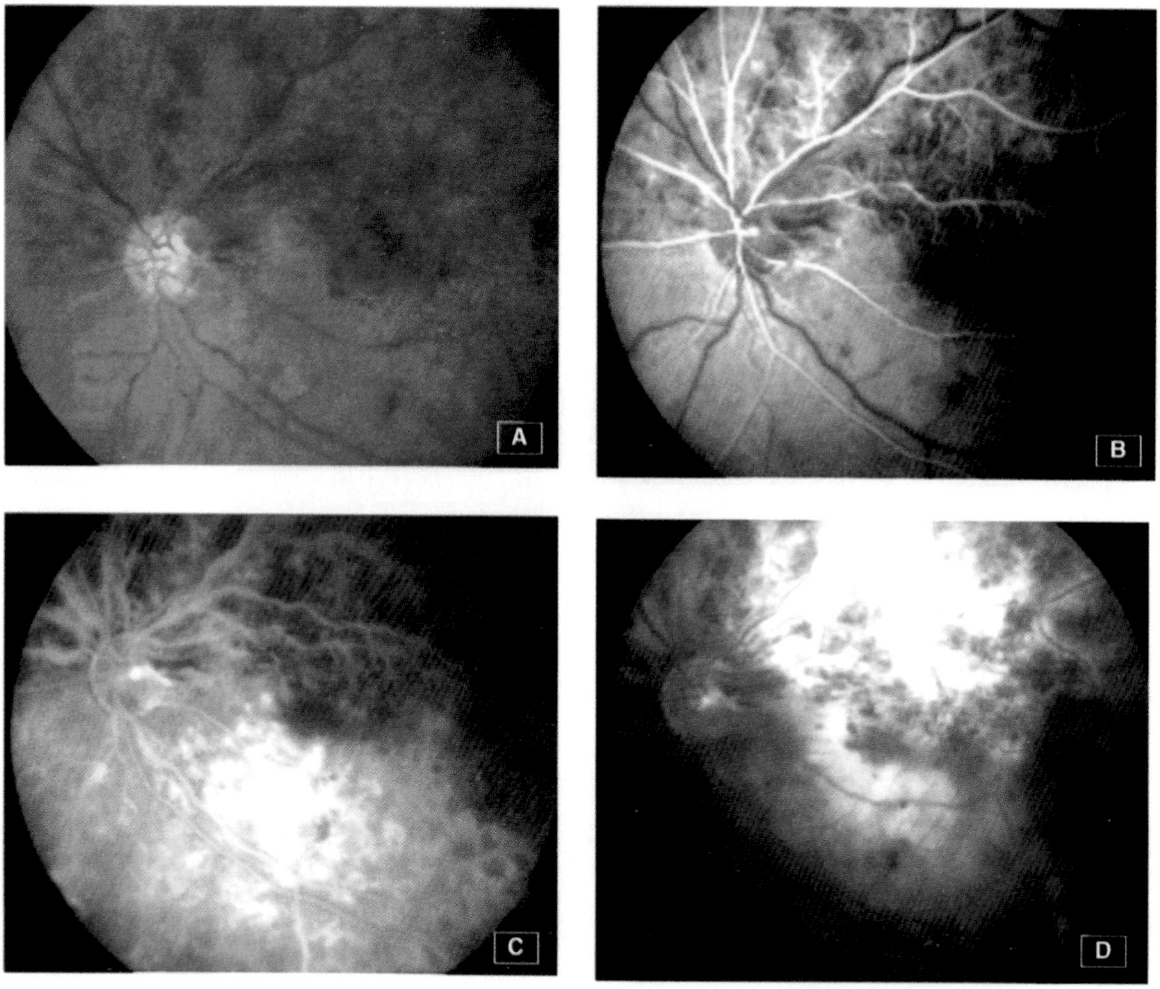

A

B

C

D

Optical Coherence Tomography

OCT scan at different angles (E) showed loss of foveal contour with central foveal thickness measuring 560 microns. There were hypo-reflective areas seen in the neurosensory retina; those under the fovea were full thickness while those in the extrafoveal region were present mostly in the outer retinal layers. In addition, there was a hyper-reflective band at the vitreoretinal interface anteriorly suggestive probably of posterior hyloid membrane attachment (arrow).

The patient had elevated homocystein levels and was treated for the same.

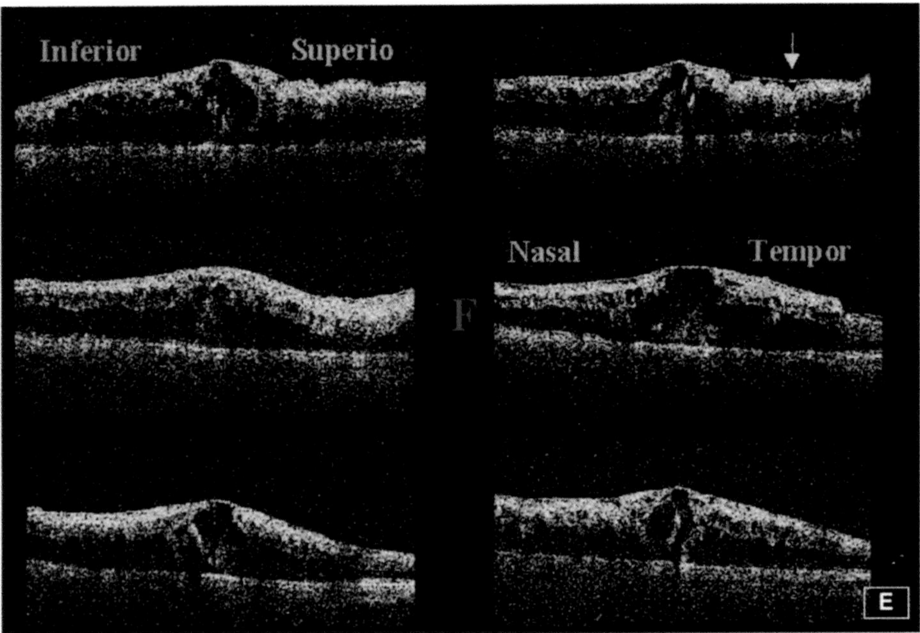

One month later, patient developed fresh upper temporal vein occlusion with occlusion of branch retinal artery supplying the macula (arrow) (F-I).

Over next three months, the visual acuity deteriorated to 20/300. Repeat OCT (J) at various angles showed foveal thickness increased to 690 microns with enhanced reflex from the posterior hyloid membrane at the vitreoretinal interface. This edema failed to respond to oral corticosteroids.

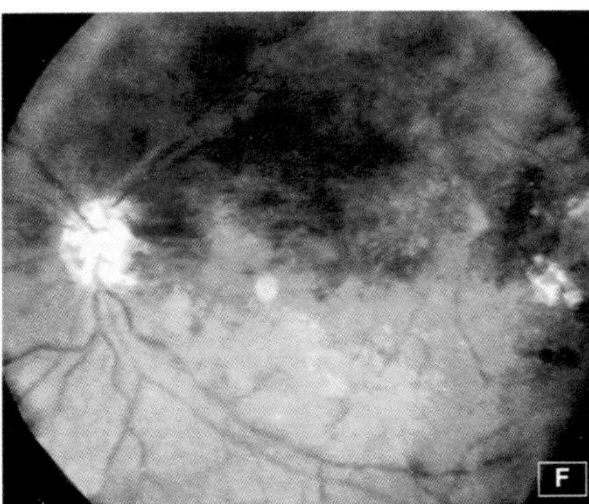

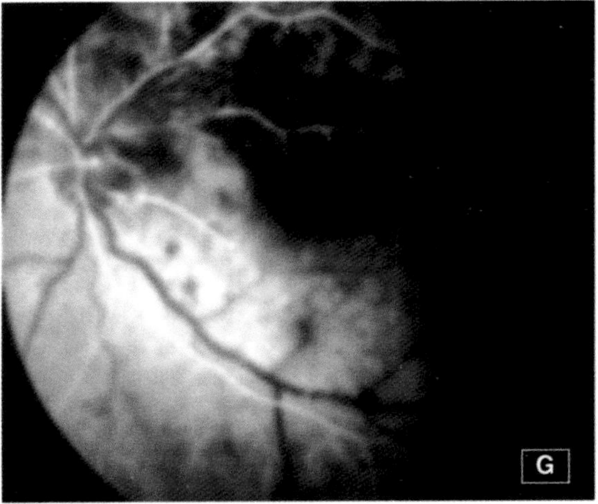

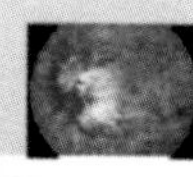

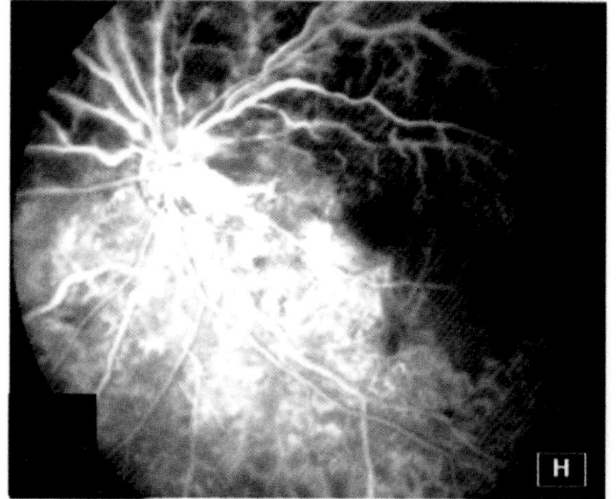

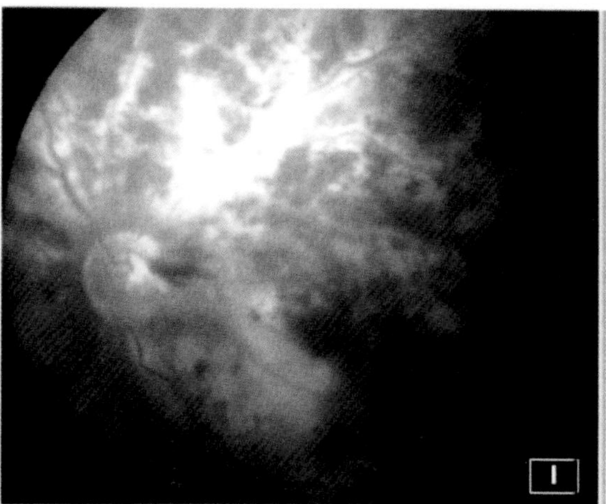

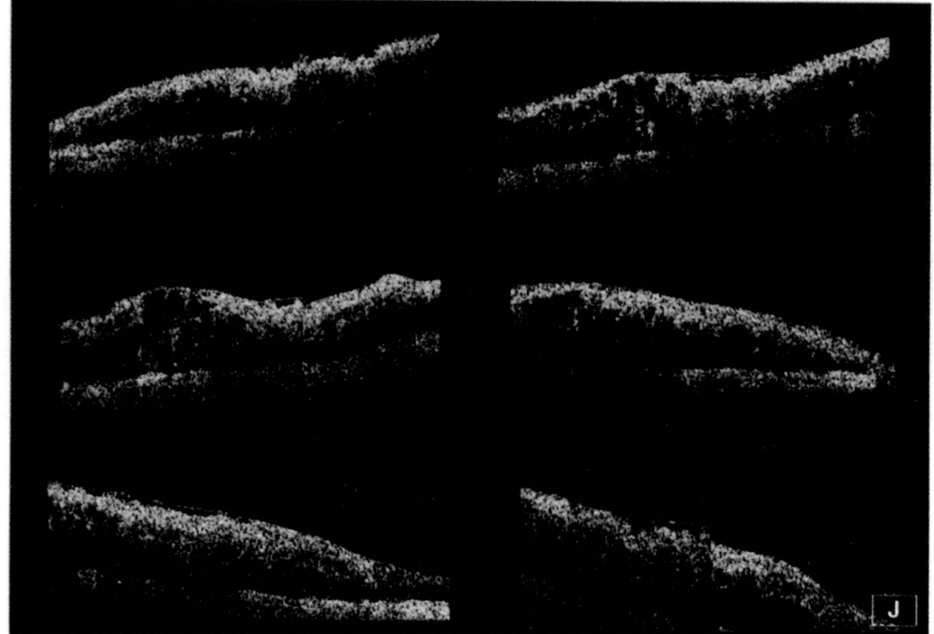

CONCLUSIONS

The development of macular edema is quite common in venous occlusions. Fluorescein angiography is an important tool in the management of retinal vascular occlusions as it helps in delineating the extent of occlusion, capillary non-perfusion and neovascularization. OCT is complementary to fluorescein angiography in these patients that helps in quantifying the macular edema and is helpful in monitoring response to therapy. Also it helps in depicting epiretinal membranes as well as taut posterior hyloid membrane that might merit surgical removal.

SUGGESTED READING

1. Spaide RF, Lee JK, Klancnik JM, Gross NE. Optical coherence tomography of branch retinal vein occlusion. Retina 2003; 23;343-347.

Chapter 9

Retinal Vasculitis

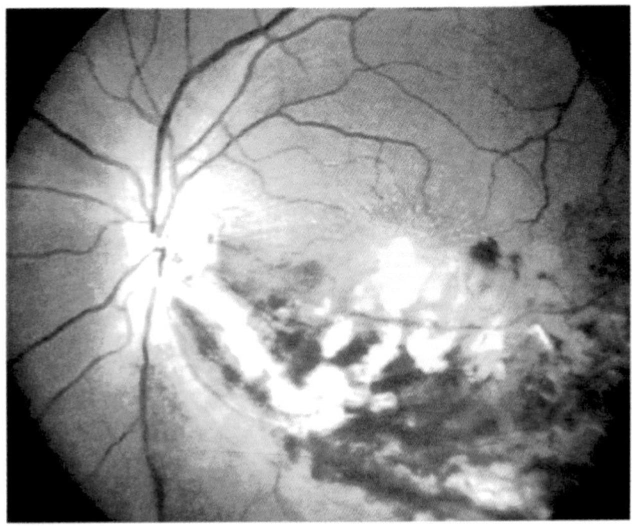

Retinal vasculitis is a common cause of visual loss in young adults. It has characteristic clinical and angiographic features. Optical Coherence Tomography is helpful in evaluating the macula in these patients. Macular edema including cystoid macular edema is known to occur in retinal vasculitis. OCT is helpful in diagnosing macular edema, cystoid macular edema, epiretinal membranes, pseudo macular hole and tractional retinal detachment. It also is helpful in monitoring response to treatment objectively.

Case 9.1: Retinal Vasculitis

Case Summary

A 40-year-old man presented with decreased vision in his left eye of one month duration. His best corrected visual acuity was 20/60 in the left eye. Fundus left eye showed vasculitis along the lower temporal vessel with hemorrhages and cotton-wool spots along the lower temporal vessels and macular edema (A). Fluorescein angiography showed hypofluorescence corresponding to retinal hemorrhages and staining of retinal vessel walls (B).

Optical Coherence Tomography

OCT of the left eye (C) showed increased retinal thickening with loss of foveal contour and reduced backscattering with hyporeflective space in the outer retina suggestive of fluid accumulation.

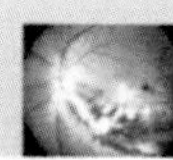

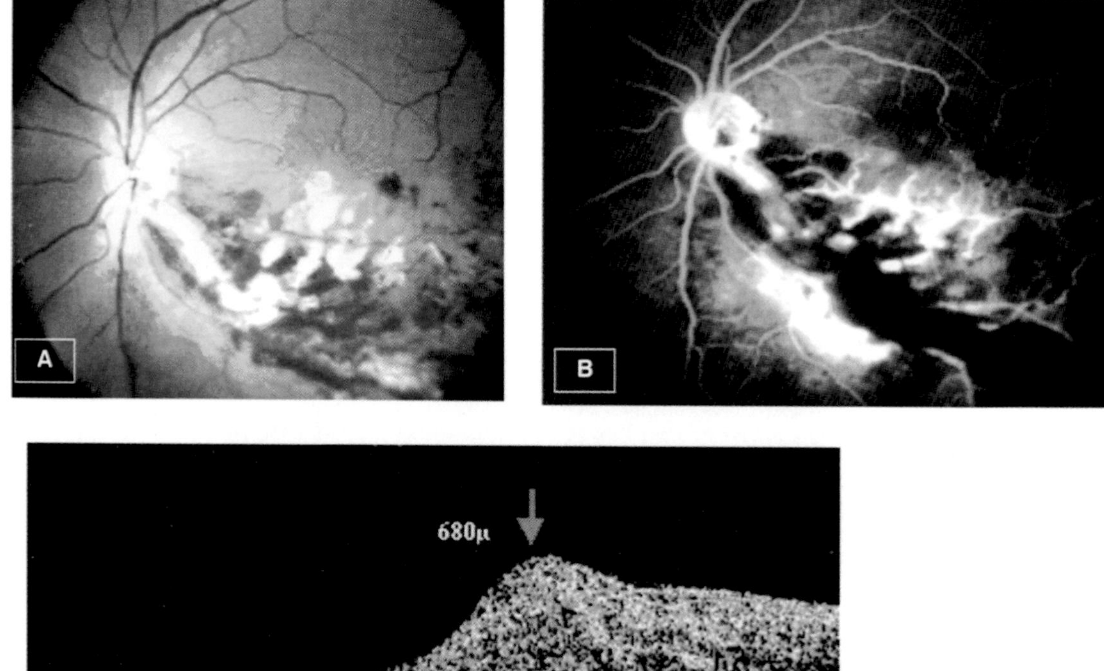

The patient had isolated idiopathic vasculitis for which he was treated with oral corticosteroids. Six weeks later, his visual acuity had improved to 20/60 and OCT showed reduction of edema (D, E).

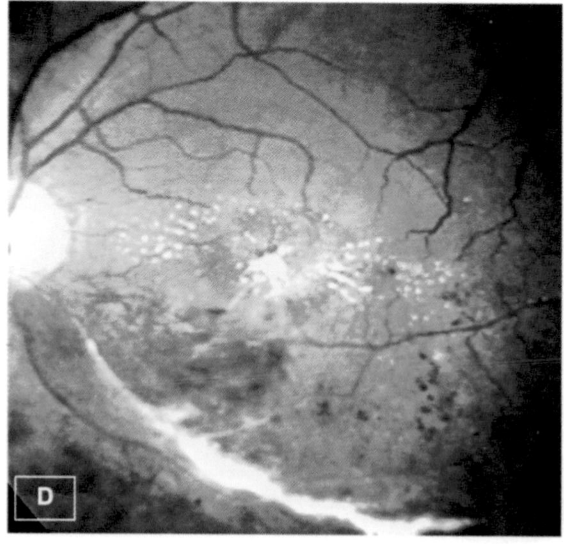

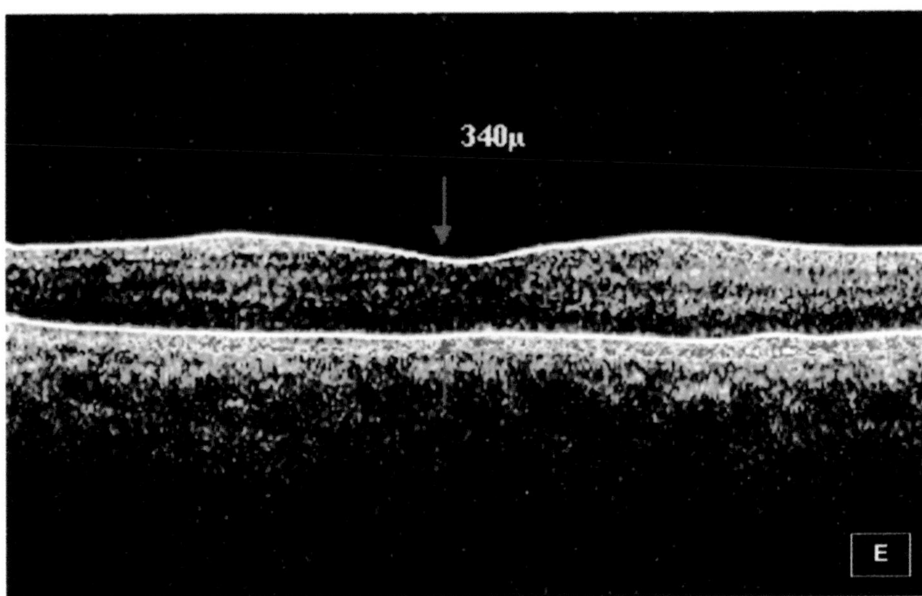

The oral corticosteroids were tapered at this stage that led to deterioration of vision in this eye. Clinical picture did not show any activation of the vasculitis but OCT showed the reappearance of macular edema with cystoid spaces (F). Detached posterior hyaloid membrane could be seen anteriorly. The oral corticosteroids were re-started following which the edema resolved again and repeat OCT done 8 months later maintained resolution (G).

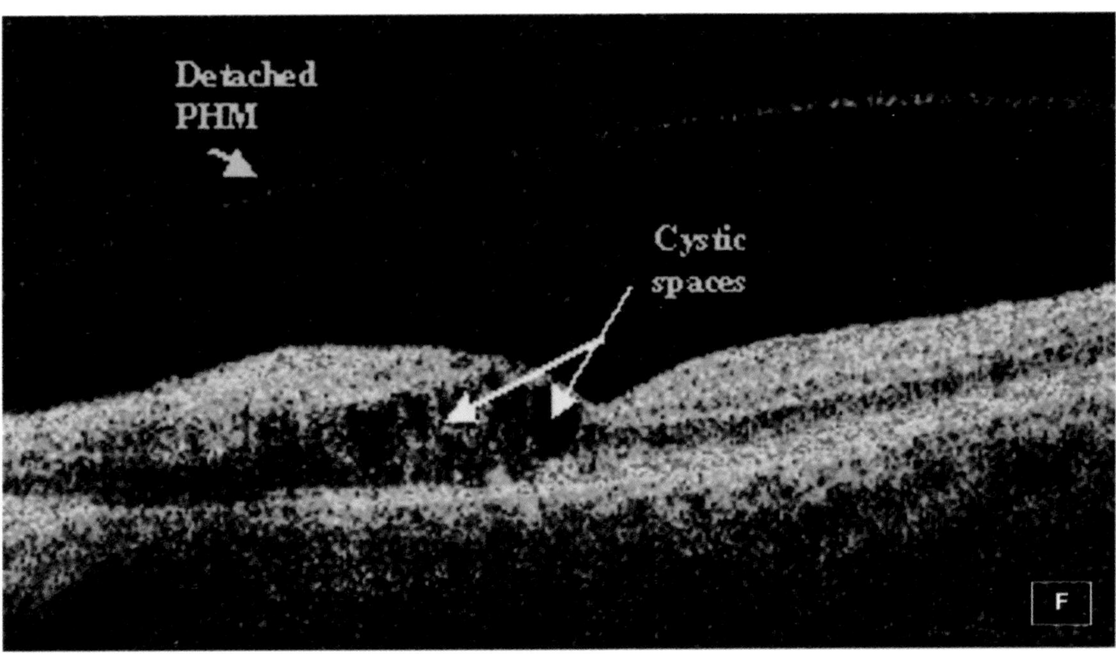

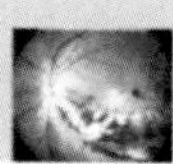

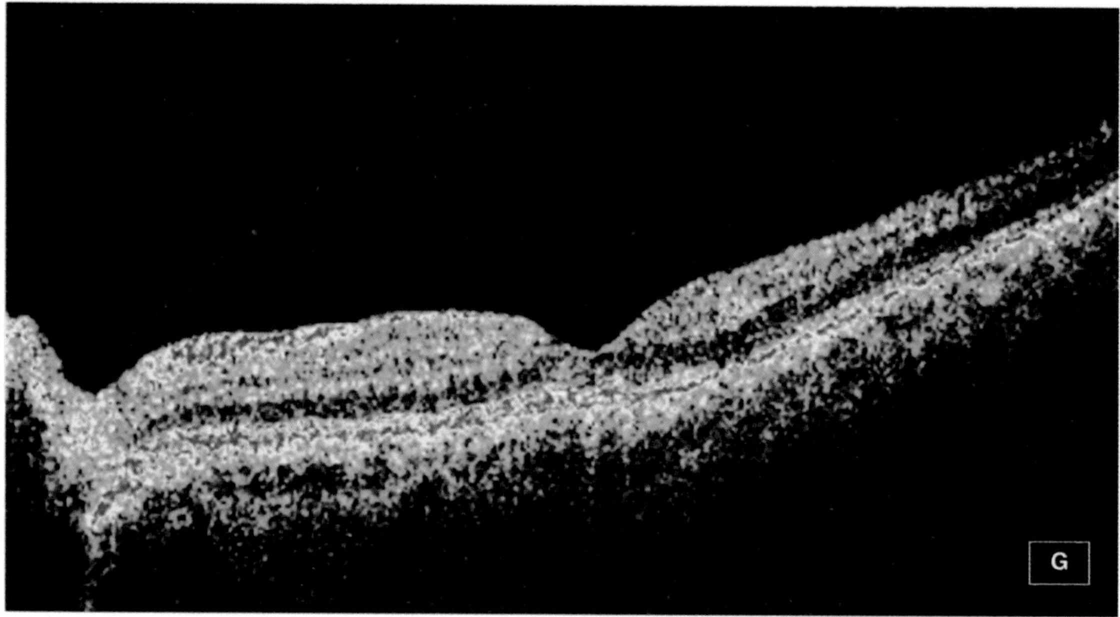

CONCLUSIONS

The macula in retinal vasculitis can show either macular edema or ischemia. OCT is helpful in the diagnosis and quantification of macular edema. It also helps in identifying cystoid macular edema and is a great non-invasive tool in monitoring response to an intervention.

Chapter 10

Epiretinal Membranes

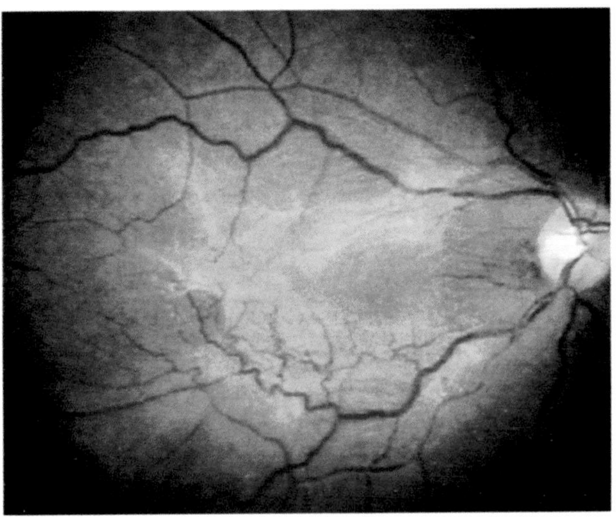

Epiretinal membranes comprise of thin, translucent membranes that are seen on the inner retinal surface in the macular area. These membranes can become semi-translucent over a period of time and their contraction might produce edema, degeneration or cystoid spaces in the underlying retina. According to the severity of retinal distortion, they can be classified as Grade 0: cellophane maculopathy, Grade 1: Crinkled cellophane maculopathy, Grade 2: macular pucker. These membranes may have associated with pseudo or true macular hole. Development of choroidal neovascular membrane may be another sequelae.

OCT helps by giving the cross-sectional view of the macula in these eyes that helps in assessing the severity of changes in the underlying retina and the adhesiveness of the membrane to the retina. OCT demonstrates the extent of the membrane, vitreoretinal interface, status of posterior hyloid membrane, associated changes like cystoid macular edema, vitreofoveal traction, macular hole, etc. This helps in prognosticating the outcome of surgery in these eyes.

The epiretinal membranes have been classified as: a) clearly separable where a clear space is visible between the epiretinal membrane (ERM) and inner retinal surface and; b) globally adherent where no area of separation can be seen easily between the ERM and inner retinal surface.

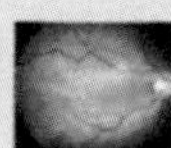

Case 10.1: Grade 1 Crinkled Cellophane Maculopathy

Case Summary

A-64-year-old man was seen with complaints of distorted vision in his right eye of one month duration. His best corrected visual acuity was 20/30. Fundus showed fine, superficial radiating retinal folds suggesting the presence of an epiretinal membrane (A).

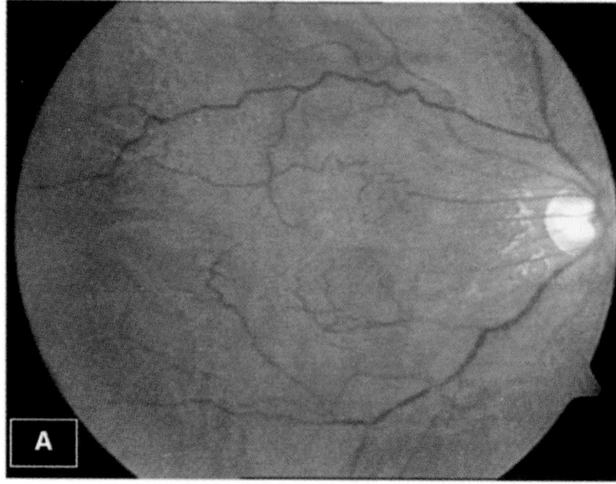

Optical Coherence Tomography

The OCT scan (B, C) through various angles showed the presence of hyperreflective band at the vitreo-retinal interface with traction on the underlying retina resulting in distortion of neurosensory retinal layers. The membrane caused traction on the underlying retina that was seen as in-foldings. **OCT helped in giving information regarding the status of underlying retinal traction in this patient that would justify surgery at this stage.**

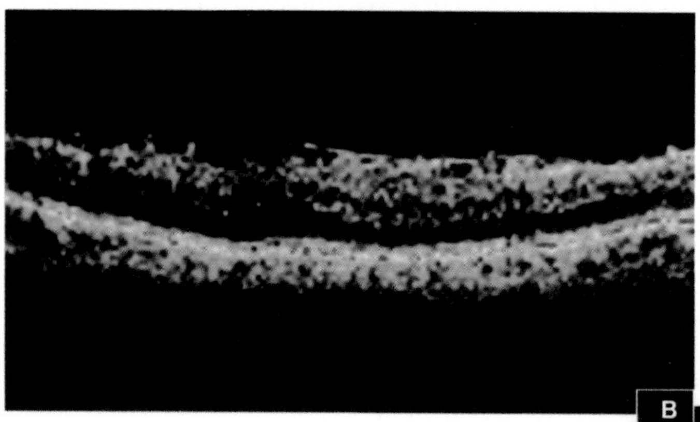

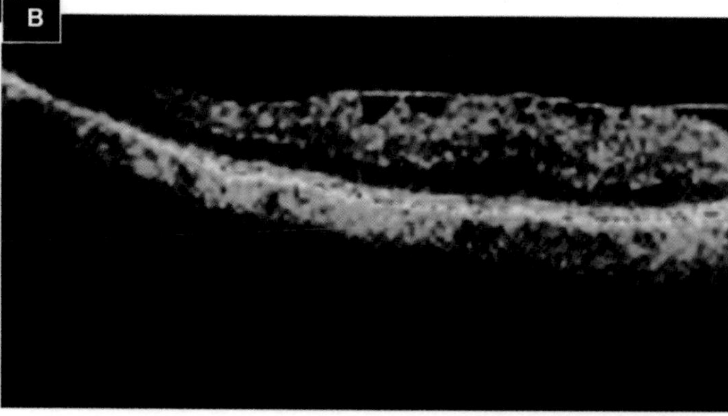

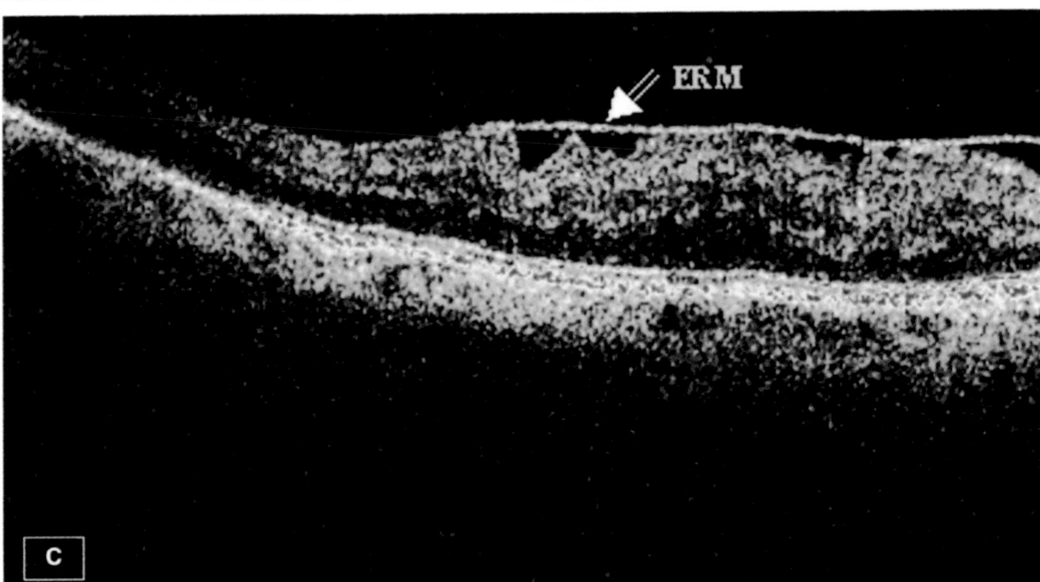

Case 10.2 Grade 2 ERM: Macular Pucker

Case Summary

A 30-year-old-man was seen with decreased vision in his right eye of 2 months duration. Clinically, a greyish membrane was seen on the inner retinal surface (arrows) (A). Fluorescein angiography showed dye leakage from the underlying retina (B).

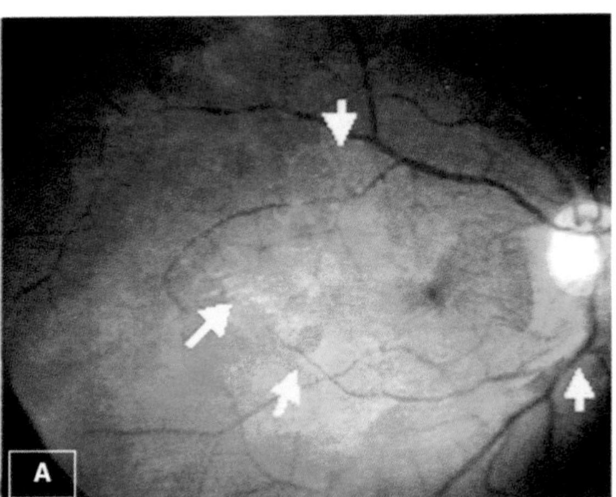

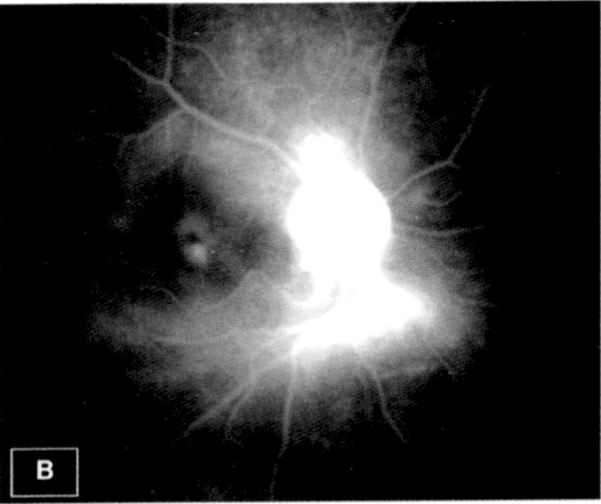

Optical Coherence Tomography

OCT line scan through the fovea (C) showed the presence of a hyper-reflective membrane extending from optic disc both nasally and temporally causing peripapillary traction as well as traction on the underlying retina (arrow). The temporal edge of the membrane could be well delineated. **OCT in this patient helped in identifying the edge of the membrane that could help the surgeon to enter the right plane of cleavage during surgery.**

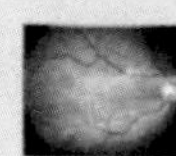

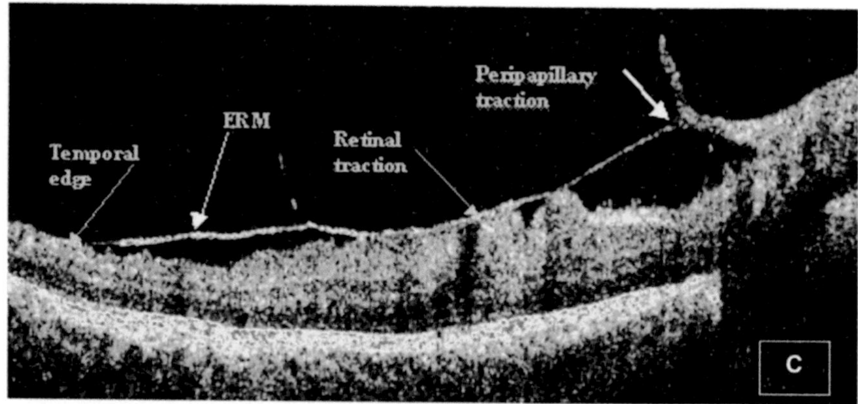

Case 10.3: Epiretinal Membrane with Underlying Retinal Edema

Case Summary

A-59-year-old man was seen as a case of ERM right eye with a visual acuity of 20/200. Fundus and fluorescein angiography confirmed epiretinal membrane (A-D).

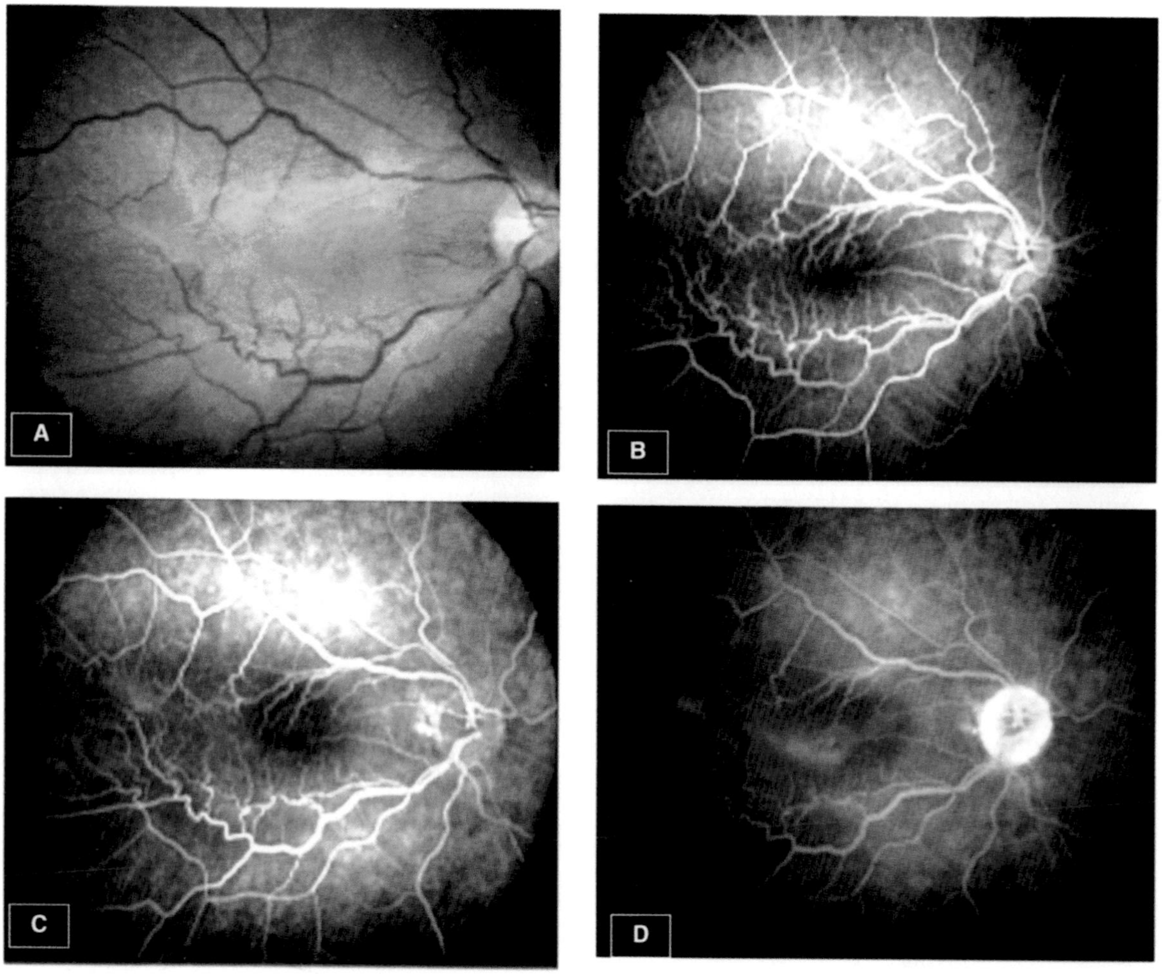

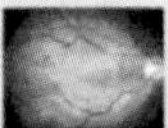

Optical Coherence Tomography

OCT line scan through the fovea (E) showed the presence of a hyper-reflective membrane on the surface of retina bridging across the fovea. In addition, there was reduced backscatter from the outer retinal layers suggesting underlying retinal edema that corresponded to the hyperfluorescence seen on fluorescein angiography.

OCT was helpful in diagnosing underlying retinal edema that could help in prognosticating the outcome following surgery.

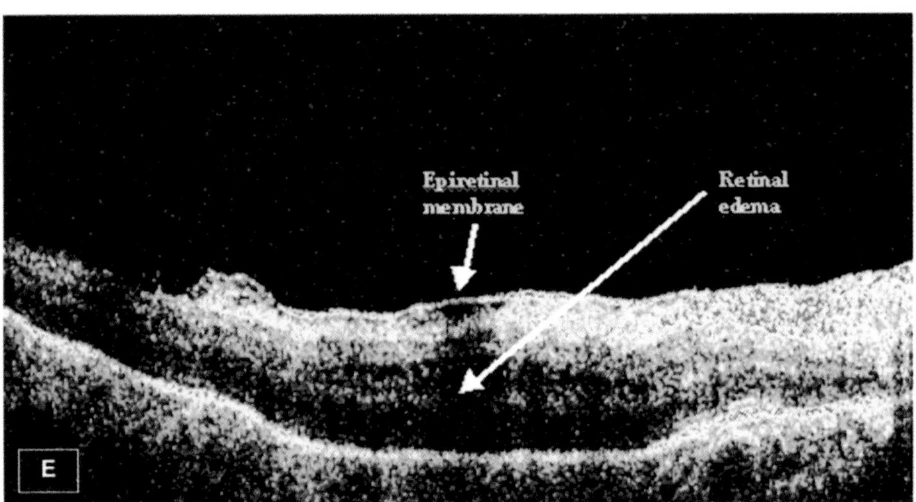

Case 10.4: ERM: Crinkled Cellophane Maculopathy

Case Summary

A 51-year-old man was seen with distortion of vision in his left eye of 6 months duration. His best corrected visual acuity was 20/40 in the left eye. Fundoscopy and red free photo showed the presence of cellophane membrane over the retinal surface (A, B). The fluorescein angiography showed staining in the late phase (C, D).

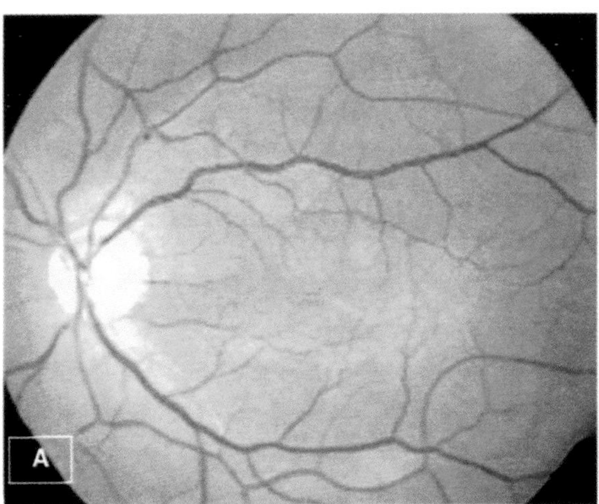

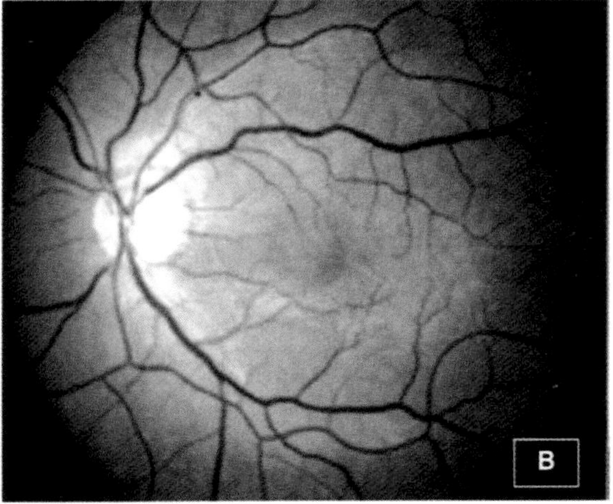

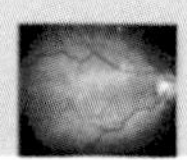

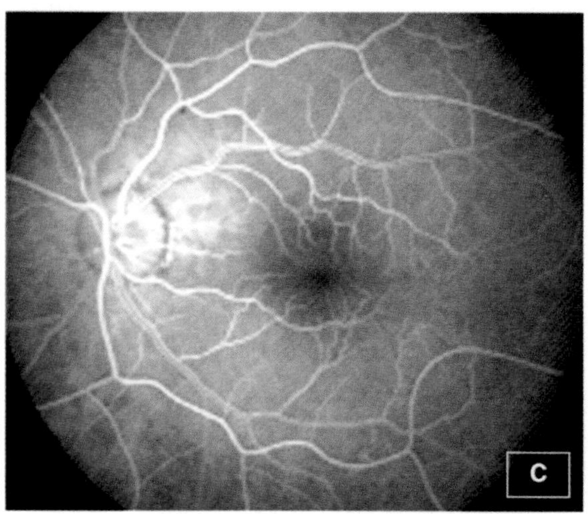

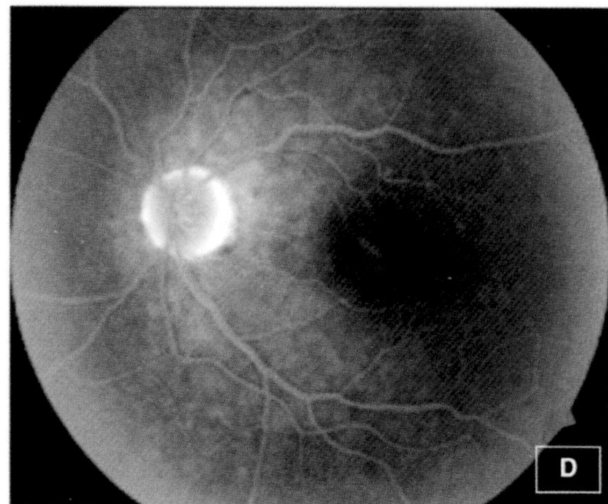

Optical Coherence Tomography

OCT of the left eye (E) showed a hyper-reflective membrane intimately adherent to the underlying retina with distortion of underlying inner retinal layers only. The patient regained a visual acuity of 20/30 following PPV (F). **Note the absence of underlying structural changes that indicate a better prognosis following surgery.**

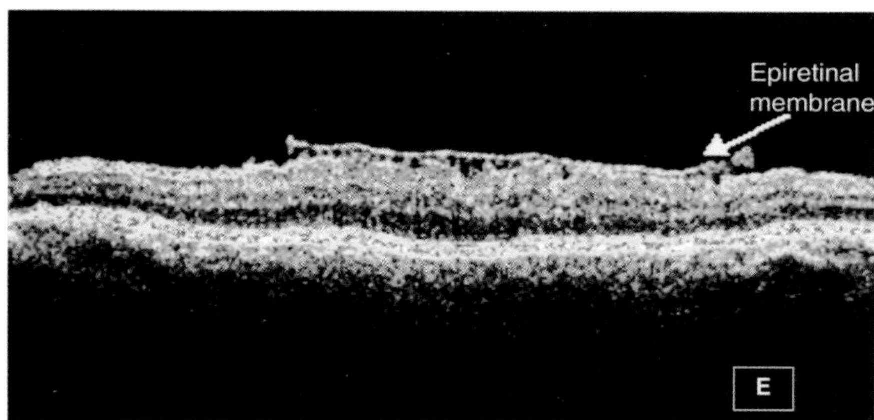

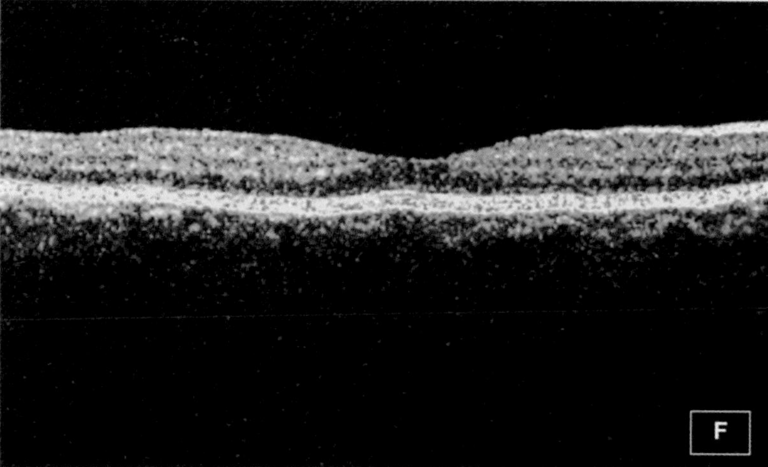

Case 10.5: ERM with PVD and True Macular Hole

Case Summary

A 56-years-old woman was seen with epiretinal membrane, stage III macular hole left eye and positive Watzke's sign (A).

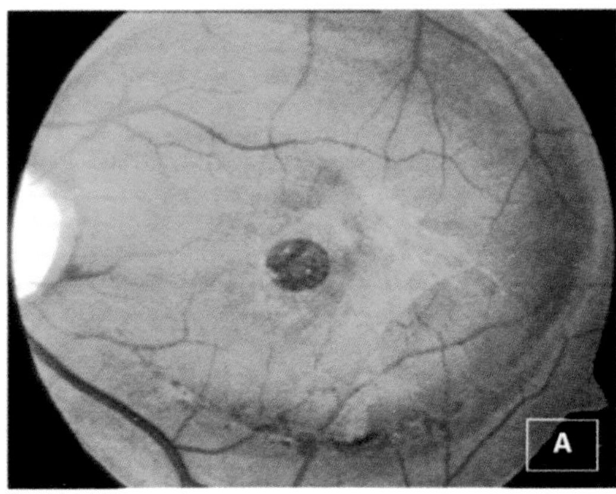

Optical Coherence Tomography

Horizontal OCT line scan (B) demonstrated stage III macular hole with complete posterior vitreous detachment. The posterior hyloid membrane was seen situated approximately 540 microns from the bottom of the hole. Following pars plana vitrectomy (PPV), the hole showed partial closure with persistent cystic spaces (C).

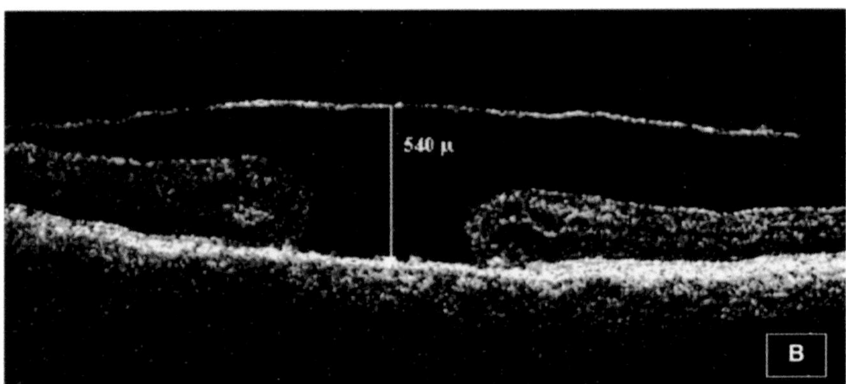

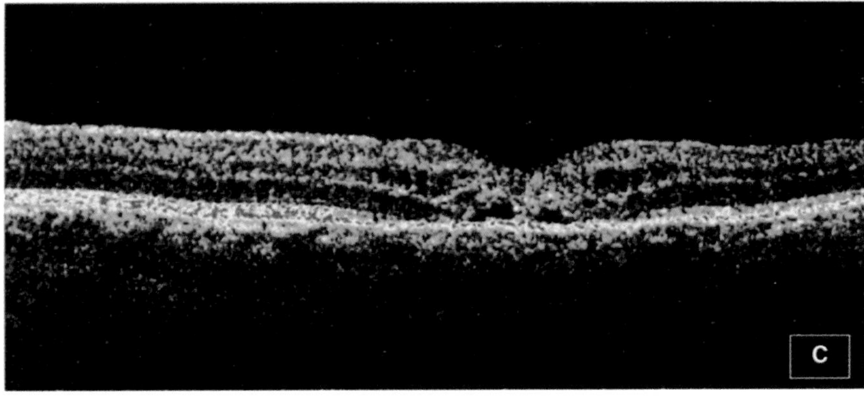

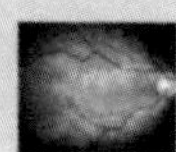

Case 10.6: Globally Adherent ERM

Case Summary

A 48-year-old woman was seen with ERM in her right eye (A). Her best corrected visual acuity was 20/200 in this eye.

Optical Coherence Tomography

OCT line scan of the right eye passing above the fovea (B) showed a hyper-reflective membrane that was intimately adherent to the underlying retina with no intervening space in between.

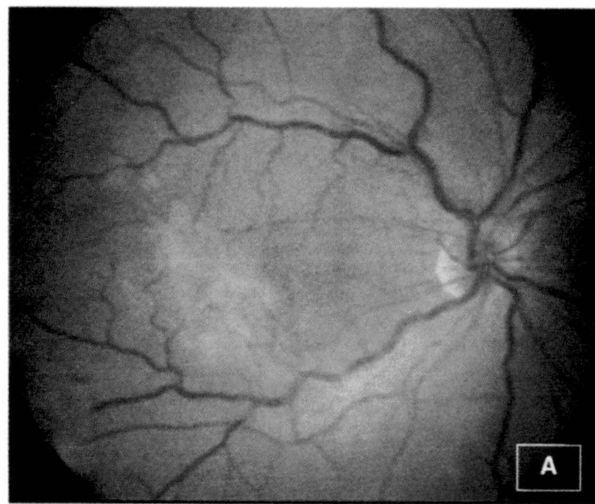

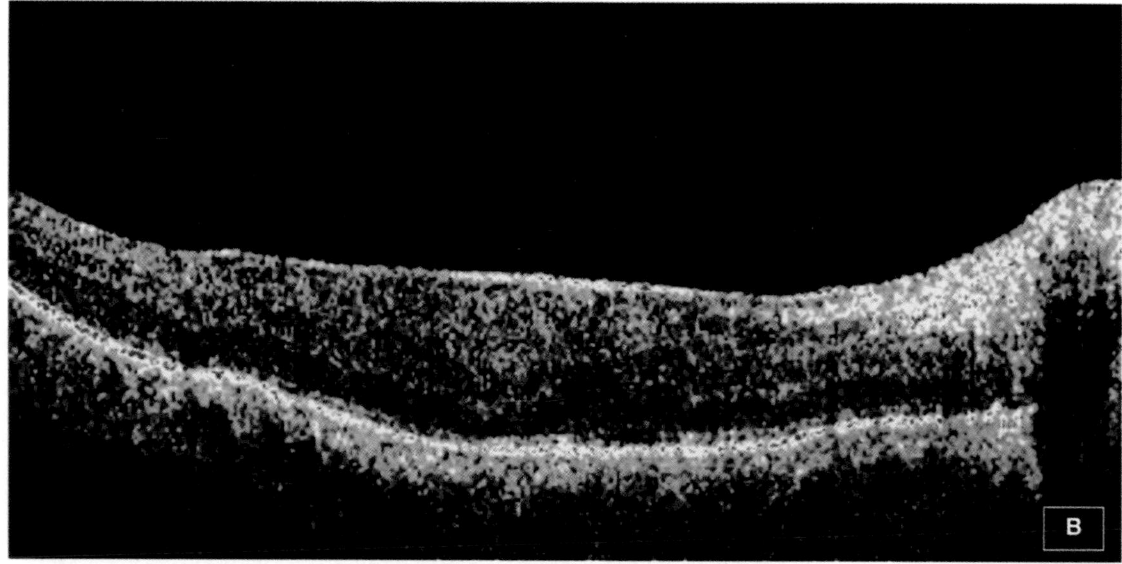

The patient underwent pars plana vitrectomy with ERM peeling. Two weeks later, her best corrected visual acuity was 20/80 (C). Repeat OCT scan through the same area (D) showed the absence of ERM.

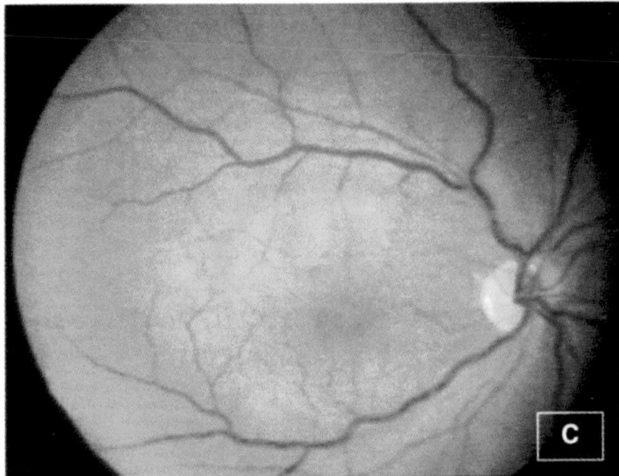

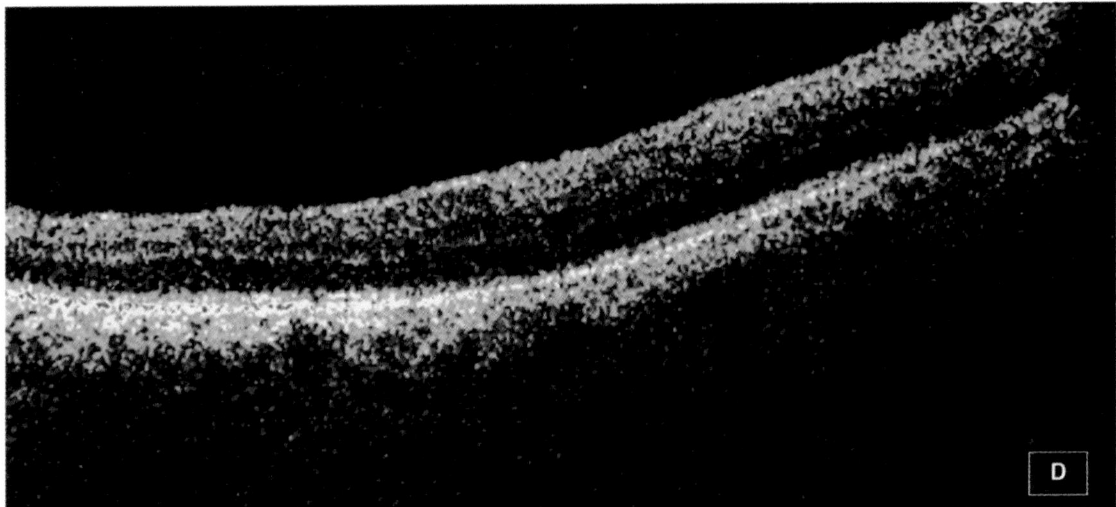

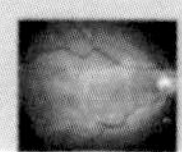

Case 10.7: Secondary ERM following Scleral Buckle Surgery

Case Summary

A 60-year-old woman had undergone retinal reattachment surgery in the right eye two years ago following which she had poor visual gain. Her best corrected visual acuity in this eye was counting fingers. Fundus right eye (A) showed a yellowish-grey membrane on the retinal surface with straightening of retinal vessels towards the membrane. The fluorescein angiography (B) showed corresponding hyperfluorescence.

Optical Coherence Tomography

OCT line scan (C) showed increased retinal thickness with hyper-reflectivity at the vitreoretinal interface. The innermost retinal layer was thrown in the folds suggesting probably internal limiting membrane folds.

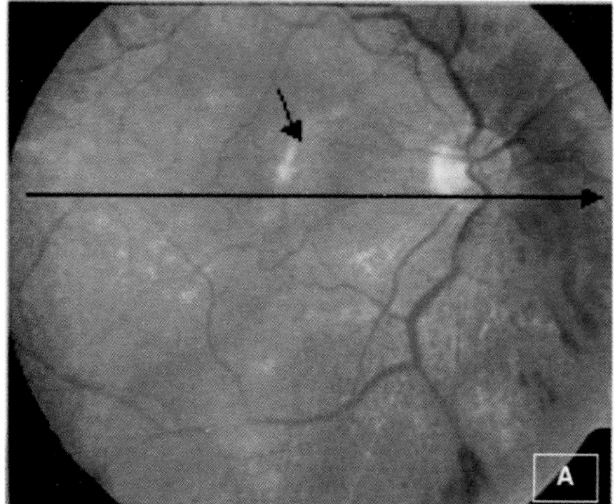

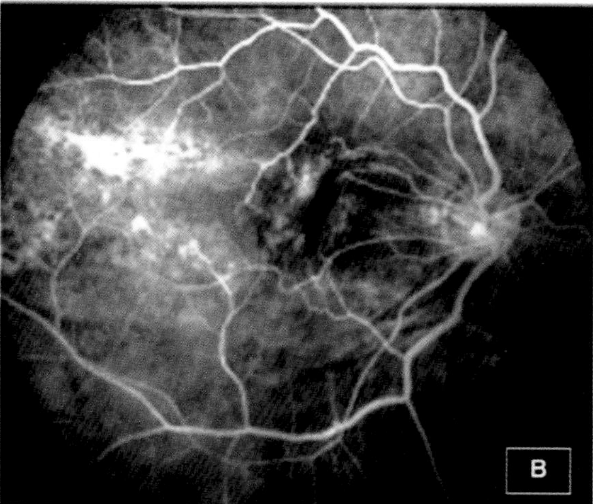

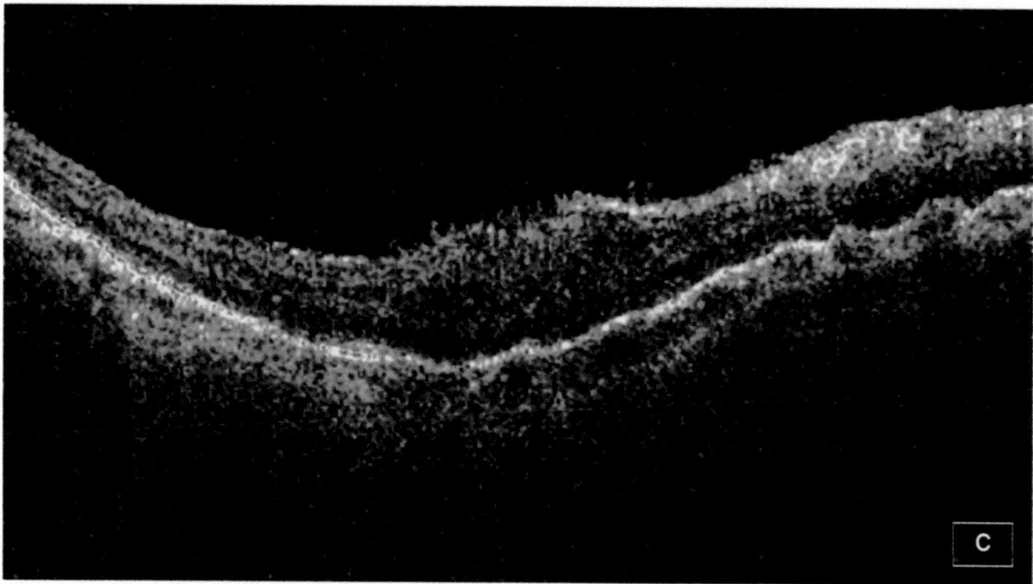

The patient underwent PPV for ERM peeling. Three weeks later, her visual acuity was improved to 20/100 (D). Repeat OCT scan (E) showed a near-normal foveal contour with few residual folds temporal to fovea.

OCT helps in tracking longitudinal follow-up following surgery.

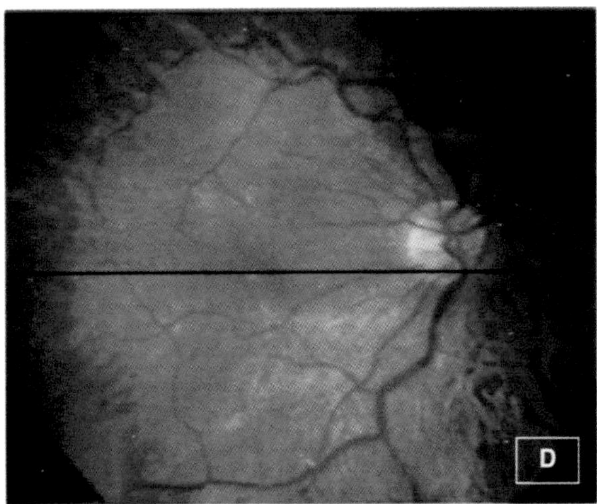

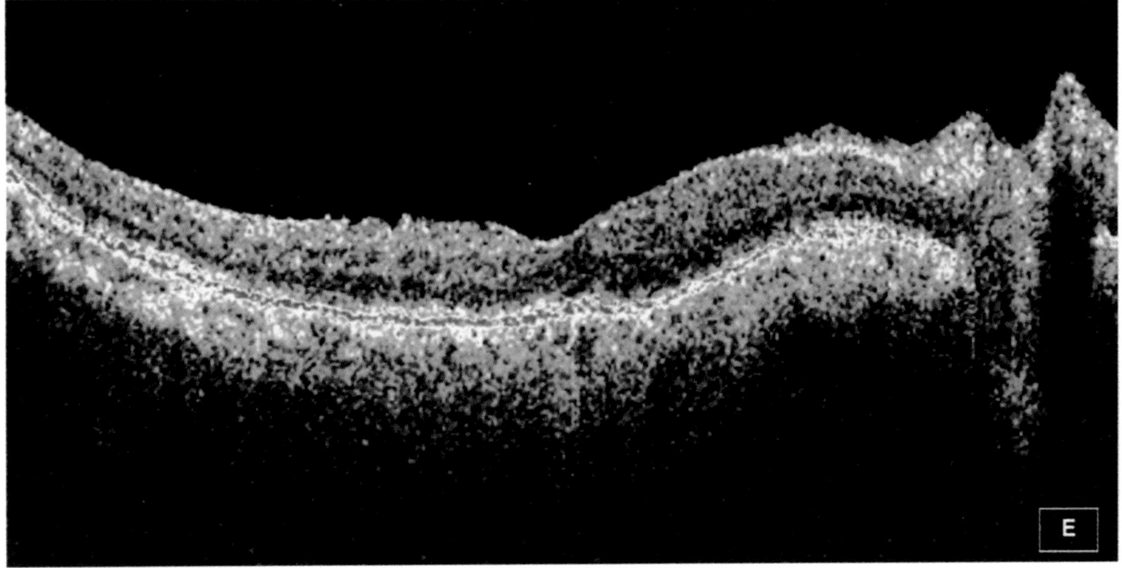

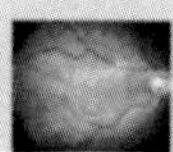

Case 10.8: Secondary ERM with lamellar macular hole following endogenous endophthalmitis

Case Summary

A 60-year-old man underwent pars plana vitrectomy in the right eye for pseudomonas endogenous endophthalmitis. Two months following surgery, he showed a fine cellophane membrane on the surface of retina with a residual retinal abscess associated with retinal hemorrhage seen temporal to the fovea (A).

The OCT scan passing through the center of the fovea (B) showed some loss of foveal contour with an overlying epiretinal membrane.

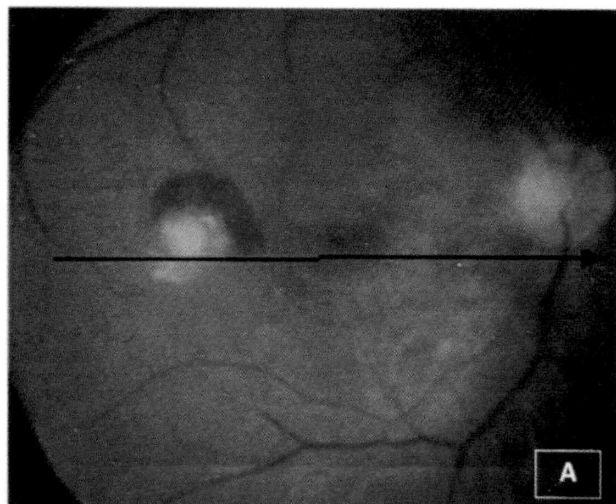

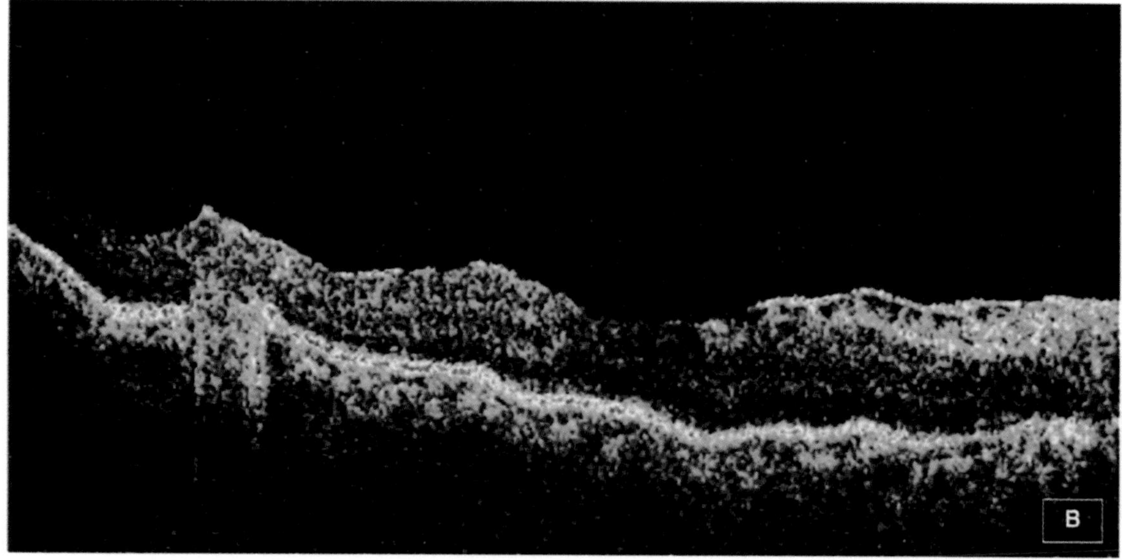

Three months later, the fundus showed clearer media with residual scar temporal to the fovea and an epiretinal membrane (C). Repeat OCT scan (D) demonstrated the presence of lamellar macular hole that was not seen clinically. **In this patient, OCT helped in demonstrating an inner lamellar hole that was not seen clinically.**

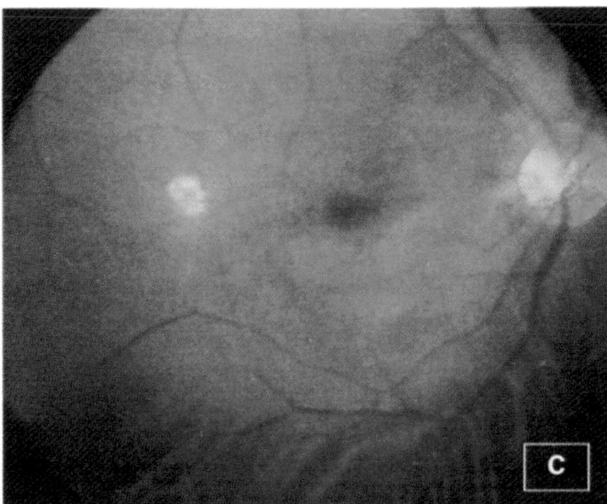

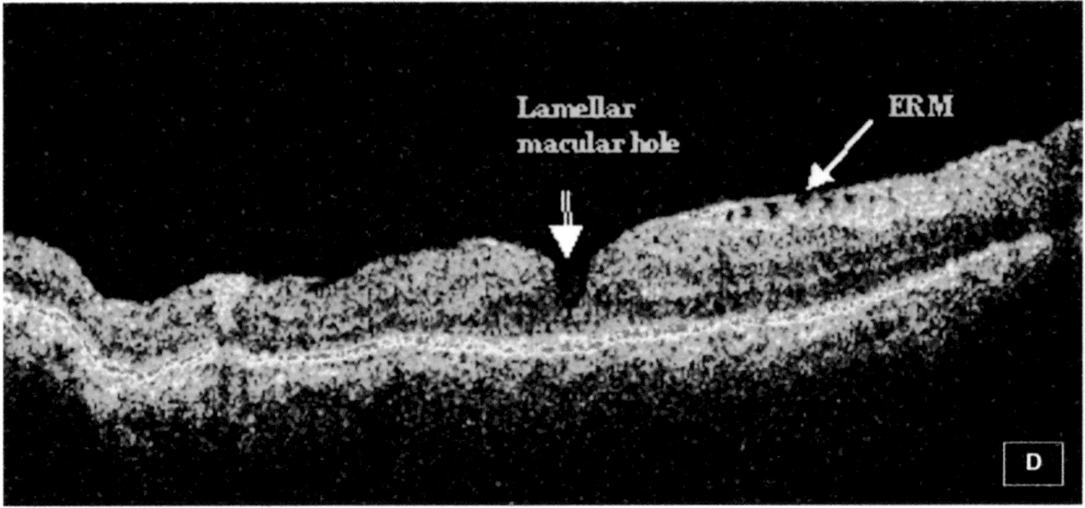

CONCLUSIONS

In epiretinal membranes, OCT helps in the following ways:

1. It helps in confirming the diagnosis of the epiretinal membranes.
2. This is a useful tool to identify the structural alterations in the underlying retina that could play a role in making decision regarding the surgical intervention as well as prognosticating the outcome.
3. It also helps in longitudinal tracking of these eyes following pars plana vitrectomy, thus obviating the need for repeat fluorescein angiography.

SUGGESTED READING

1. Wilkins JR, Puliafito CA, Hee MR et al. Characterization of epiretinal membranes using optical coherence tomography. Ophthalmology 1996;103:2142-51.

Chapter 11

Age Related Macular Degeneration

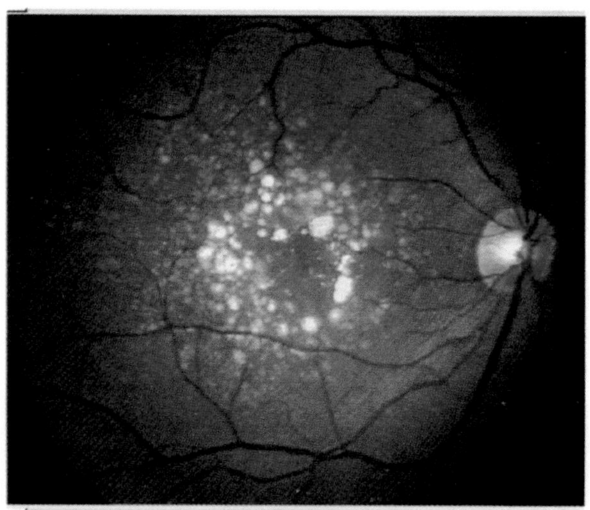

OCT IN AGE RELATED MACULAR DEGENERATION

Age related macular degeneration (ARMD) is a disease that primarily affects choriocapillaris, Bruch's membrane and retinal pigment epithelium (RPE). It can be categorized as:

NON-NEOVASCULAR ARMD

Drusens

The drusens may be hard or soft. Soft drusens, on OCT, are seen as areas of focal elevation of RPE. These appear as modulations in the RPE associated with shallow borders with no optical shadowing underneath. These findings are consistent with the belief that drusens result due to accumulation of material under the neurosensory retina and within Bruch's membrane.

These drusens can be differentiated from serous pigment epithelium detachments (PED) as the latter show optical shadowing of choroid under the PED.

Geographic Atrophy

Geographic atrophy is an advanced stage of non-neovascular ARMD characterized by well demarcated pigment epithelial/choriocapillaris atrophy. OCT shows increased optical reflectivity from the choroid due to increased penetration of the light through overlying atrophic retina.

Neovascular ARMD

Neovascular ARMD is characterized by classic or occult choroidal neovascular membrane or mixed form, serous/hemorrhagic detachment of neurosensory retina/pigment epithelium or fibrovascular scar.

1. *Classic Choroidal Neovascular Membrane (CNVM):* The normal RPE-choriocapillaris form a highly reflective continuous band. In well defined CNVM, there is disruption/thickening of this band with the thickened edges demarcating the boundaries of CNVM.
2. *Occult CNVM:* This is characterized by the disruption in RPE-choriocapillaris complex where the boundaries are poorly defined. These membranes also have accompanying subretinal fluid/ retinal edema that helps them to be differentiated from pigmentary atrophy.
3. *Serous PED:* These are seen as elevation of RPE with an optically clear space underneath. The underlying choroid shows reflection/optical shadowing.
4. *Fibrovascular Pigment Epithelial Detachment (PED):* This is seen as elevation of RPE with a clear demarcation between RPE and underlying structures that appear as yellow/green. In this, the optical shadowing from the underlying choroid is absent.
5. *Hemorrhagic PEDs:* The findings are same as serous PED except that the backscattering from RPE attenuates towards the outer retina with absent choroidal reflections.

   OCT helps in the management of ARMD in the following ways:

   A. *Disease categorization:* OCT gives an insight into the localization of pathology with changes occurring at the ultra structural level that helps in categorizing the disease. Since the management protocol in these patients depends on the category, OCT in addition to fundus photography and fluorescein angiography helps in disease categorization that is the most crucial step in the management. However, it must be noted that OCT is complementary to clinical examination, fluorescein angiography and indocyanin green angiography; it alone cannot establish the diagnostic category.
   B. *Early occult CNVM:* In patients with soft confluent drusens, occult CNVM can often be missed on fluorescein angiography. OCT is a very helpful device in picking up the CNVM in these patients. We, in our experience, found OCT very useful in diagnosing these occult CNVMs as a step between fluorescein angiography and indocyanine green angiography.
   C. *Associated changes:* OCT helps in depicting additional features like cystoid macular edema, RPE rip, neurosensory atrophy of retina, etc.
   D. *Response to treatment:* OCT helps in monitoring response to thermal laser photocoagulation, transpupillary thermotherapy (TTT) and photodynamic therapy (PDT). Following PDT, 5 stages have been described :

      Stage I: This is seen within one week of therapy and is an acute response to treatment characterized by acute inflammatory response with increase in subretinal fluid.

      Stage II: This is seen between 1-4 weeks of treatment and is characterized by resolution of serous fluid with restoration of foveal contour.

      Stage III: This is seen between 4-12 weeks of treatment and is characterized by the presence of either greater subretinal fluid to fibrous tissue suggestive of active choroidal neovascularization CNV (Stage III a) or more fibrous tissue with minimal subretinal fluid suggesting inactivity (Stage III b).

      Stage IV: Is characterized by the presence of cystoid spaces.

      Stage V: Is the final stage showing resolution of subretinal fluid and finally the retina becomes thin and fibrous tissue also merges with it.

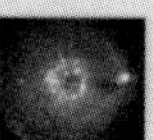

DISEASE CATEGORIZATION

Case 11.1: Intermediate-risk Non-neovascular ARMD

Case Summary

A 59-year-old man was seen with bilateral drusens. His best-corrected visual acuity was 20/30 in the right eye. The fundus in the right eye showed extensive medium sized drusens, with few large drusens (≥125 microns) and few calcified drusens and some areas of RPE atrophy (A). The drusens as well as the area of RPE atrophy were hyperfluorescent on fluorescein angiography (B).

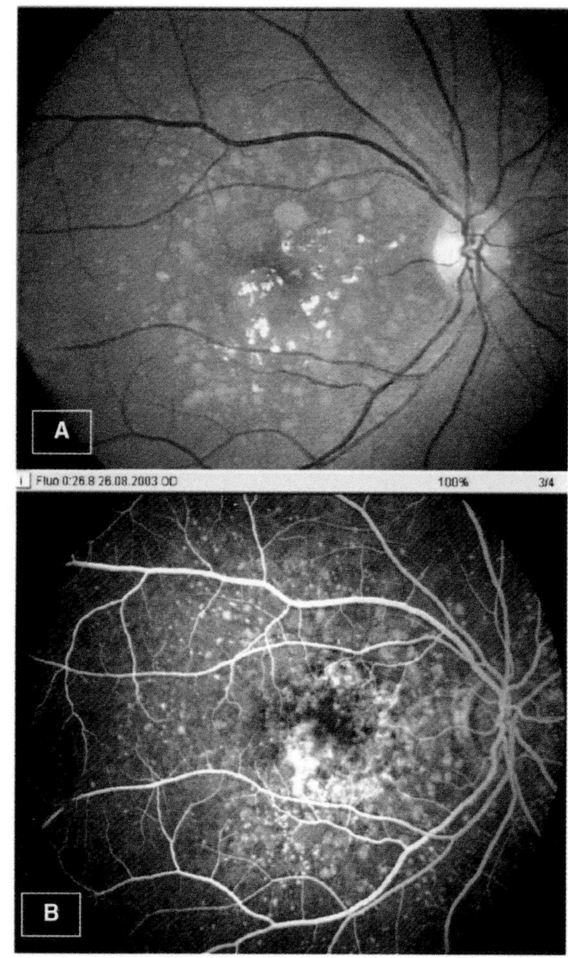

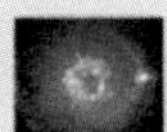

Optical Coherence Tomography

OCT line scan inferior to the fovea passing through the area of RPE atrophy and calcified drusens (C) showed hard drusens as small disruptions in the RPE projecting into the overlying photoreceptor layer. The area of RPE atrophy showed hyper-reflectivity from underlying choroid.

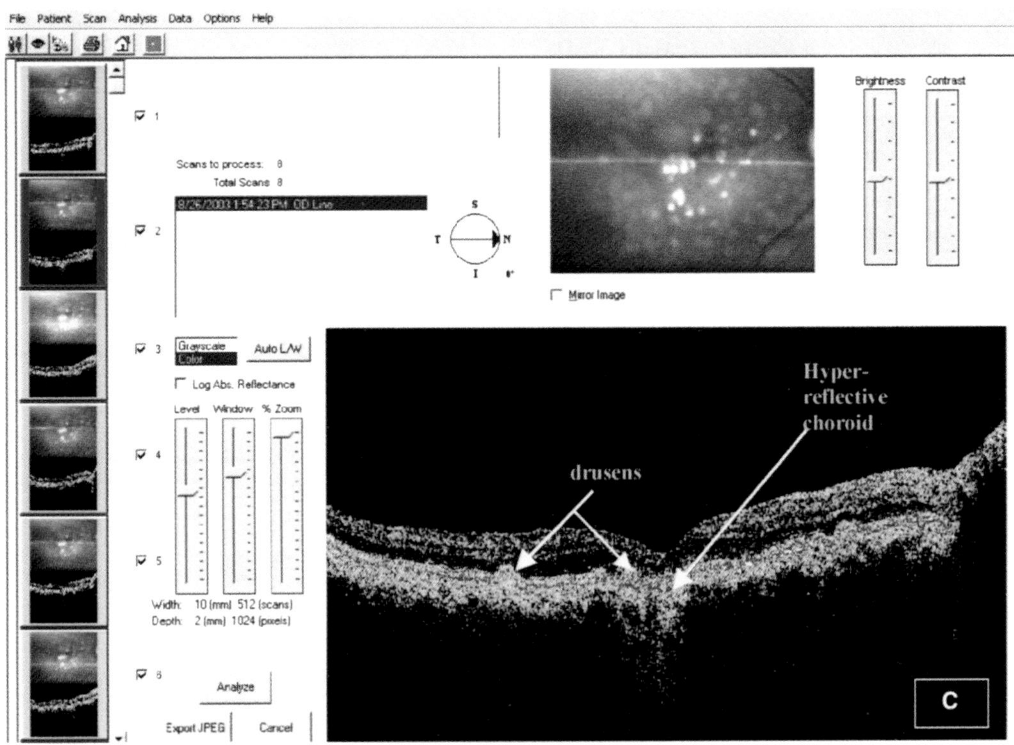

Case 11.2: Soft Drusens, High Risk Non-neovascular ARMD

Case Summary

A 56-years-old man was seen with drusens in the right eye with a visual acuity of 20/40. Fundus showed soft drusens that were predominately indistinct and > 125 microns in size (A). This eye has 18-20% risk of developing CNV over next 3-5 years.

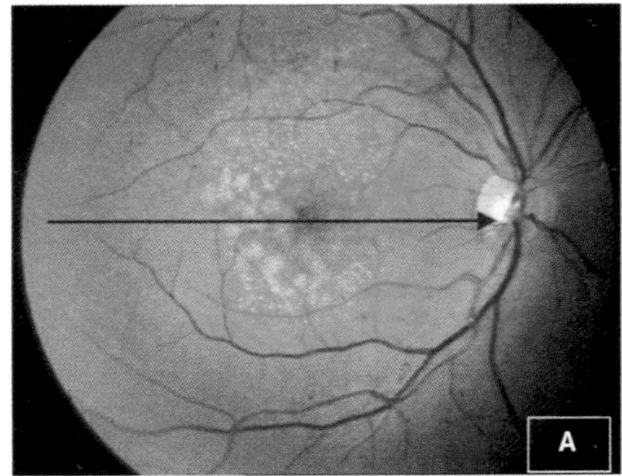

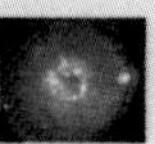

Optical Coherence Tomography

OCT line scan through the drusens (B) showed irregular elevations of RPE (arrows) with no shadow from the underlying choroid. These drusens carry high-risk of CNV.

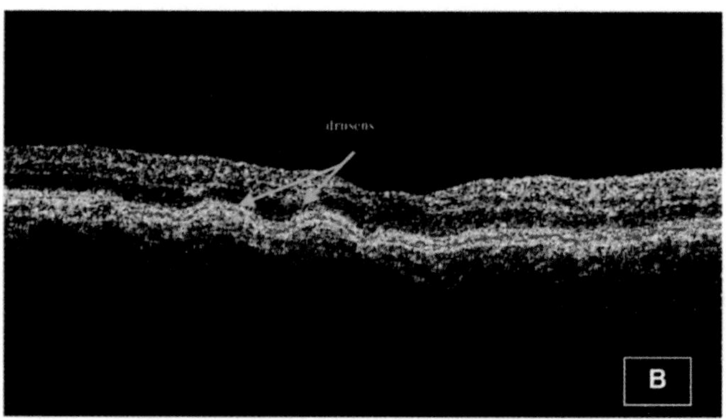

Case 11.3: CNVM Contiguous to Geographic Atrophy

Case Summary

A 56-year-old woman was seen with an area of geographic atrophy with a choroidal neovascular membrane developing adjacent to the area of atrophy (A). On fluorescein angiography (B), the membrane showed early hyperfluorescence that increased in the late phase (C).

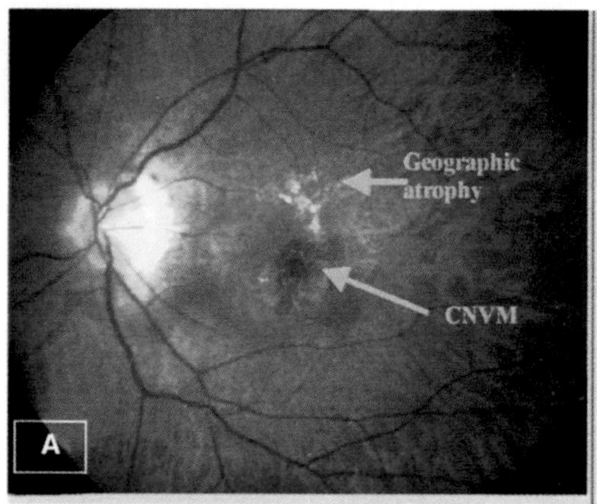

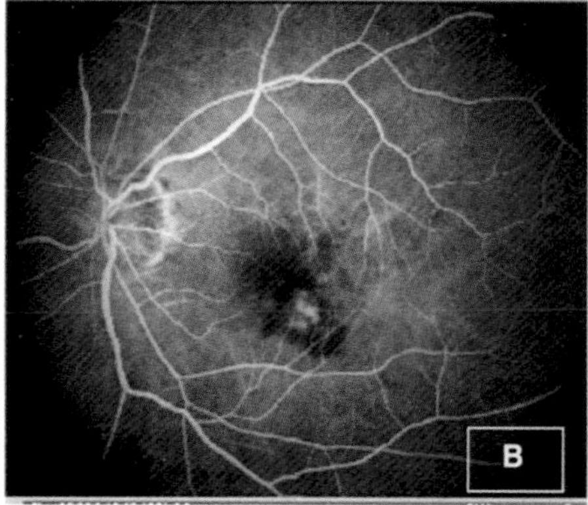

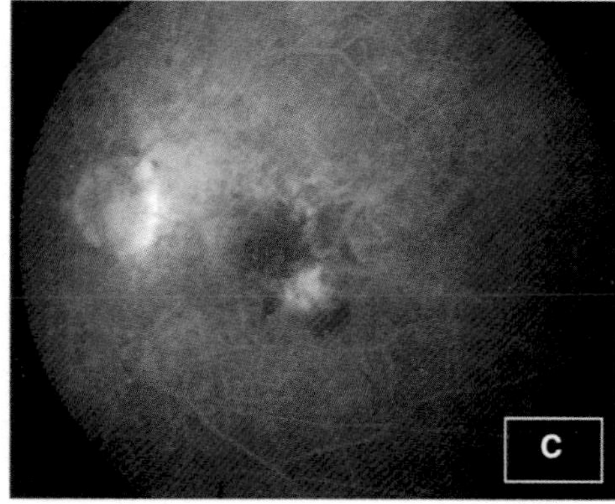

Optical Coherence Tomography

The horizontal OCT line scan through the CNVM showed increased retinal thickness temporal to the fovea with increased reflectivity from the outer retinal layers suggesting a fibrovascular complex of a classic CNVM (D, E).

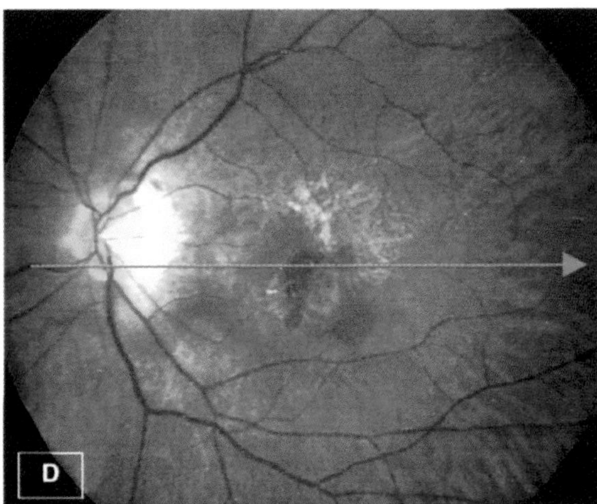

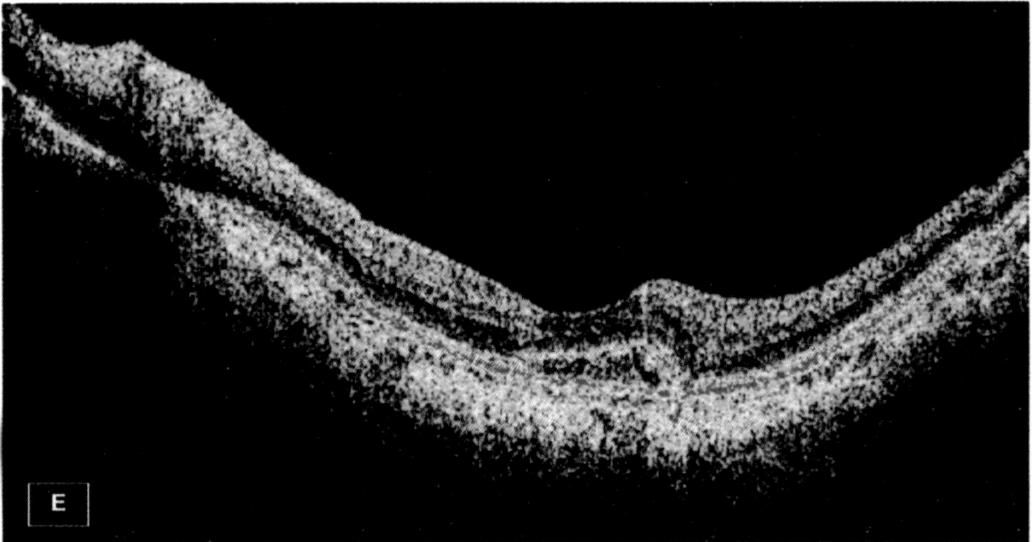

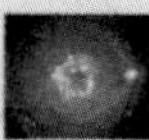

Case 11.4: Fibrovascular PED

Case Summary

A 57-year-old man was seen with a visual acuity of 20/80 in the left eye. His fundus showed a small yellowish, pigment epithelium detachment (A).

Optical Coherence Tomography

Horizontal line scan passing through the center of the PED (B) showed elevation of the hyper-reflective band corresponding to RPE with moderate-high backscatter beneath suggesting the presence of either cloudy exudates or a fibrovascular PED.

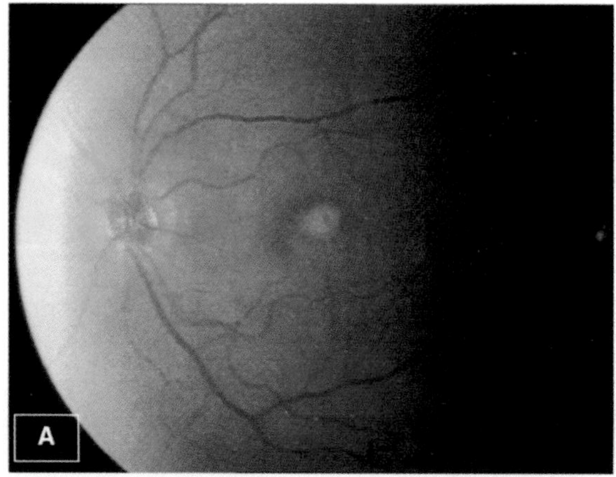

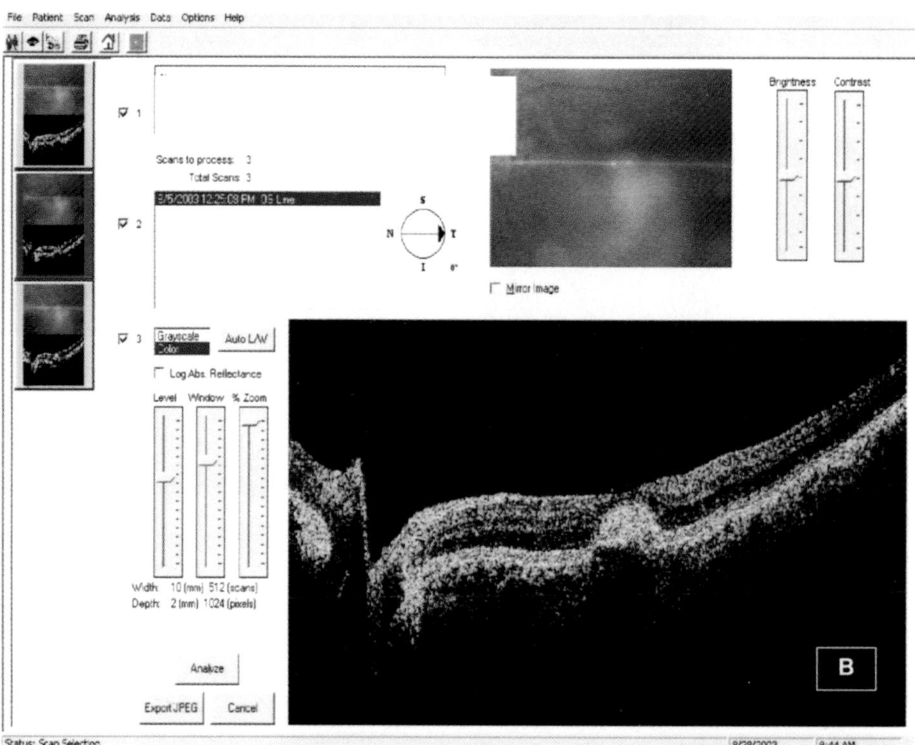

Case 11.5: Fibrovascular Pigment Epithelial Detachment

Case Summary

A 76-year-old man was seen with fibrovascular pigment epithelial detachment (PED) in the left eye (A). The fluorescein angiography showed hyperfluorescence only in the late phase (B). Indocyanine green angiography showed hyperfluorescence corresponding to the area of PED (C, D).

Optical Coherence Tomography

The OCT line scan through the center of the lesion (E) showed the presence of fibrovascular pigment epithelial detachment with adjoining serous fluid.

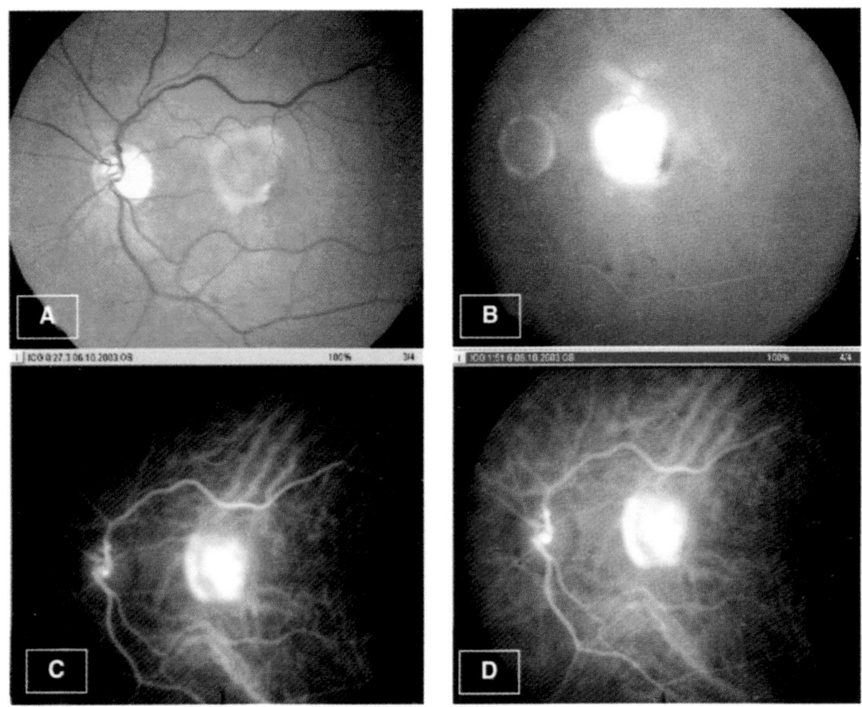

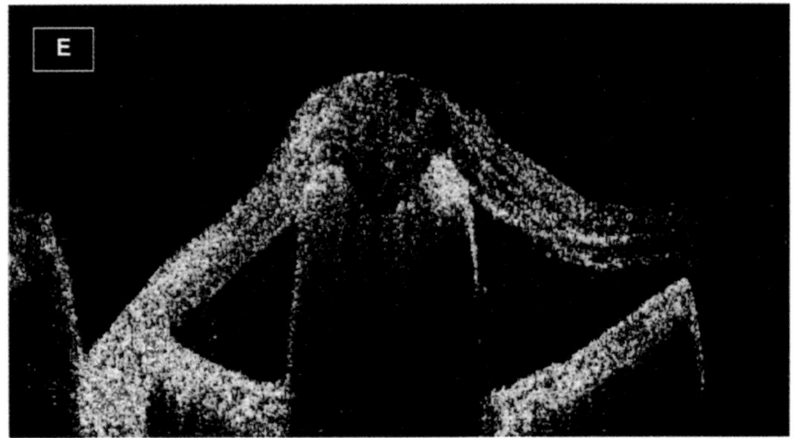

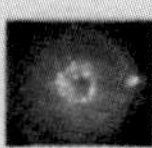

Case 11.6: Disciform Scar in ARMD

Case Summary

A-65-year-old woman was seen with a visual acuity of counting fingers in the right eye. Fundus right eye showed a well demarcated area of disciform scar with drusens surrounding the atrophic area (A).

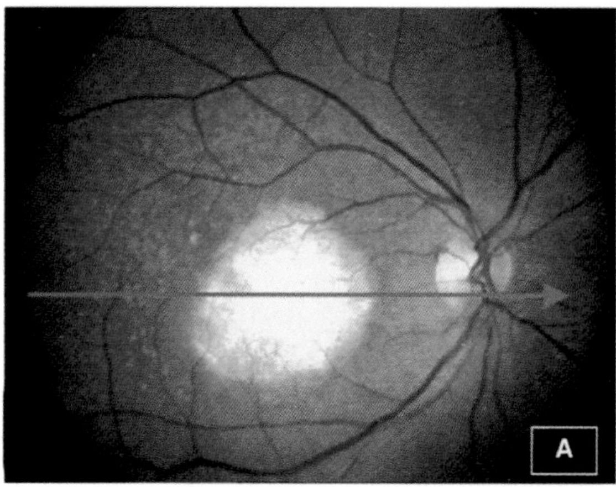

Optical Coherence Tomography

OCT scan (B) showed an area of increased reflectivity from underlying choroid that was consistent with the atrophy of overlying RPE. There was no associated subretinal fluid.

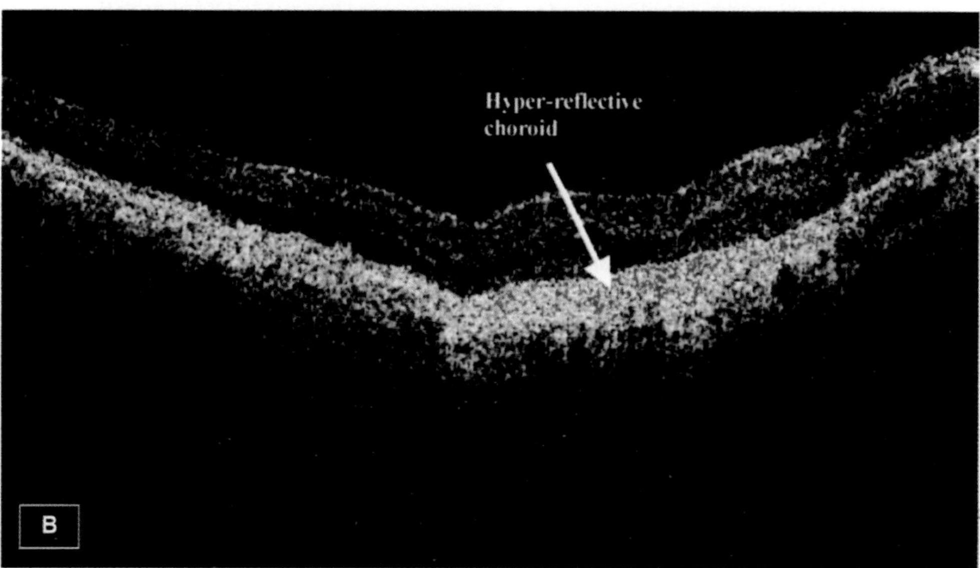

The left eye of the patient showed multiple small- medium sized drusens with only one large drusen ≥ 125 microns in size (C).

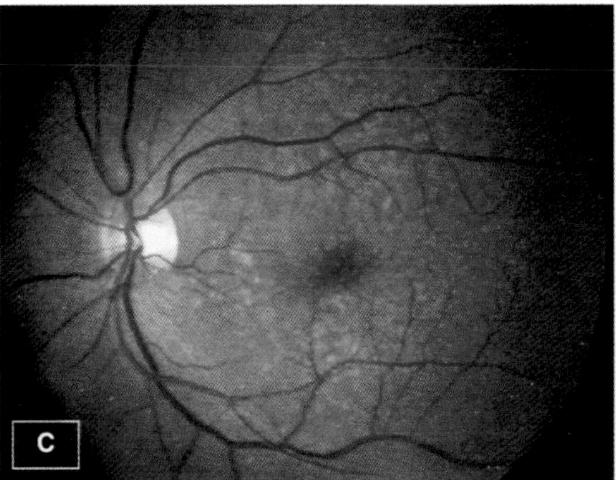

Optical Coherence Tomography

OCT line scan (D) showed multiple areas of irregular retinal pigment epithelium consistent with small, hard drusens.

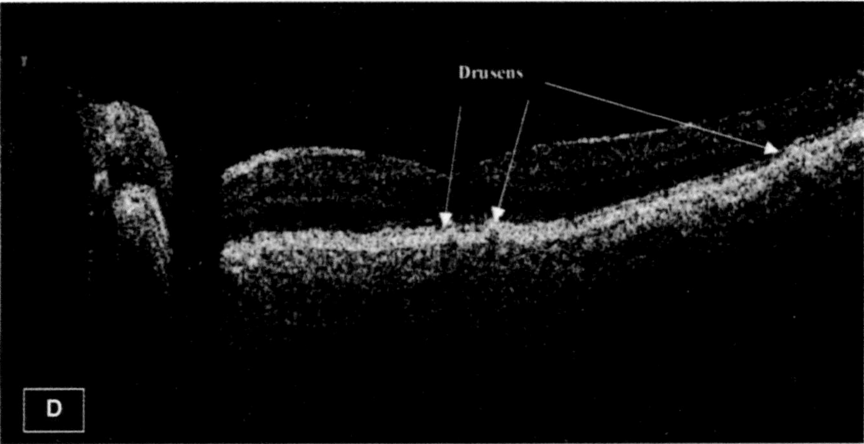

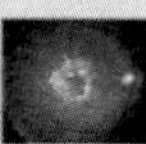

B. EARLY OCCULT CNVM

Case 11.7: Confluent, Soft Drusens with OCCULT CNVM

Case Summary

A 62-year-old woman was seen with complaints of diminished vision in both her eyes of one year duration. Her best corrected visual acuity was 20/60 in the right eye. Fundus showed the presence of soft confluent drusens , majority being >125 microns (A). The drusens were hyperfluorescent on fluorescein angiography. In addition there was an area of hyperfluorescence suggesting an underlying CNVM (B).

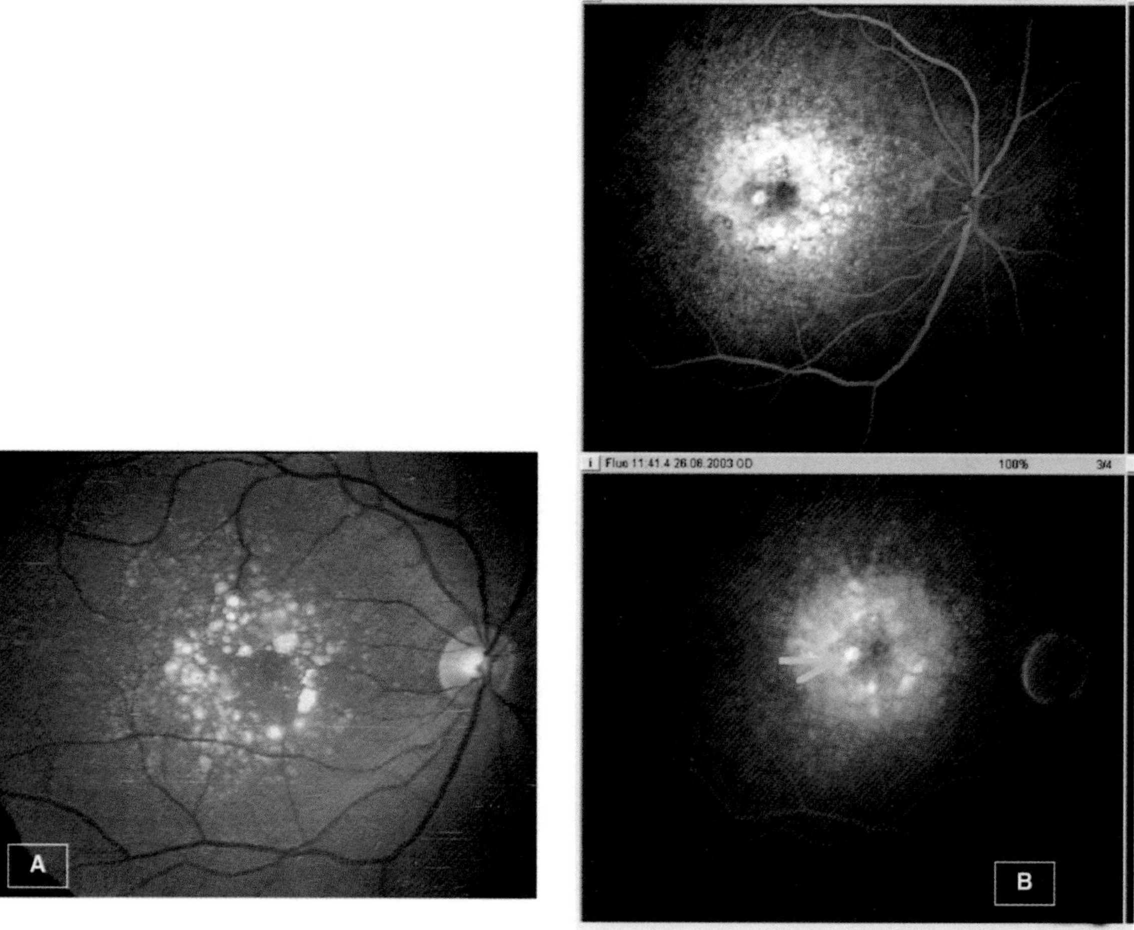

Optical Coherence Tomography

OCT (C, D) showed soft drusens as areas of focal elevation of RPE that appeared as modulations in the RPE. There was no optical shadowing from underlying choroid. There was also an area of hyporeflectivity under the fovea suggestive of subretinal fluid. The reflections from the choroid underlying RPE detachment were not attenuated and optical backscatter was seen in the sub-RPE space suggestive of an underlying CNVM.

OCT helped in diagnosing an underlying occult CNVM in this patient.

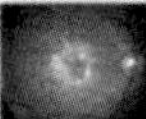

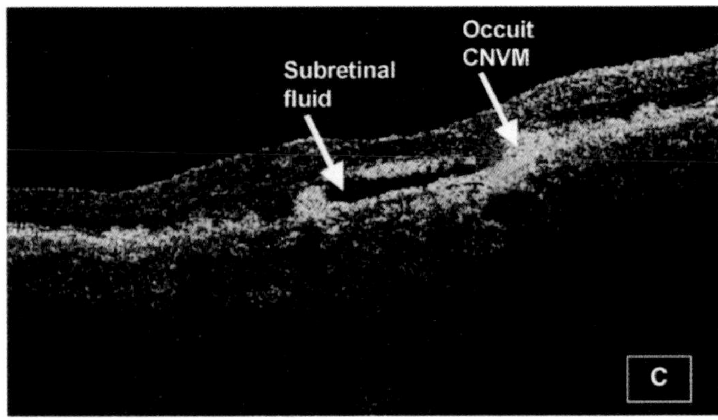

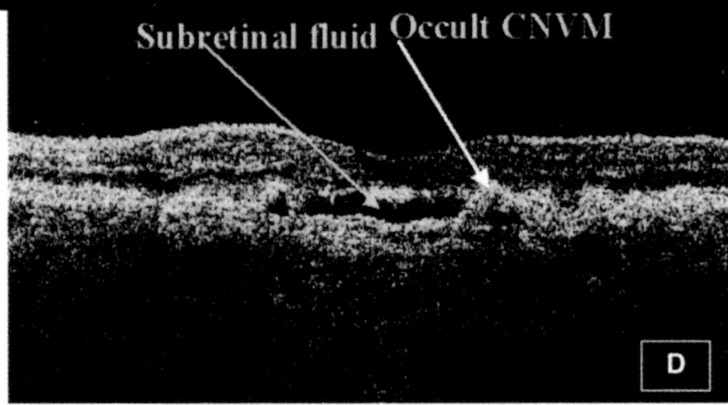

In the left eye (E), the patient had drusens with a small greenish-grey area in the center suggesting an underlying occult CNV (arrow). This area was hyperfluorescent on fluorescein angiography.

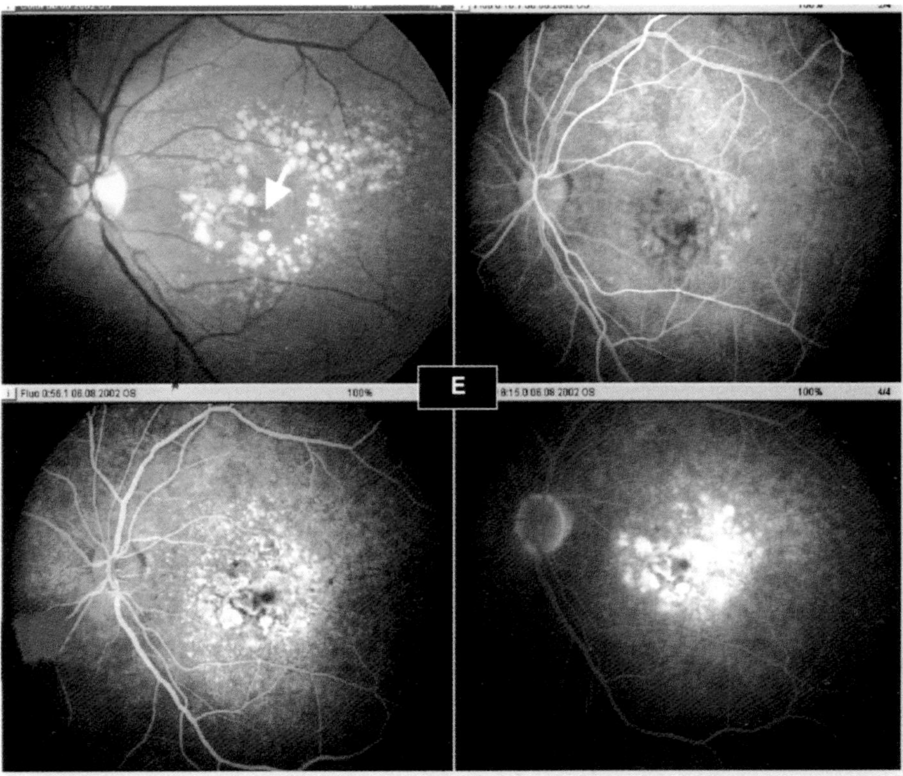

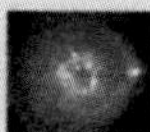

Optical Coherence Tomography

OCT scan just below the fovea (F) showed modulations in the RPE suggestive of drusens. The reflective band corresponding to the RPE was detached and an optical backscatter was seen extending from the underlying choroid into the sub-RPE space suggestive of occult CNV.

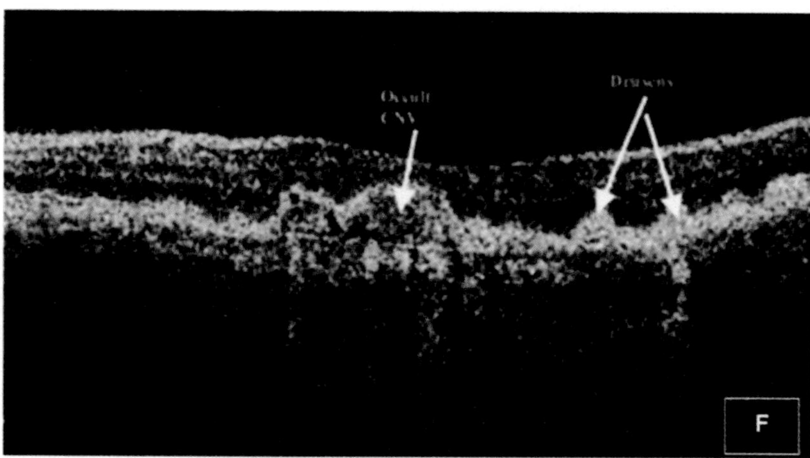

C. Associated Changes

Case 11.8: CNVM with Cystoid Spaces

Case Summary

A 56-year-old man was seen with a visual acuity of counting fingers and a large subfoveal predominately classic membrane in the left eye (A).

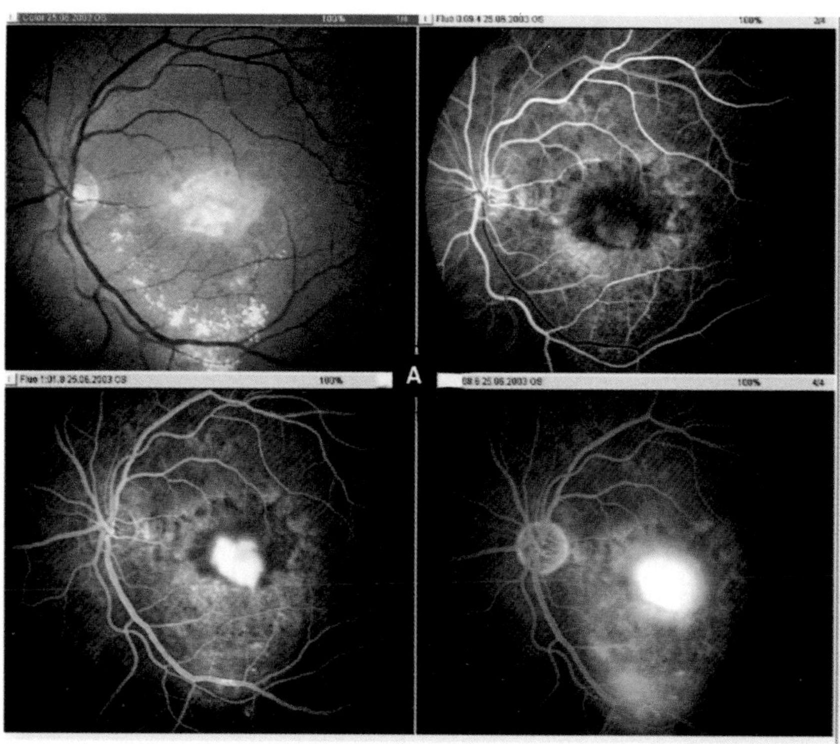

Optical Coherence Tomography

OCT left eye through 45° angle (B) showed the presence of a large fibrovascular complex with accumulation of serous fluid in the adjoining retina and the presence of cystoid spaces in the overlying retina. **These cystoid spaces were better defined on OCT and were not so well appreciated on fluorescein angiography due to hyperfluorescence in the late phase.**

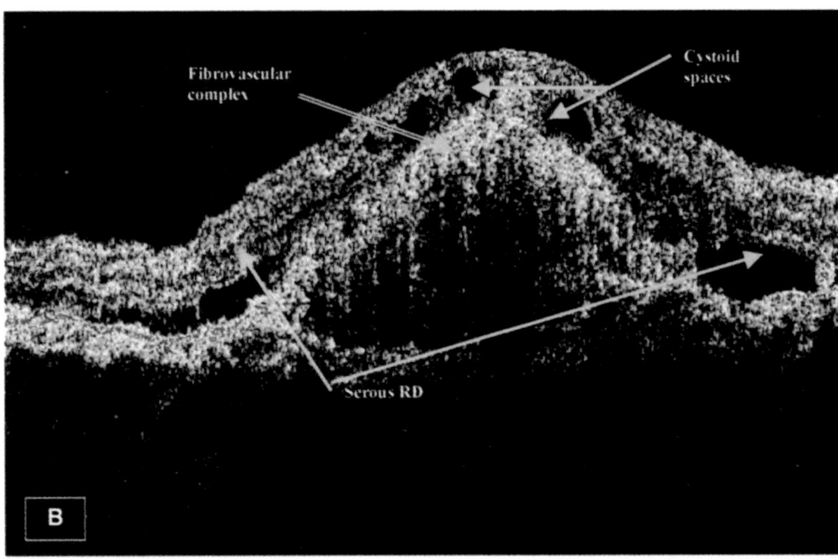

D. RESPONSETOTHERAPY

Case 11.9: Transpupillary Thermotherapy for Occult CNVM

Case Summary

A 62-year-old man complained of blurring of vision in his left eye of 2 months duration. The fundus of the left eye (A) showed few drusens with subretinal hemorrhage inferior to the fovea with central greyish-yellow exudation. The visual acuity was 20/70. Fluorescein angiography (B) showed an area of hyperfluorescence with hypofluorescence in the area of bleed. ICG (C) showed the extent of the CNV (arrows).

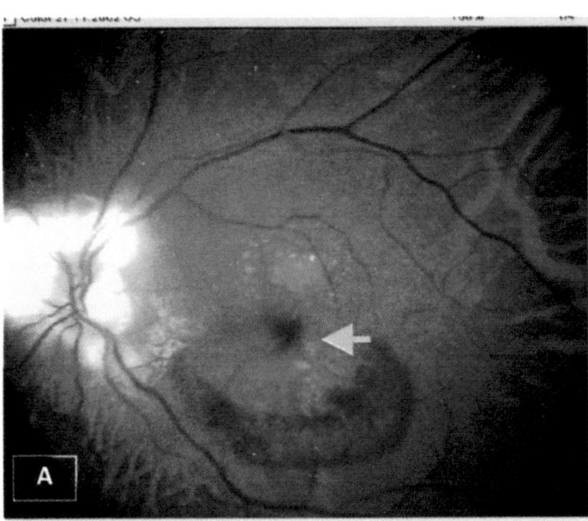

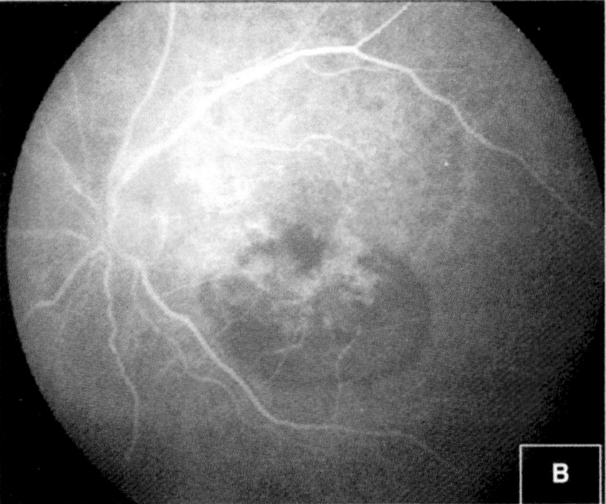

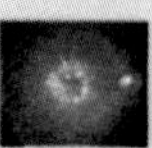

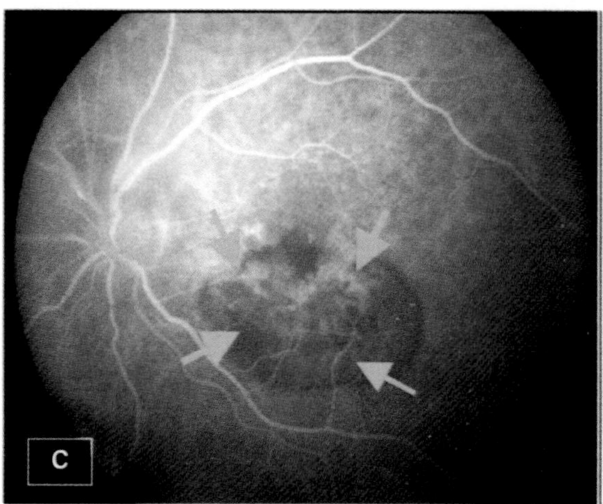

Optical Coherence Tomography

The vertical line scan through the fovea (D) showed an area of elevated retinal pigment epithelium (RPE). The overlying neurosensory retina showed thickening. The underlying choroid did not show any backscatter. However, the space beneath the elevated RPE showed mild backscatter suggestive of exudation or fibrovascular proliferation. Because of the sub-RPE location of the CNVM, the diagnosis of occult CNVM was made and patient was offered transpupillary thermotherapy (TTT).

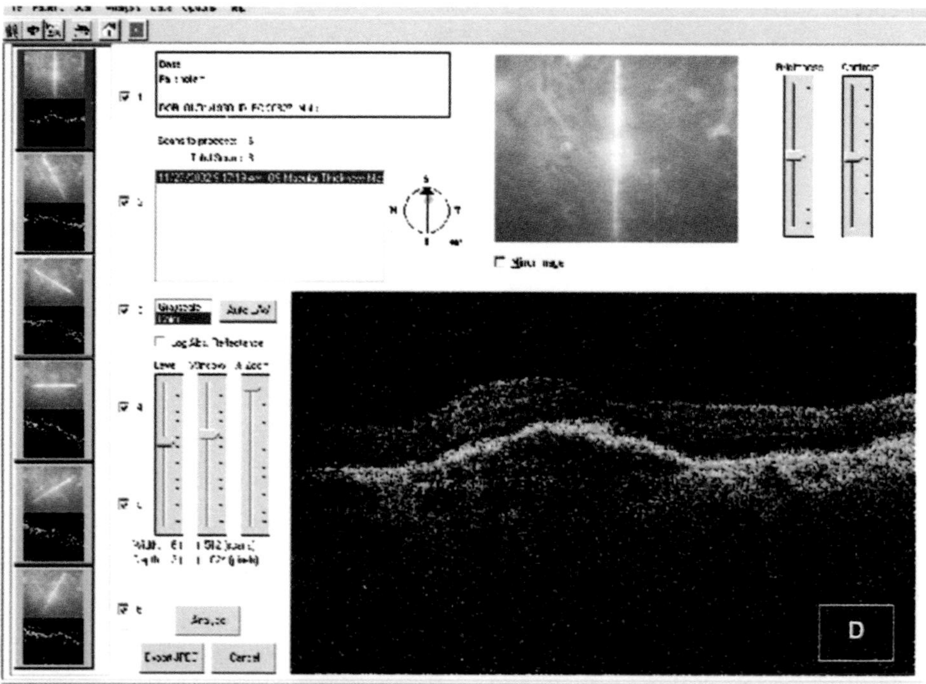

Three weeks following TTT (E), his visual acuity in this eye was 20/60. The hemorrhage was absorbed and minimal scar could be seen. Six weeks later (F), his visual acuity had improved to 20/30. The patient has maintained the same status over 7 months follow-up with no recurrences.

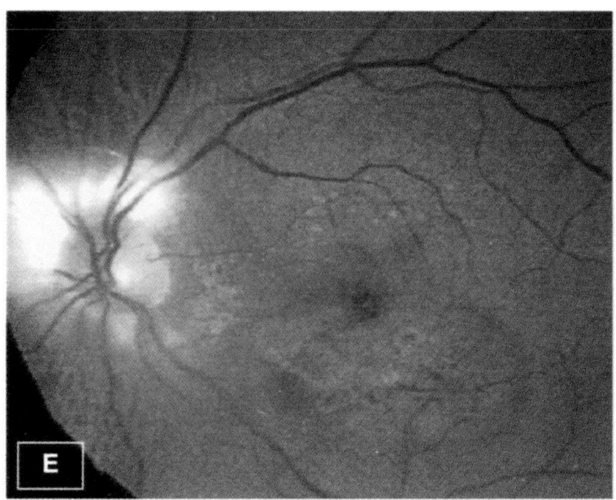

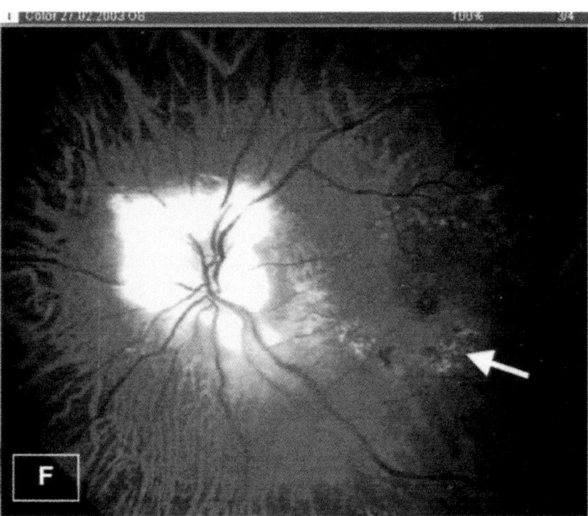

Repeat OCT scan done 3 weeks after TTT (G) showed an increase in the hyper-reflectivity overlying the area of CNV with few overlying cystoid spaces, representing probably the reactionary edema following TTT. Repeat scan at 6 weeks (H), however, showed disappearance of this reaction with almost near-normal contour of RPE.

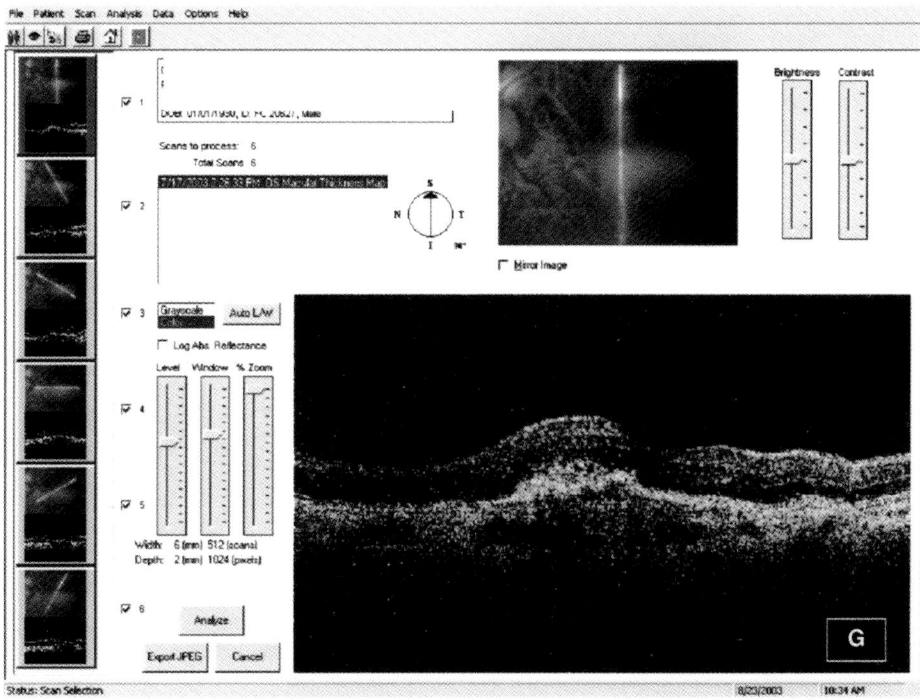

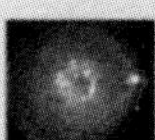

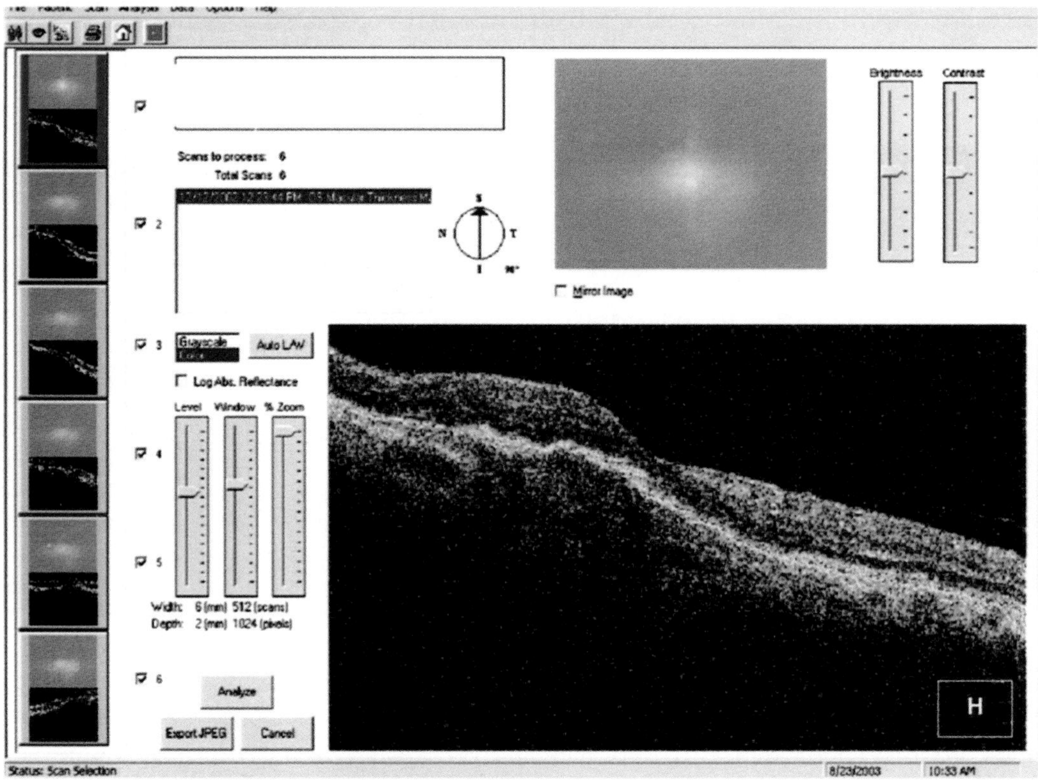

Case 11.10: Transpupillary Thermotherapy for Subfoveal Occult CNVM with Minimally Classic Component

Case Summary

A 58-year-old man was seen with micropsia in his left eye of 20 days duration. The fundus (A) showed a greyish-yellow area inferonasal to the fovea (arrow). On fluorescein angiography (B), the CNVM showed mixed hyperfluorescence with an area of increased hyperfluorescence suggestive of the classic component (arrow). The ICG (C) showed the entire membrane.

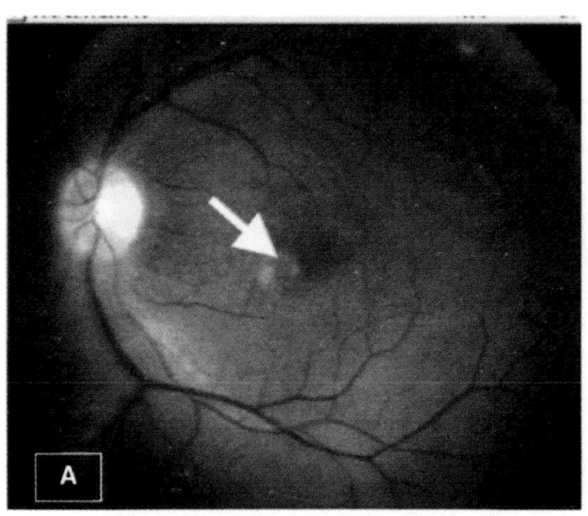

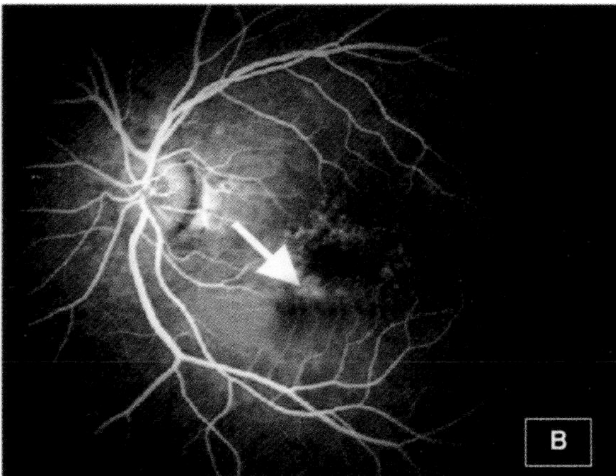

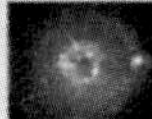

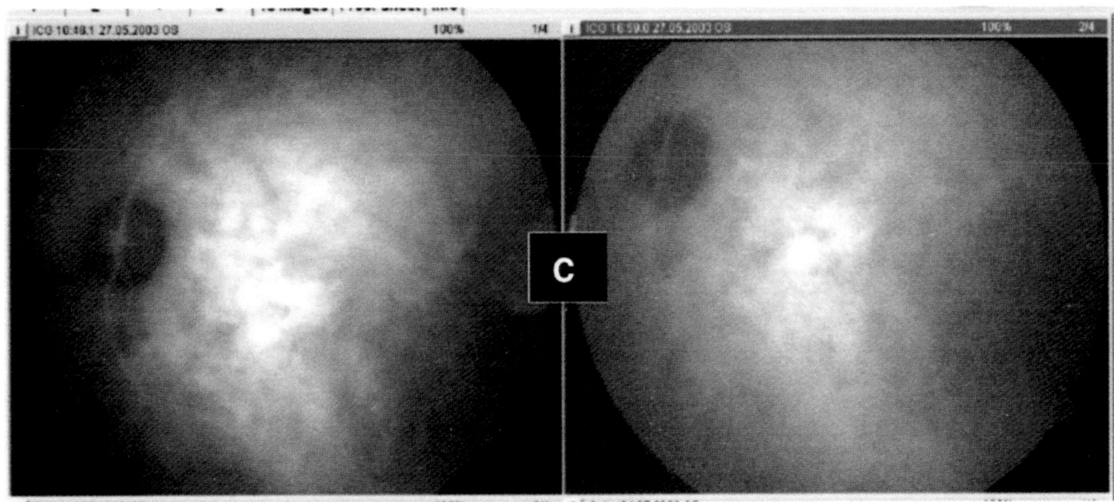

Optical Coherence Tomography

The horizontal OCT scan through the CNVM (D) showed disruption in the RPE layer with patchy reflections from choriocapillaries suggesting fibrovascular proliferation. The outer retina nasal to this showed reduced optical backscattering suggesting intraretinal fluid accumulation. The scan line passing below the fovea (E) showed a serous PED.

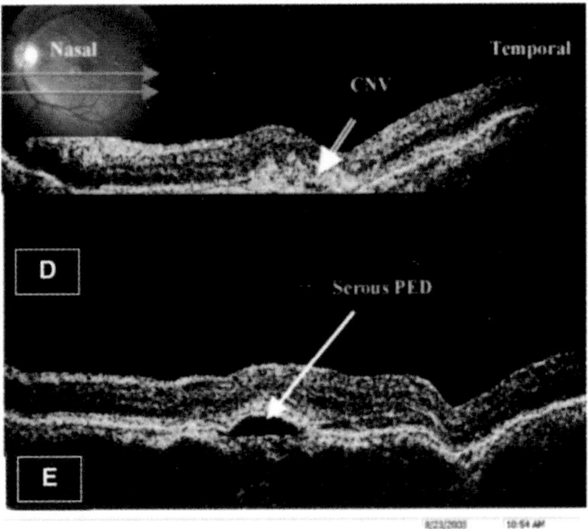

The patient elected to receive TTT for this CNVM. Two months later, his best corrected visual acuity was 20/30. Fundus did not show any CNVM or scar (F).

Optical Coherence Tomography

Repeat OCT done at 2 months following TTT (G) showed return of retinal thickness to normal. The RPE in the area of CNVM showed mild disruption (arrow). The PED seen inferiorly was however, persistent (not shown).

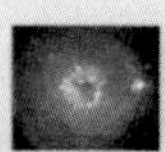

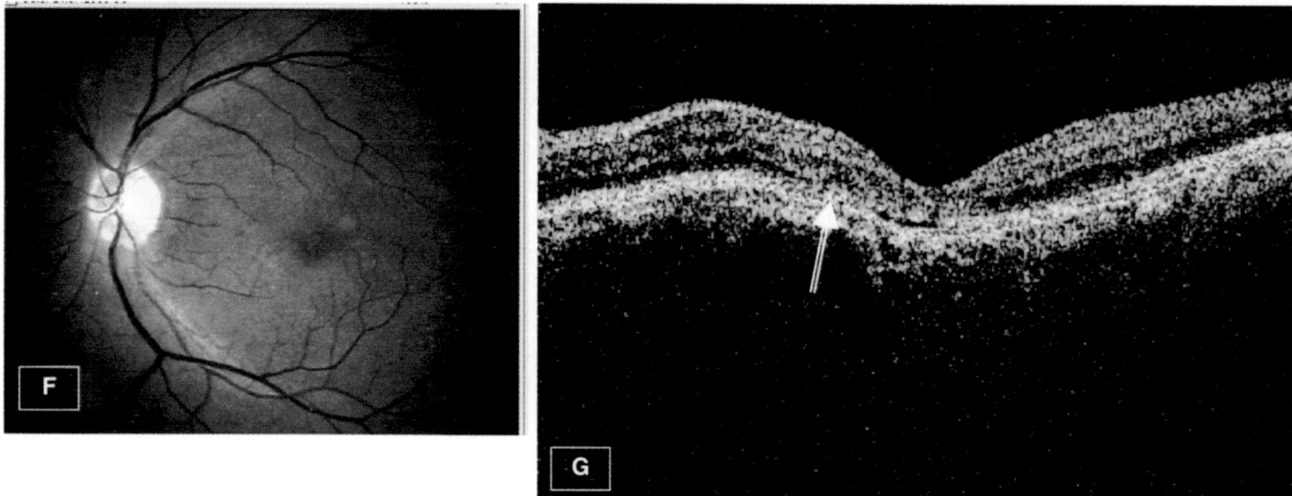

Case 11.11: Classic CNVM: Worsening on TTT

Case Summary

A 52-year-old man was seen with a visual acuity of 20/200 in the left eye with subfoveal CNVM (A). The fluorescein angiography showed a well-defined area of discrete hyperfluorescence (B)

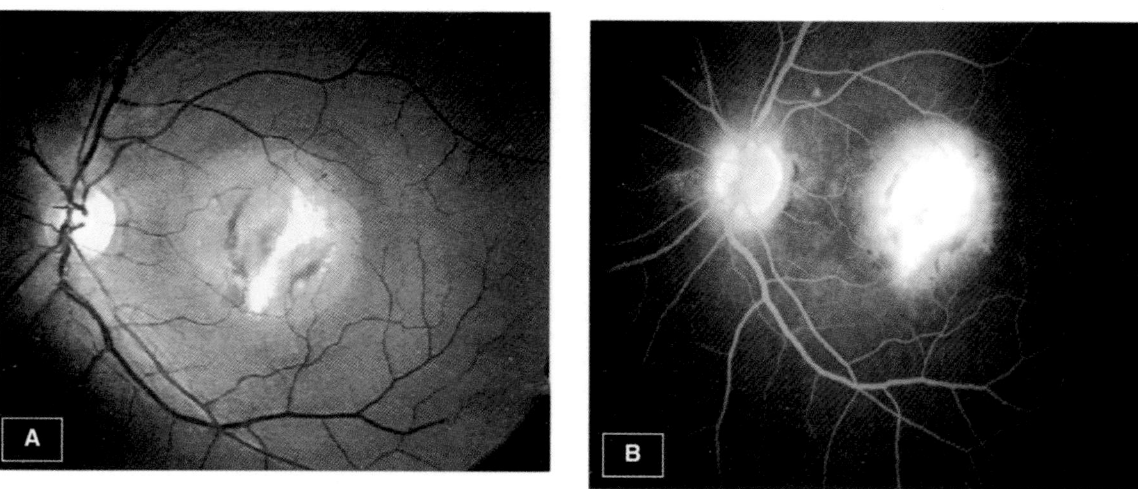

Optical Coherence Tomography

OCT scan (C) showed disruption in the RPE with focal area of enhanced reflectivity seen beneath the foveal center within the retinal layers suggestive of a classic CNVM. The foveal retinal thickness was 480 microns. The detached posterior hyloid was seen anterior to it. The patient elected to receive transpupillary thermotherapy as he could not afford PDT.

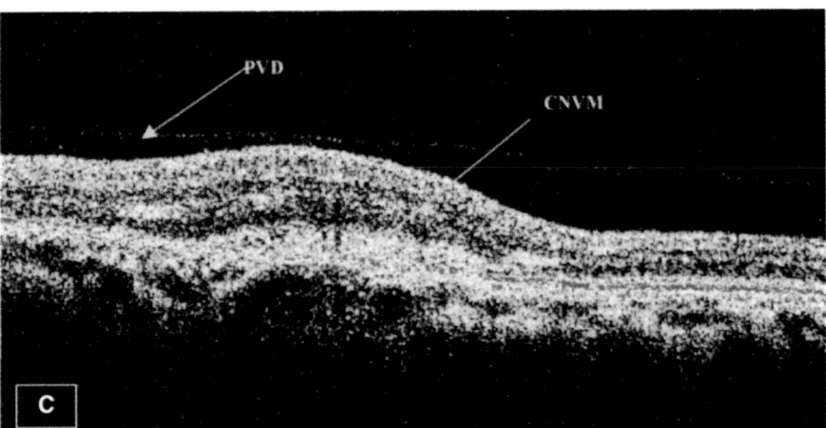

Repeat OCT scan (D) done four weeks following TTT, did not show any reduction in the classic component of the CNVM.

Three months later, repeat OCT scan (E) showed the appearance of subretinal fluid seen on either side of CNVM, indicating worsening following TTT.

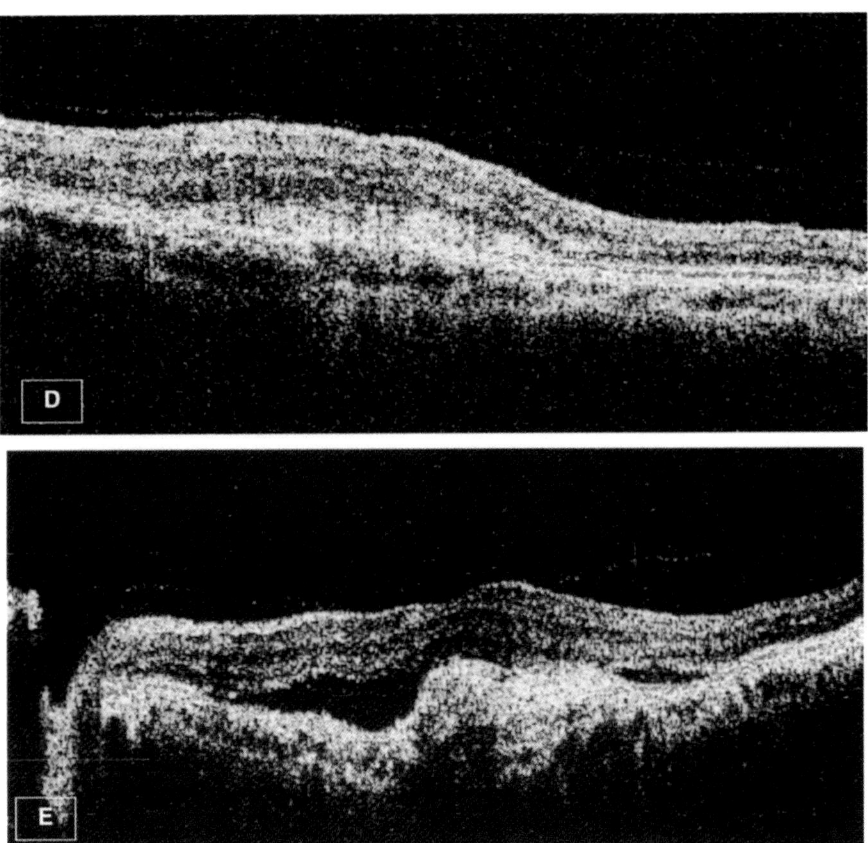

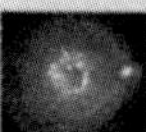

Case 11.12: Cystoid Macular Edema following Transpupillary Thermotherapy for Juxtafoveal Classic CNVM

Case Summary

A 57-year-old woman was seen with left eye juxtafoveal CNVM (A). Her visual acuity in this eye was 20/80.The fluorescein angiography showed an initial area of mixed fluorescence with late hyperfluorescence (B-D).

Optical Coherence Tomography

Horizontal OCT line scan (E) passing through the CNVM showed an area of increased hyper-reflectivity in the outer retinal layers with an overlying hyporeflective space suggesting an intraretinal cyst. These findings were consistent with classic CNVM.

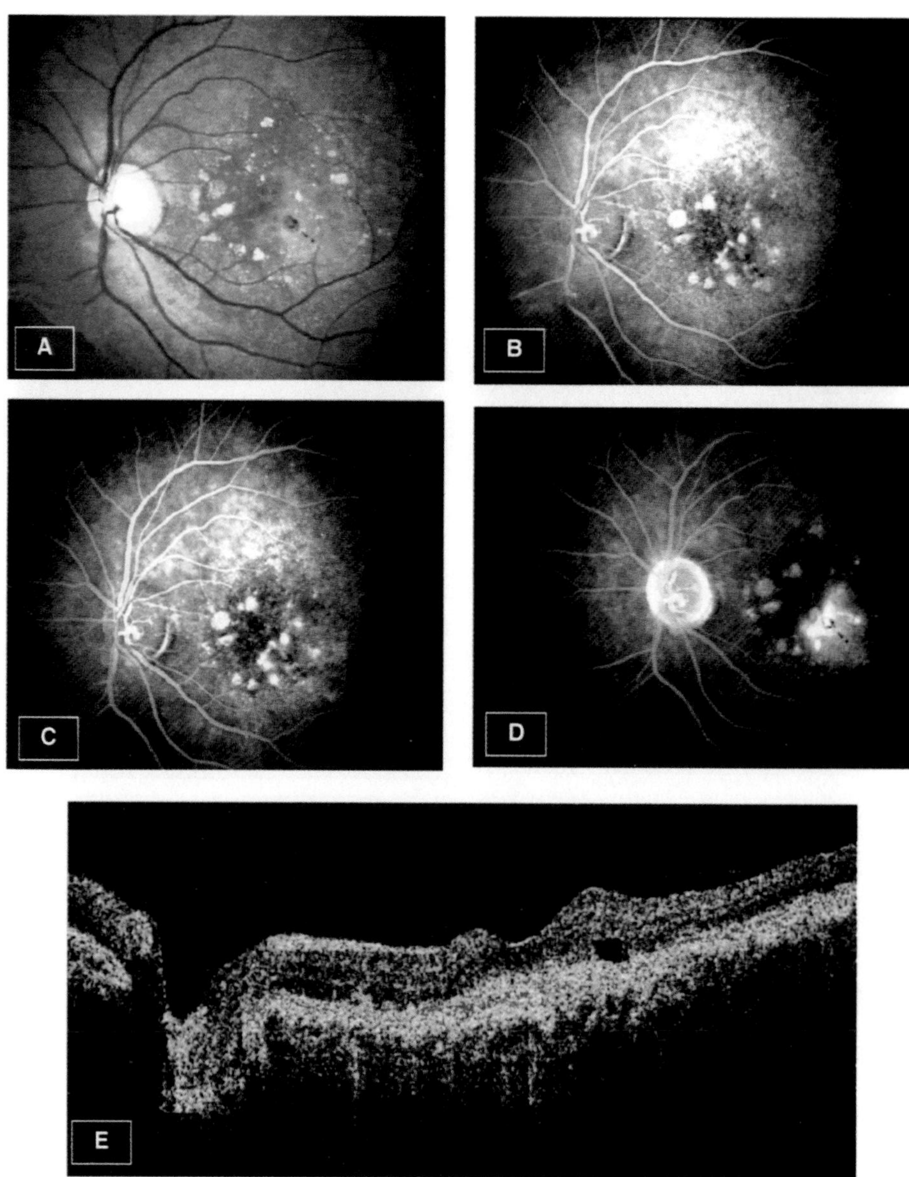

The patient underwent TTT for this CNVM. Three months later, her visual acuity was reduced to 20/100. Both fundus photograph and fluorescein angiograms showed an increase in the area of CNVM with overlying cystoid spaces (F,G).

Repeat OCT scan (H) showed the presence of large cystoid spaces seen as hyporeflective areas with intervening hyper-reflective septae suggesting the development of cystoid spaces following TTT.

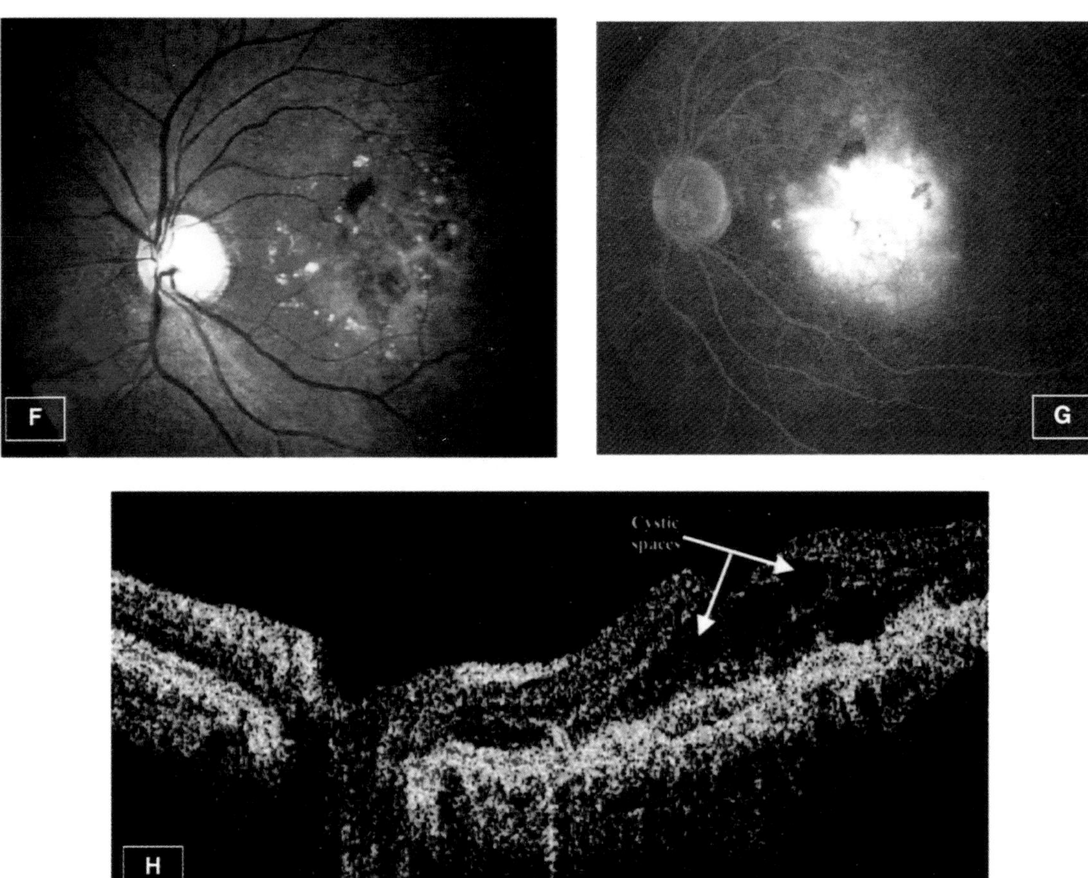

Case 11.13: Persistent CNVM following Thermal Laser for Extrafoveal Classic CNVM

Case Summary

A 60-year-old woman was seen with decreased vision in the right eye of 14 days duration. Fundus and fluorescein angiography of the right eye (A) showed a large PED (thin arrow) temporal to the fovea and a small extrafoveal classic CNVM (thick arrows).

Optical Coherence Tomography

OCT line scan through the lesions (B) showed an area of large PED with adjoining pocket of serous fluid. In addition, there was an area of moderate to intense hyper-reflectivity in the neurosensory retina suggesting a classic CNVM. The patient received thermal laser photocoagulation for the extrafoveal CNVM.

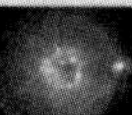

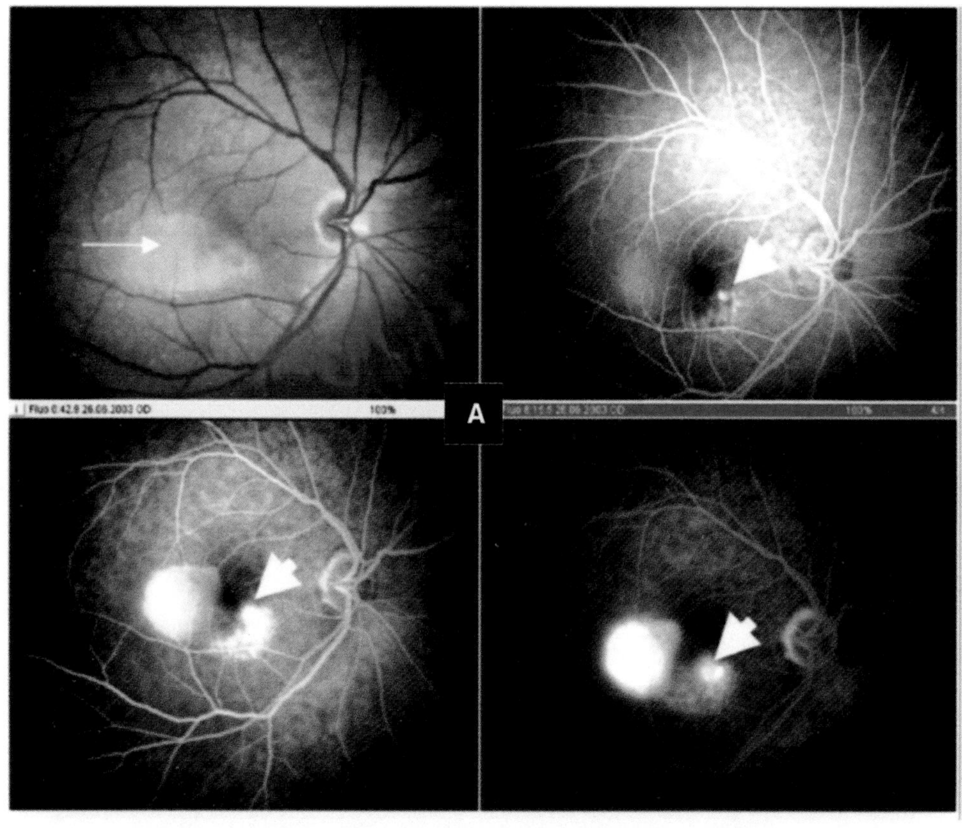
A

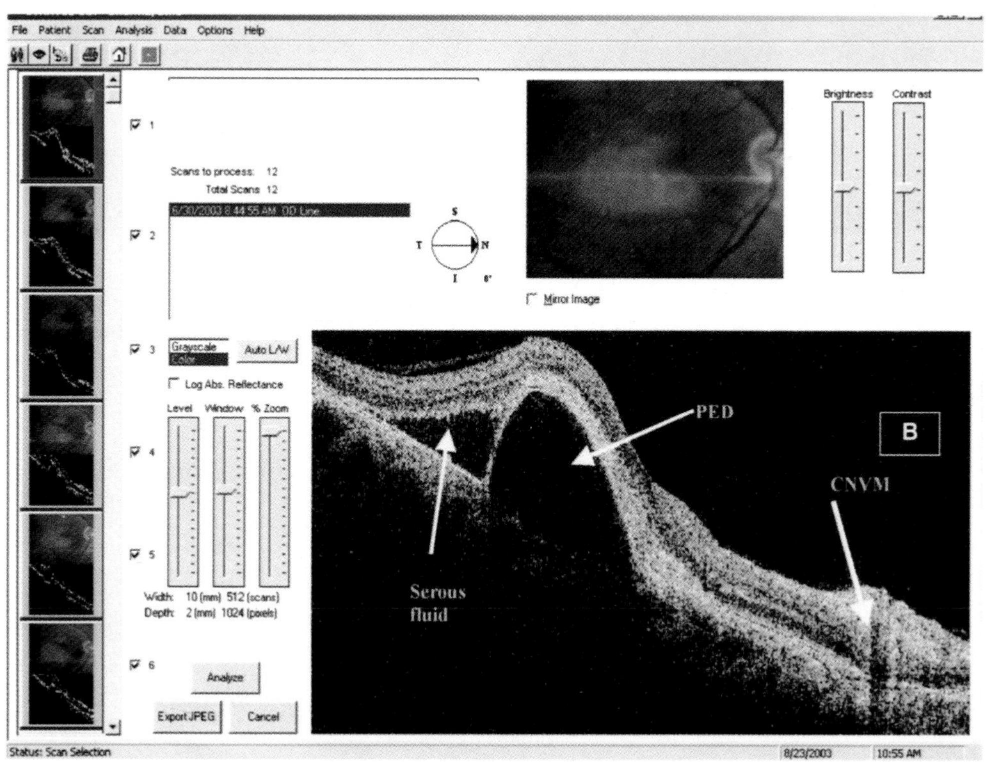
File Patient Scan Analysis Data Options Help
Scans to process: 12
Total Scans 12
6/30/2003 8:44:55 AM OD Line
S
T
N
I
Mirror Image
Brightness
Contrast
Grayscale
Color
Auto L/W
Log Abs. Reflectance
Level
Window
% Zoom
Width: 10 (mm) 512 (scans)
Depth: 2 (mm) 1024 (pixels)
Analyze
Export JPEG
Cancel
Status: Scan Selection
8/23/2003
10:55 AM
PED
B
CNVM
Serous fluid

Two weeks later, the fundus showed persistence of CNVM at the foveal edge that was confirmed on fluorescein angiography (C).

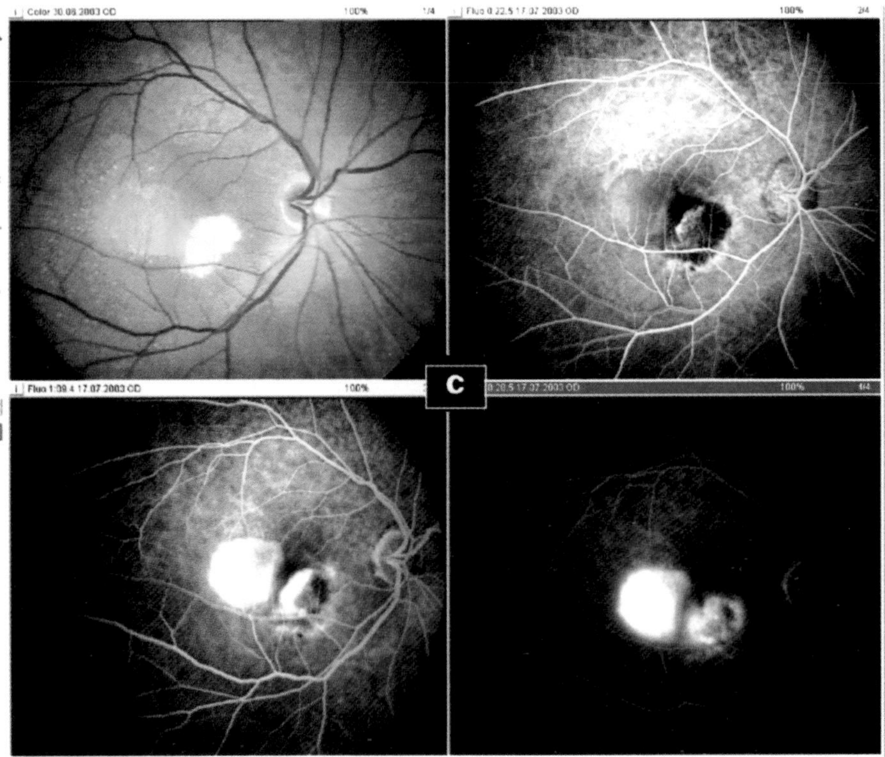

Repeat OCT scan showed the growth of CNVM towards the fovea (D).

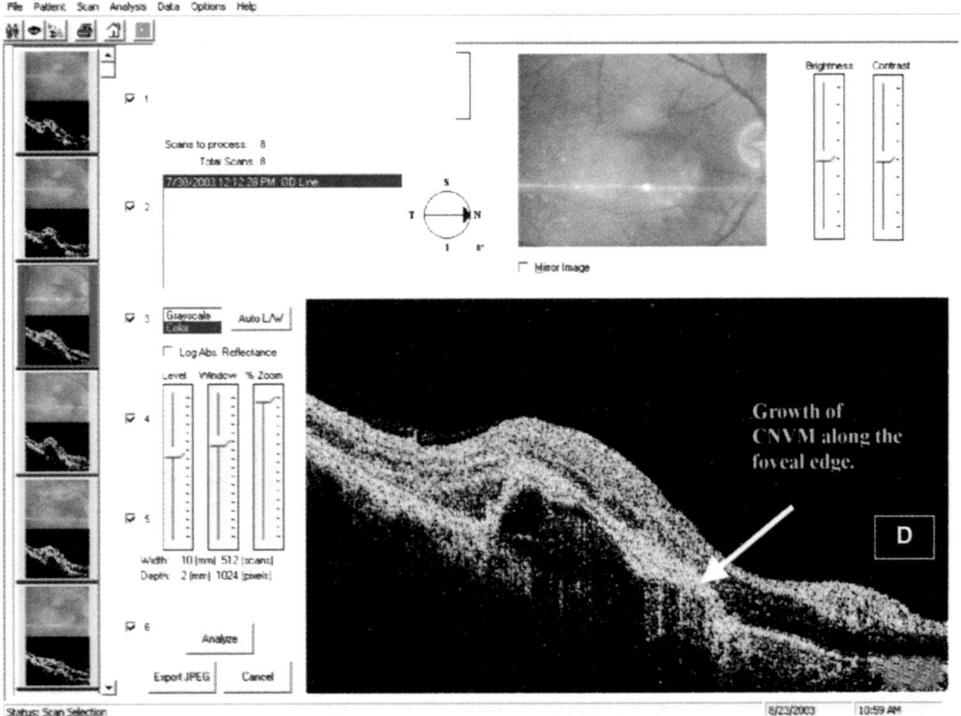

Case 11. 14 : Photodynamic Therapy for Juxtafoveal Recurrent Choroidal Neovascular Membrane

(*Courtesy* of Dr. Monique Leys, West Virginia University Eye Institute, Morgantown, USA.)

Case Summary

A 56-year-old man was seen with recurrent choroidal neovascular membrane (CNVM) with a scar of krypton laser photocoagulation done for extrafoveal CNVM (A). Fluorescein angiography (B) showed CNV at the edge of previous photocoagulation scar.

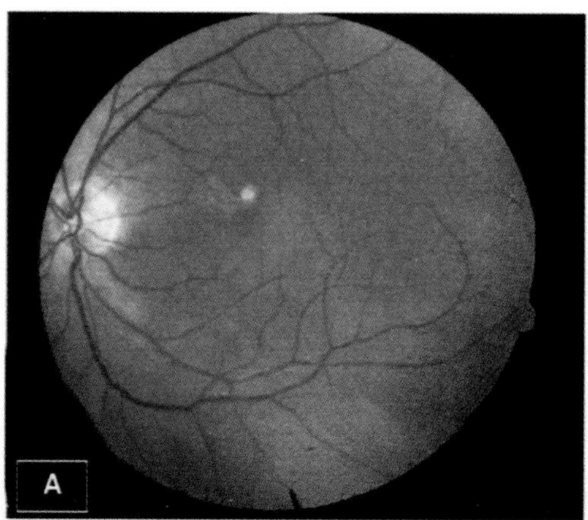

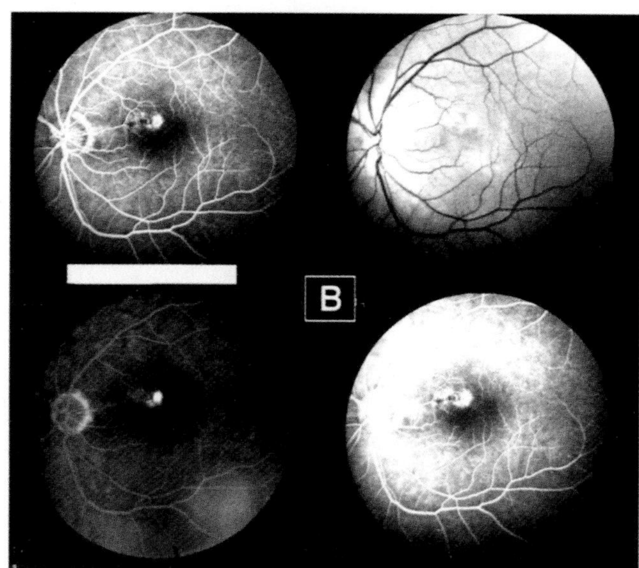

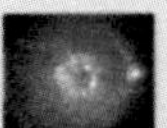

Optical Coherence Tomography

Horizontal OCT line scan through the area of CNVM (C) showed a small occult CNV with associated serous detachment (arrow). The patient received photodynamic therapy with verteporfin.

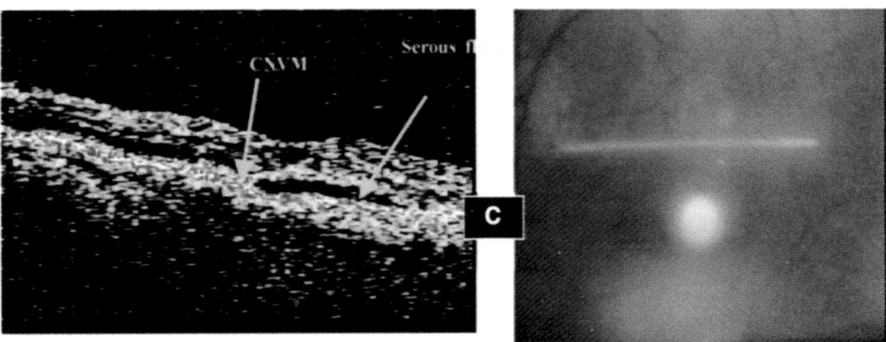

Four weeks later, repeat fundus photograph and OCT scan showed resolution of serous fluid (D, E).

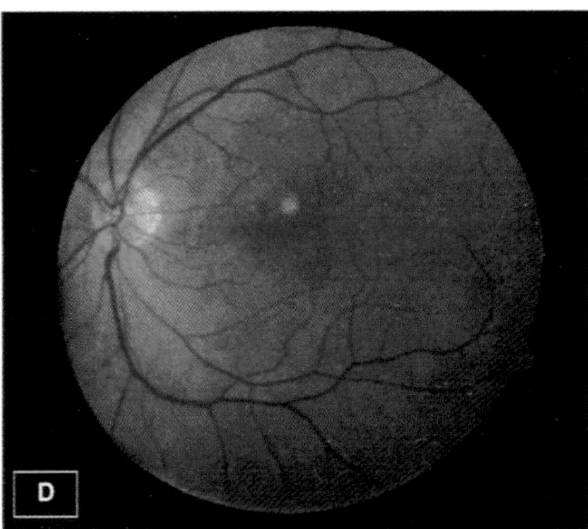

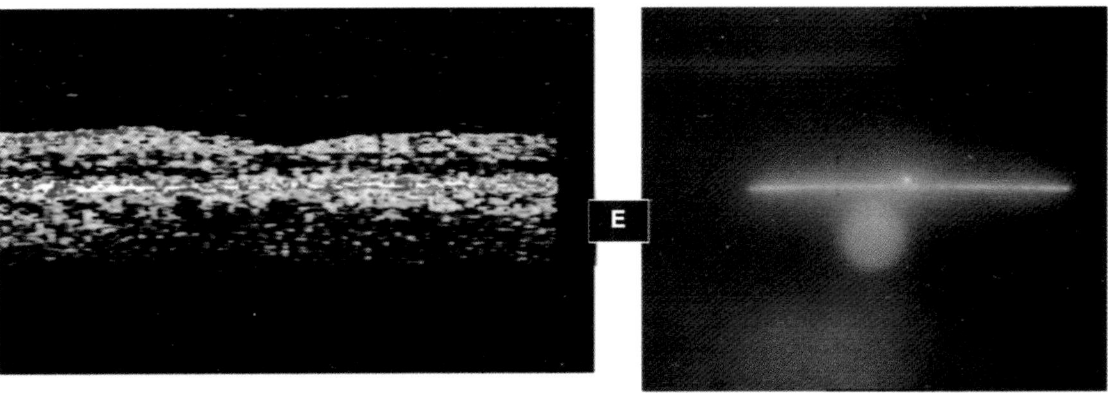

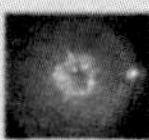

Case 11.15 : Photodynamic Therapy for Juxtafoveal CNVM

Case Summary

A 50-year-old woman was seen with floaters in the left eye of 10 days duration. Her best-corrected visual acuity was 20/20. The fundus and fluorescein angiography showed a juxtafoveal choroidal neovascular membrane (A). There were no drusens indicating that probably the membrane was idiopathic rather than age-related.

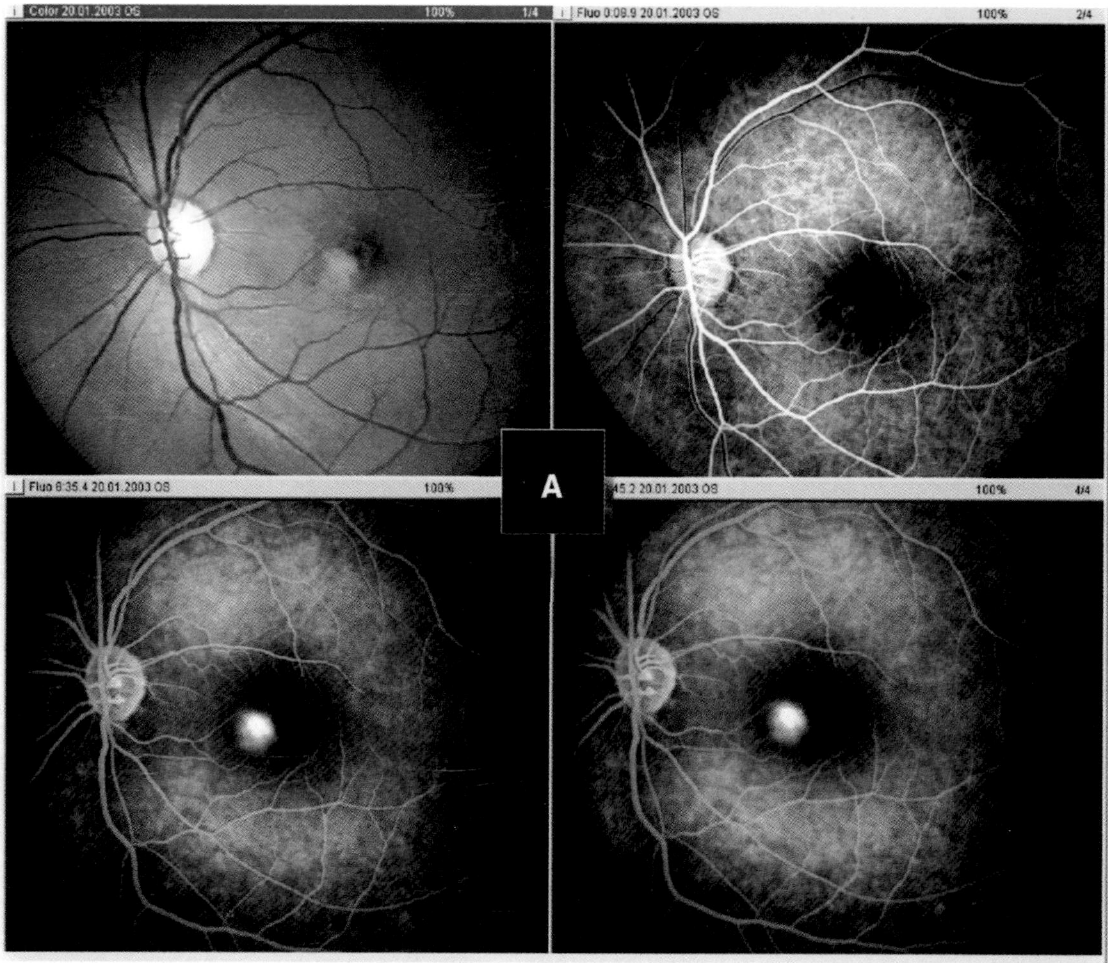

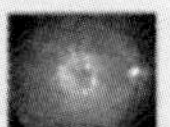

Optical Coherence Tomography

OCT scan (B) showed juxtafoveal increased retinal thickness with mild backscattering from outer retinal layers and disruption in RPE layer. Just anterior to the disrupted RPE was an area of moderate reflectivity with small cystic spaces in the overlying retina suggestive of a predominately classic CNVM.

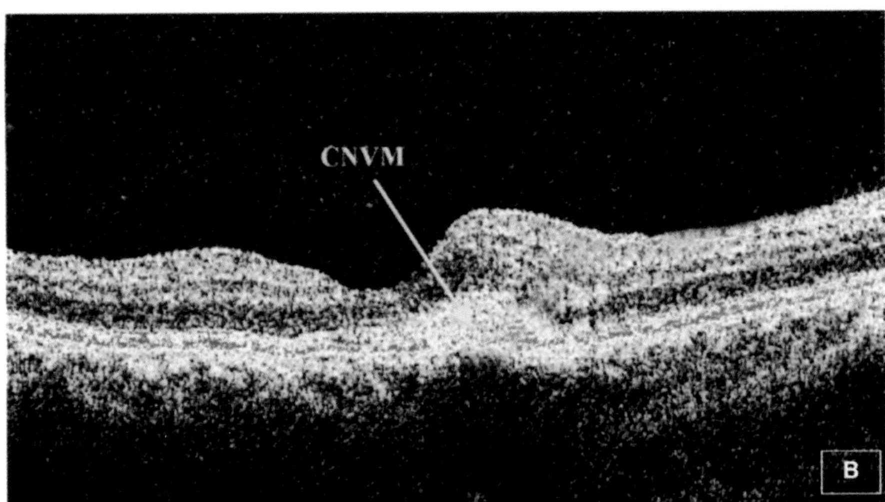

The patient received photodynamic therapy for this CNVM. Twelve weeks later, her visual acuity was 20/20 (C).

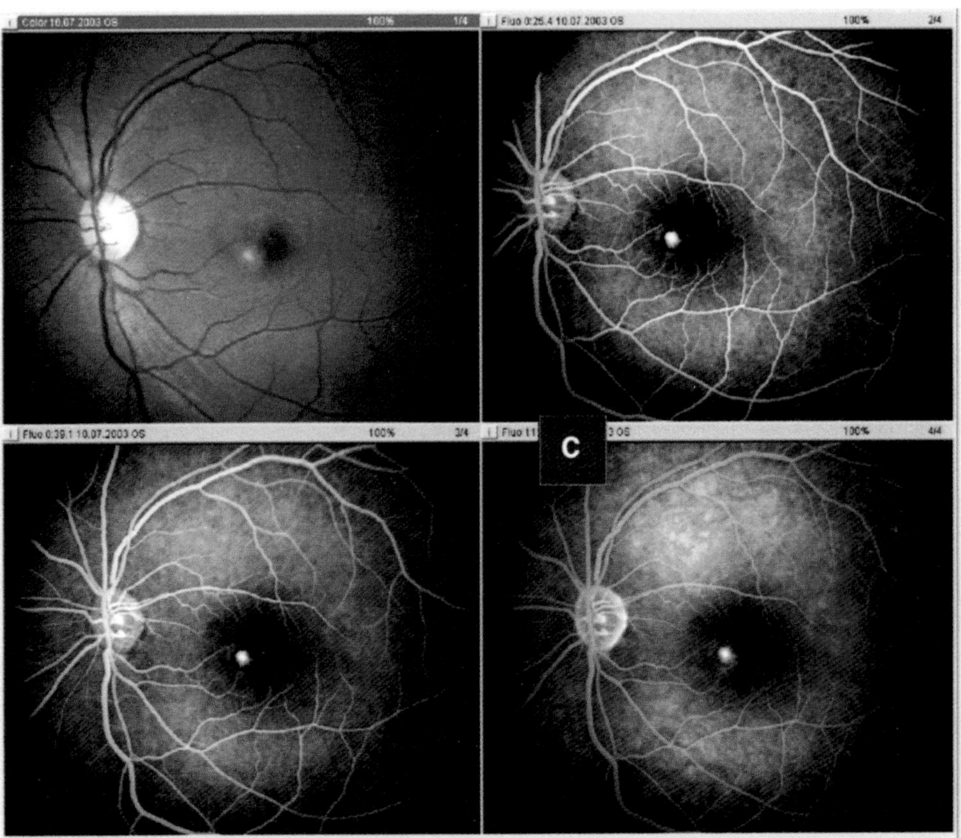

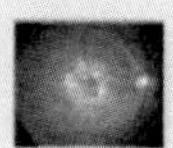

Repeat OCT (D,E) showed return of foveal thickness to normal with presence of area of moderately increased reflectivity corresponding to fibrovascular scar (arrow) and no intraretinal fluid indicating stage 3b of resolution following PDT.

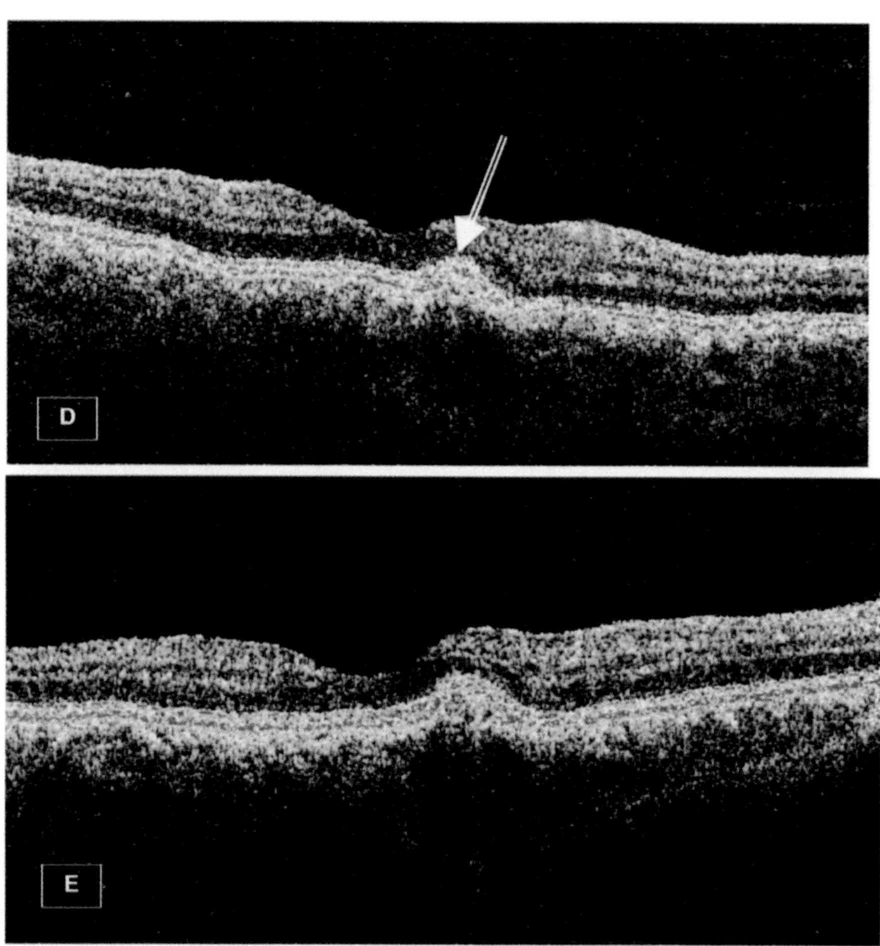

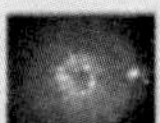

Case 11.16: Fuchs' Spot

Case Summary

A 54-year-old lady was referred as ARMD. Fundoscopy showed a Fuchs' spot and a Lacquer crack (A) that was hyperfluorescent on fluorescein angiography (B-D).

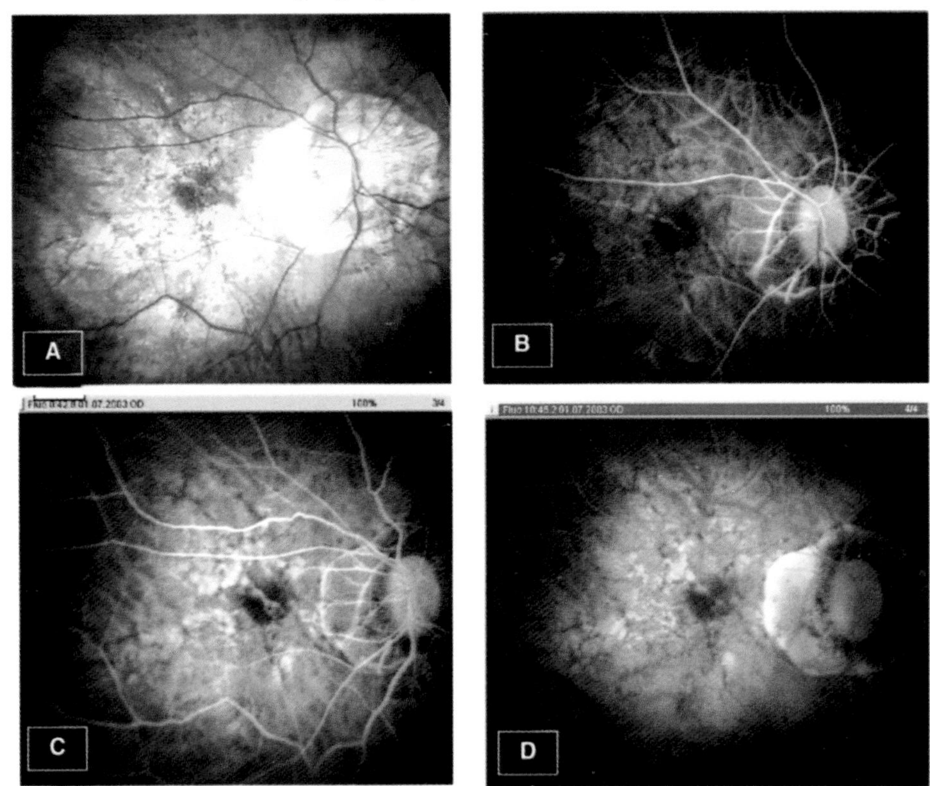

Optical Coherence Tomography

OCT line scan of the right eye (E) showed choroidal neovascular tissue just nasal to the fovea with discontinuity in the RPE-choriocapillary complex and retinal pigment epithelial hyperplasia.

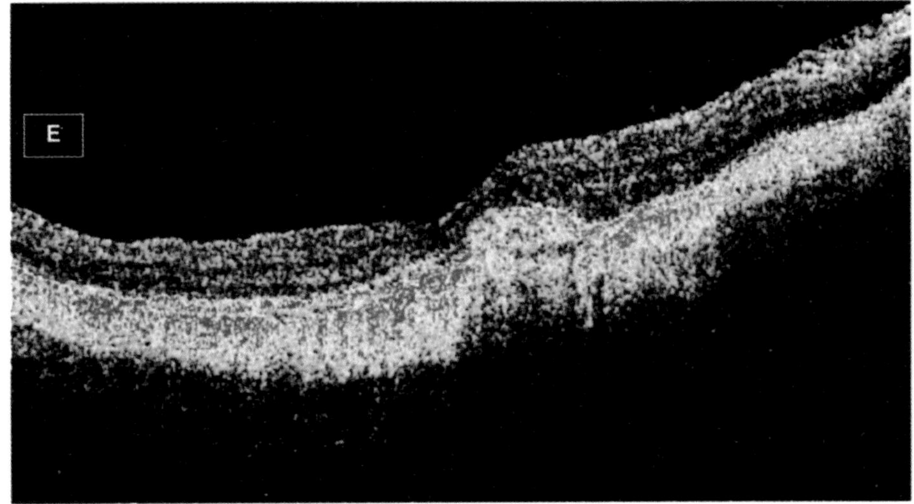

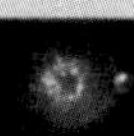

CONCLUSIONS

There are three aspects in the management of ARMD patients:

1. Disease categorization
2. Management issues that depend on the disease category.
3. Monitor response to the therapy and to define indications for retreatment.

OCT aids in the practical management of these patients by helping in categorization of ARMD, picking up the associated secondary changes and also closely monitoring response to the various therapies that are available. In our experience, we have started using it as an investigative tool between fluorescein angiography and indocyanin green angiography that helps us in prompt disease categorization.

SUGGESTED READINGS

1. Rogers AH, Martidis A, Greenberg PA, Puliafito CA.Optical Coherence Tomography findings following photodynamic therapy of choroidal neovascularization. Am J Ophthalmol 2002; 134:566-576.
2. Costa RA, Farah ME, Cardillo JA et al. Immediate indocyanine green angiography and optical coherence tomography evaluation after photodynamic therapy for subfoveal choroidal neovascularization. Retina 2003 ; 23 : 159-65.
3. Puliafito CA, Hee MR, Lin CP et al. Imaging of macular disease with optical coherence tomography. Ophthalmology 1995; 102:217-219.

Chapter 12

Choroidal Neovascular Membranes

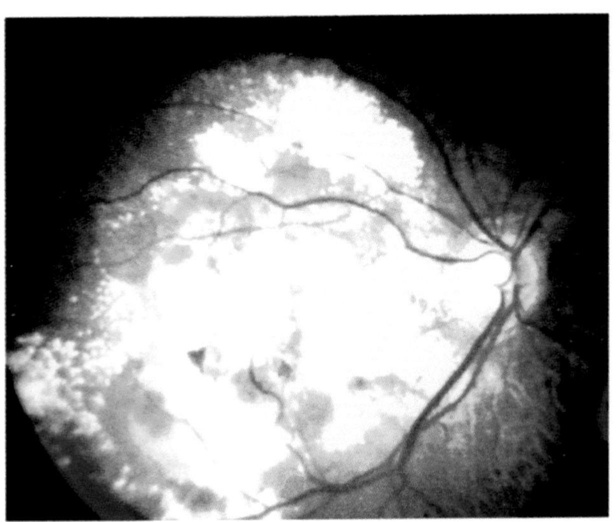

OPTICAL COHERENCETOMOGRAPHY IN CHOROIDAL NEOVASCULAR MEMBRANES

Optical coherence tomography is a very important tool in the management of choroidal neovascular membranes (CNVM). It provides *in vivo* histopathology of the retina giving information at tissue structural level. The choroidal neovascularization is seen as highly reflective, bright red band in the retina. The associated serous fluid is seen as hyporeflective spaces. There might be associated cystoid spaces in the retina. The present section deals with CNVMs other than Age-related macular degeneration. Majority of these CNVMs are of classic variety.

OCT provides the following information:

A. To rule out the presence of underlying CNVM in patients with hemorrhagic pigment epithelium detachments.
B. To study the *in vivo* characteristics of CNVM in different diseases.
C. To study response to therapy. This has already been shown in chapter 11 (Cases 11.9 to 11.15).

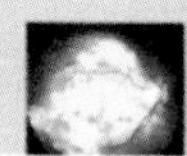

A. TO RULE OUT THE PRESENCE OF UNDERLYING CNVM IN PATIENTS WITH HEMORRHAGIC PIGMENT EPITHELIUM DETACHMENTS

Case 12.1: Hemorrhagic Pigment Epithelial Detachment

Case Summary

A 50-year-old woman was seen with decreased vision in her left eye of one month duration. Her best corrected visual acuity was 20/200. The fundus L/E showed hemorrhagic PED with hard exudates (A). Fluorescein angiography (B) showed the presence of hyperfluorescent spot in the center surrounded by a hypofluorescent ring.

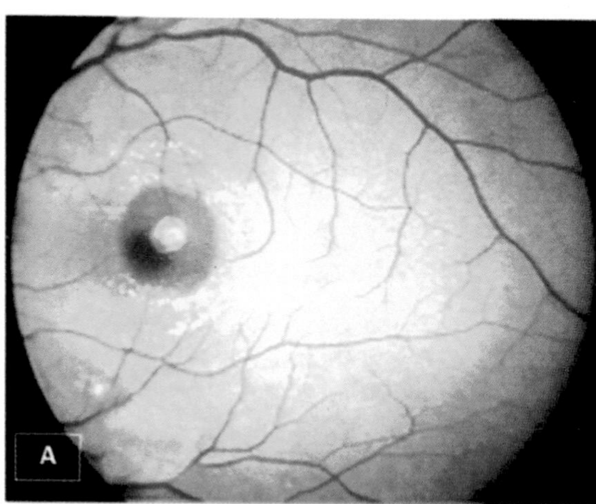

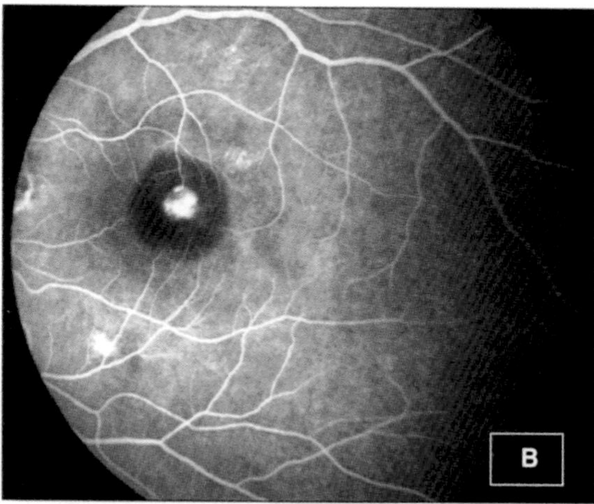

Optical Coherence Tomography

OCT scan through fovea (C) showed loss of foveal contour with PED (arrow) with attenuation of underlying choroidal reflection. No evidence of choroidal neovascularization was seen in this patient.

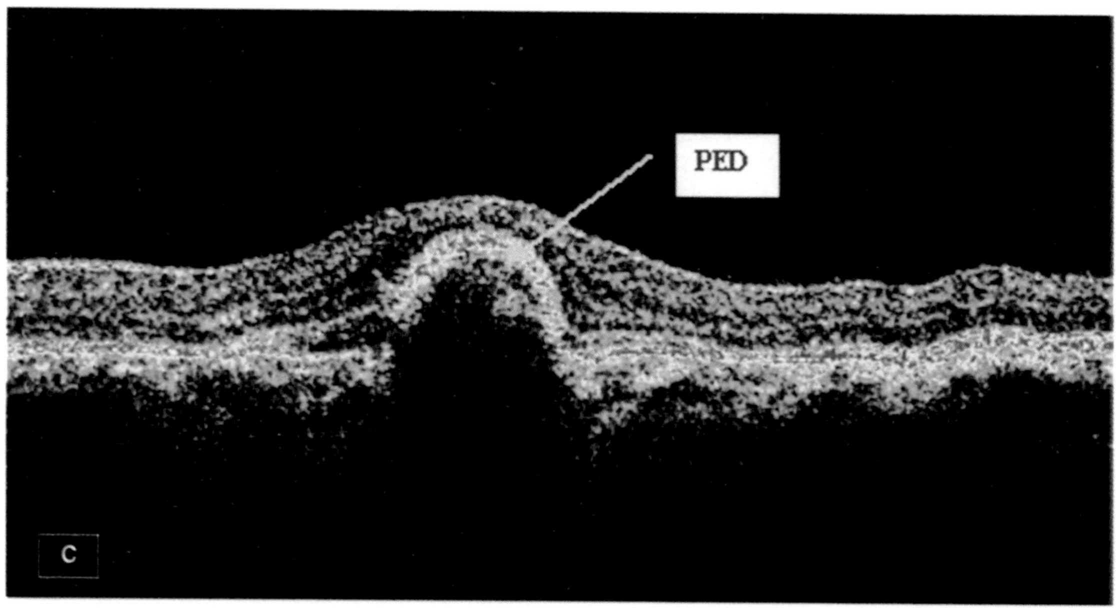

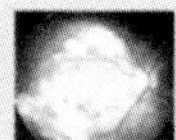

B. TO STUDY THE IN VIVO CHARACTERISTICS OF CNVM IN DIFFERENT DISEASES

Case 12.2: CNVM in Angioid Streaks

Case Summary

A 45-year-old woman was seen with the diagnosis of angoid streaks and choroidal neovascular membrane in the right eye (A). The CNVM showed mixed fluorescence in the early phase with late hyperfluorescence. The peripapillary angioid streaks too showed hyperfluorescence on angiography (B).

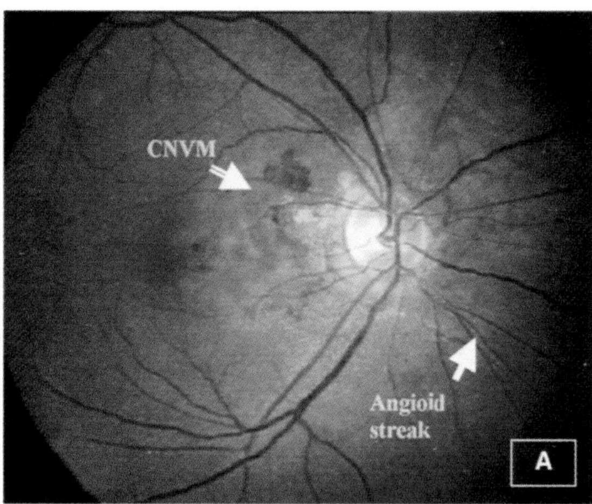

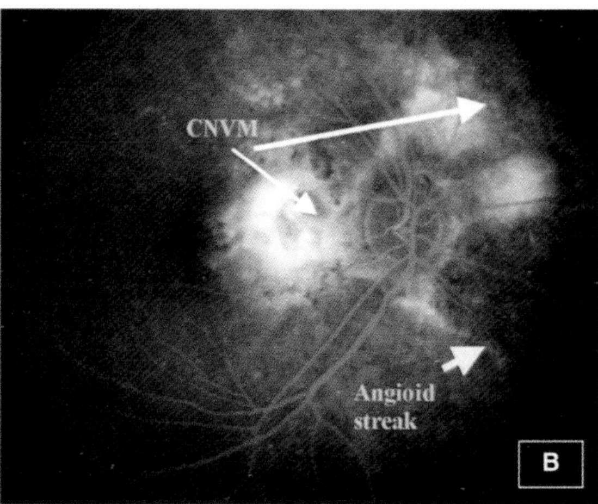

Optical Coherence Tomography

OCT scan through different angles (C, D) showed increased retinal thickness nasal to fovea with an area of moderate hyper-reflectivity in the outer retinal layers (arrow) with overlying cysts corresponding to the area of CNVM seen clinically.

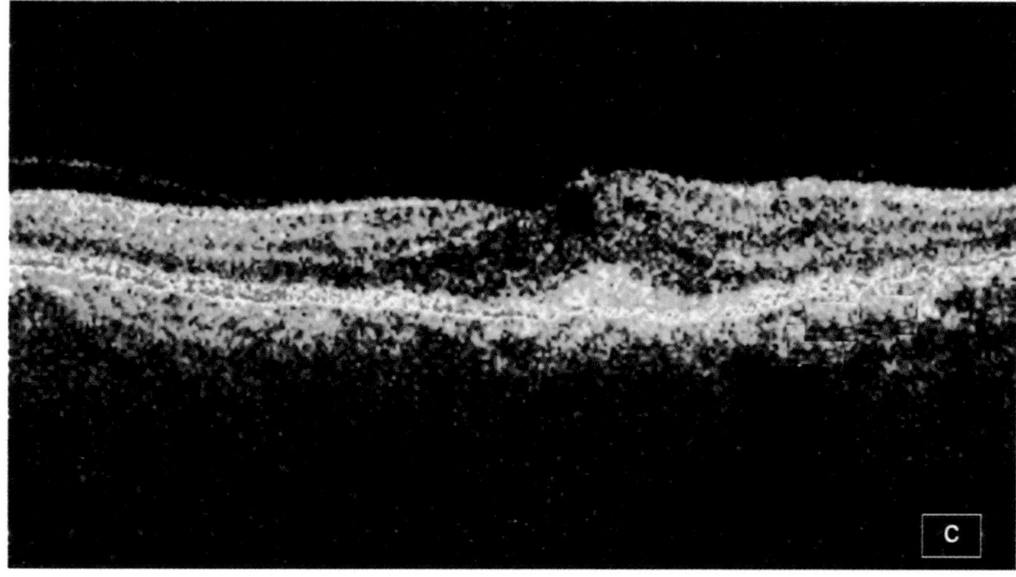

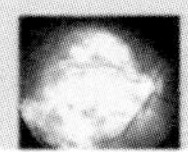

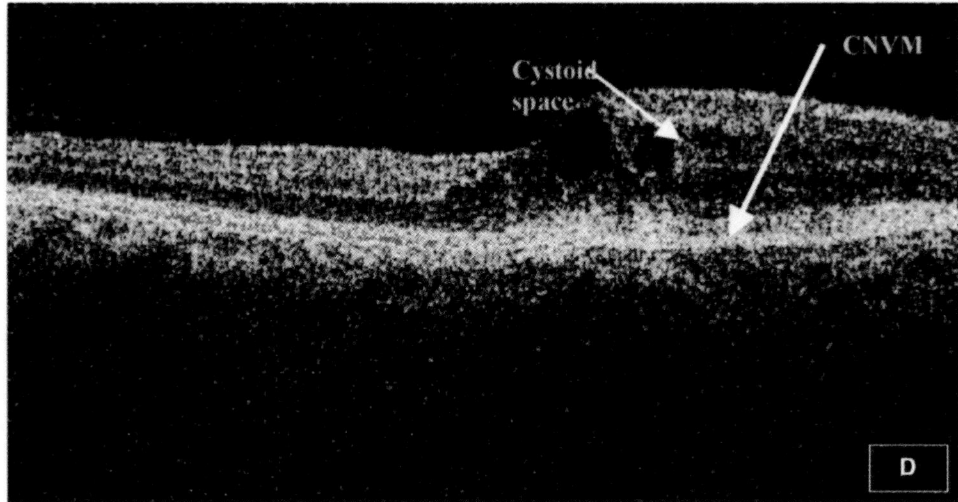

The left eye too showed the presence of peripapillary angioid streaks with CNVM that was extrafoveal (E). Fluorescein angiography (F) showed hyperfluorescence superonasal to the fovea corresponding to the CNVM seen clinically. The angioid streaks were hyperfluorescent.

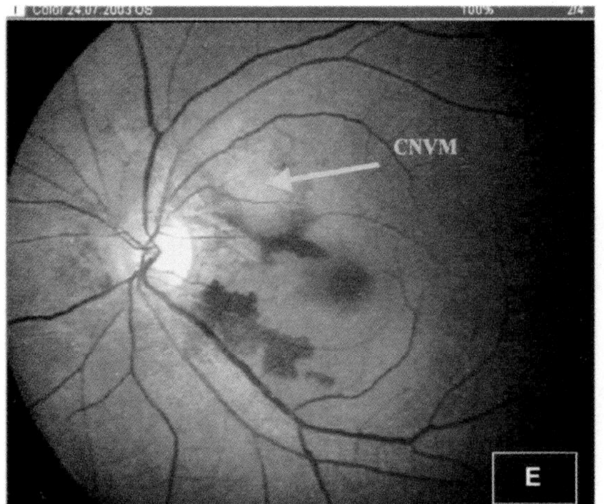

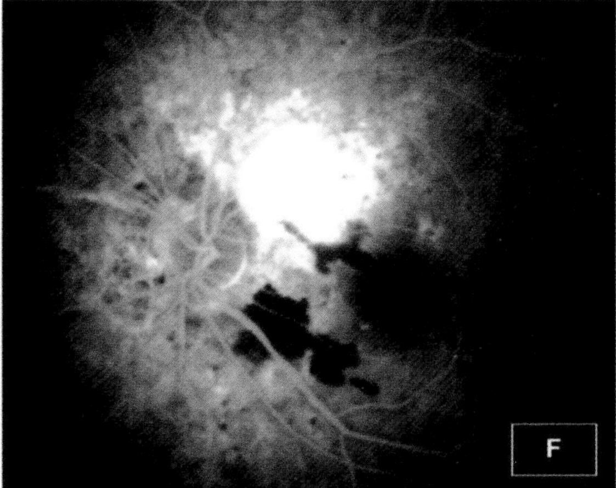

Optical Coherence Tomography

OCT scan superonasal to fovea (G, H) showed an area of moderately intense hyper-reflectivity in the outer retinal layers (arrow) corresponding to the area of CNVM seen clinically. OCT also showed hyporeflective area under the fovea suggestive of subretinal fluid. **The OCT was able to demonstrate the presence of fluid under the fovea in this patient that was not seen clinically or angiographically.**

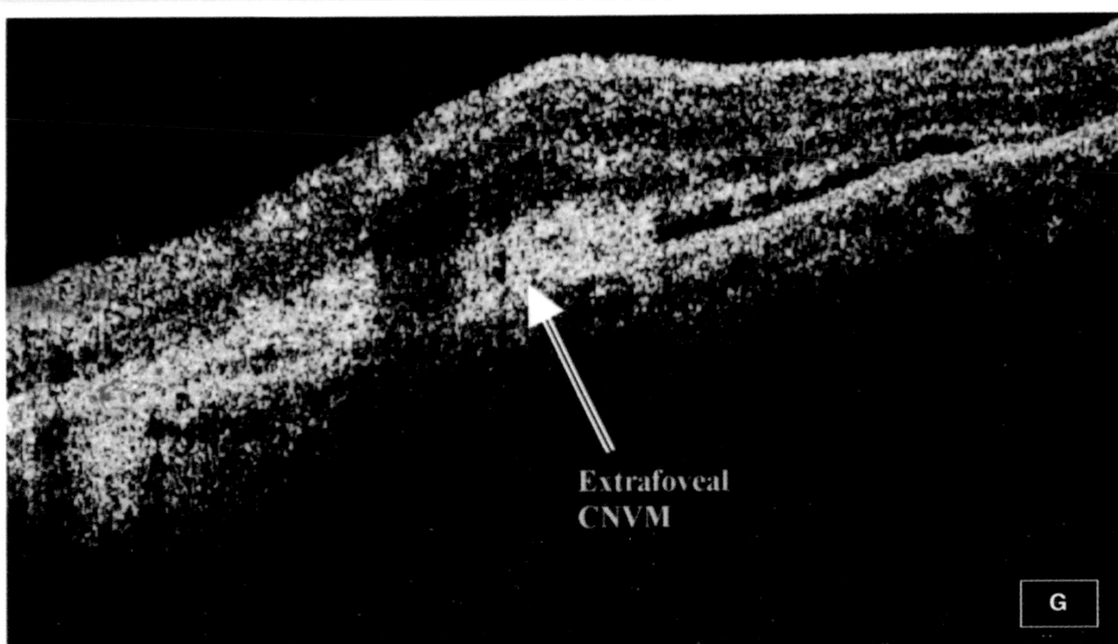
Extrafoveal
CNVM
G

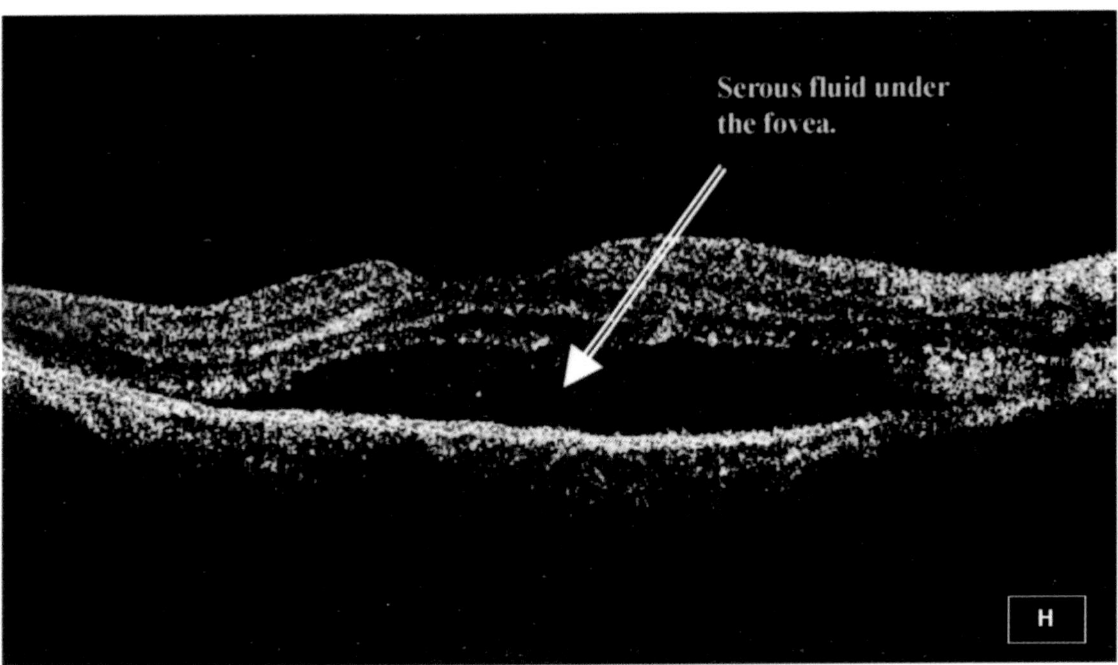
Serous fluid under
the fovea.
H

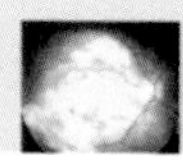

Case 12.3: Peripapillary CNVM in Retinal Vasculitis

Case Summary

A 13-year-old boy was seen with peripheral vasculitis, microaneurysms and angiomatous proliferation on disc. No areas of capillary non-perfusion were seen in the periphery. He had already received oral corticosteroids for vasculitis. His best corrected visual acuity in the right eye was 20/30. The anterior segment did not show any inflammation. Fundus showed angiomatous lesions on optic nerve head with a peripapillary yellowish-white subretinal lesion that was hyperfluorescent on angiography (A). His work-up for tuberculosis, sarcoidosis, Bartonella, syphilis, HIV, collagen vascular disorders and Toxoplasma were negative. A working diagnosis of IRVAN (Idiopathic Retinal Vasculitis, Angiomatosis and Neuroretinitis) was made.

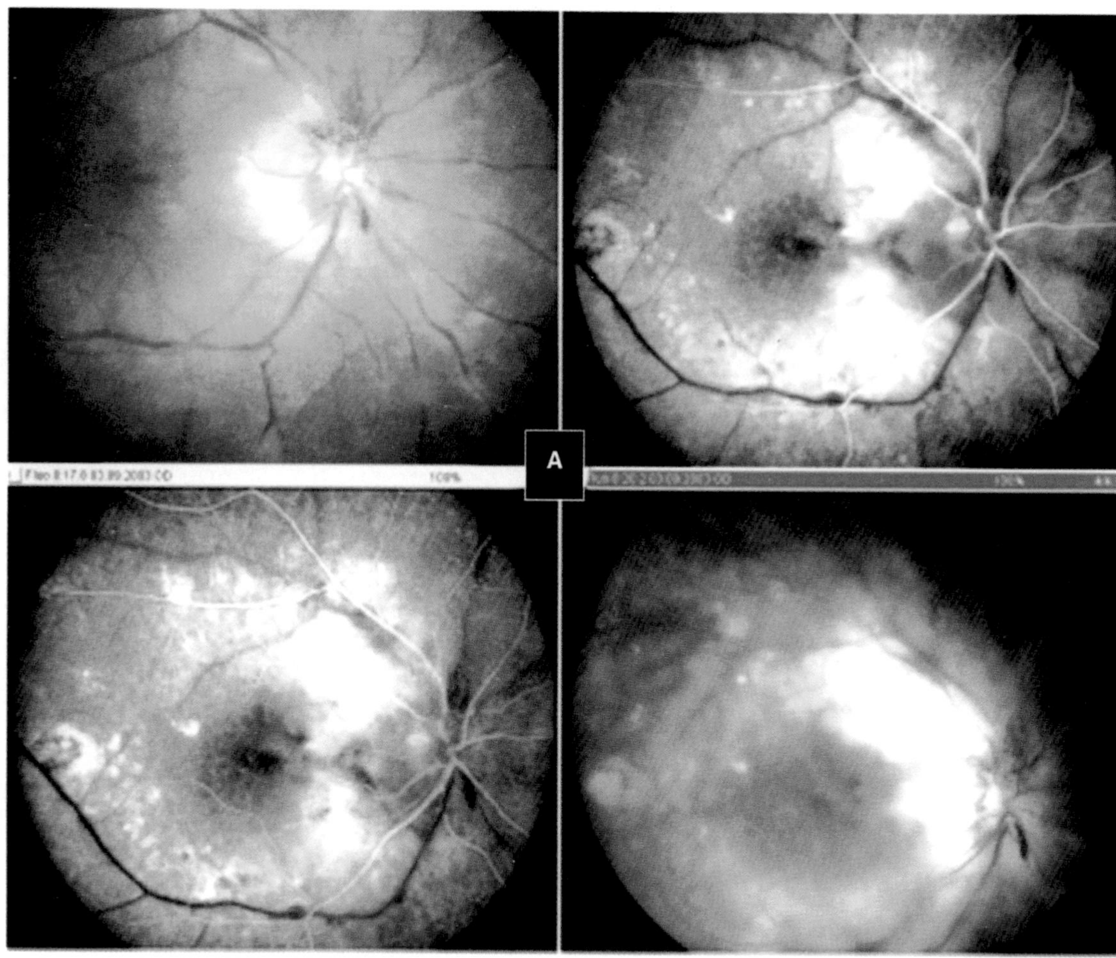

A vertical OCT line scan passing just temporal to the optic disc (B) confirmed the presence of juxtapapillary CNVM by showing the presence of moderately hyper-reflective backscatter in the neurosensory retina with adjoining hyporeflective area suggesting the presence of fluid.

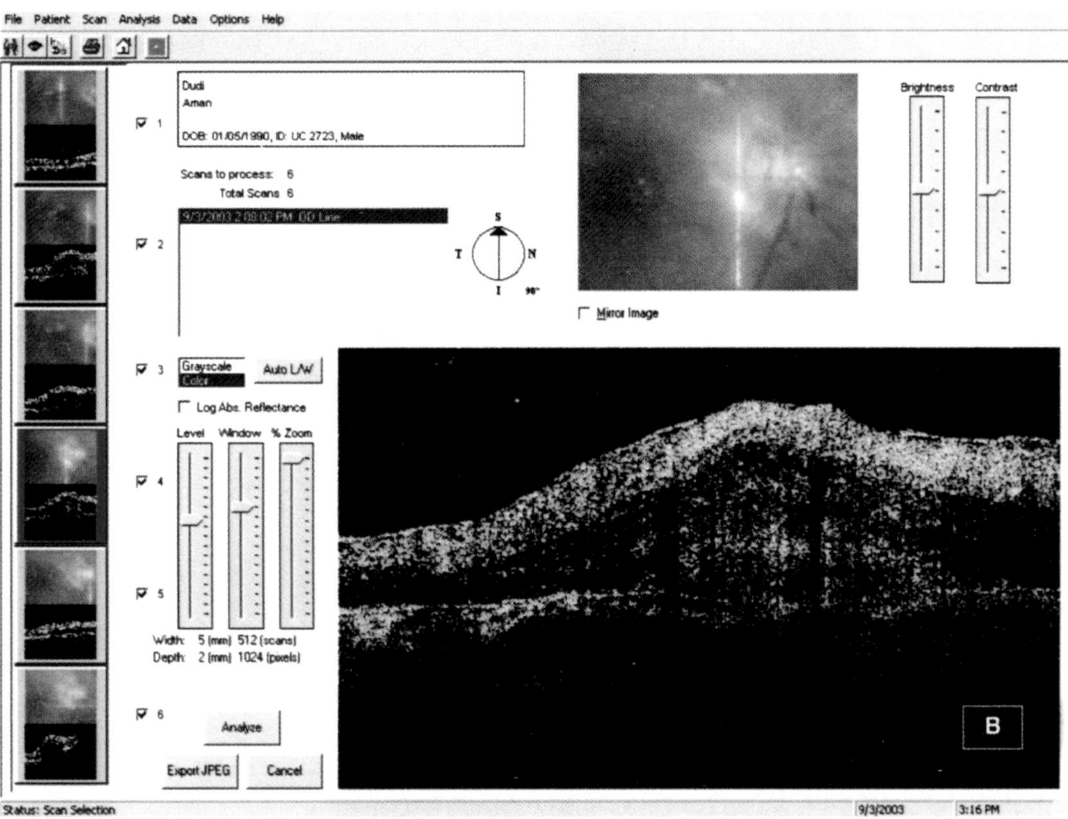

CONCLUSIONS

It has been highlighted in the previous chapter too, that OCT defines the several features of the membrane and is a good tool for monitoring response to the therapy.

Chapter 13

Juxtafoveal Telangiectasia

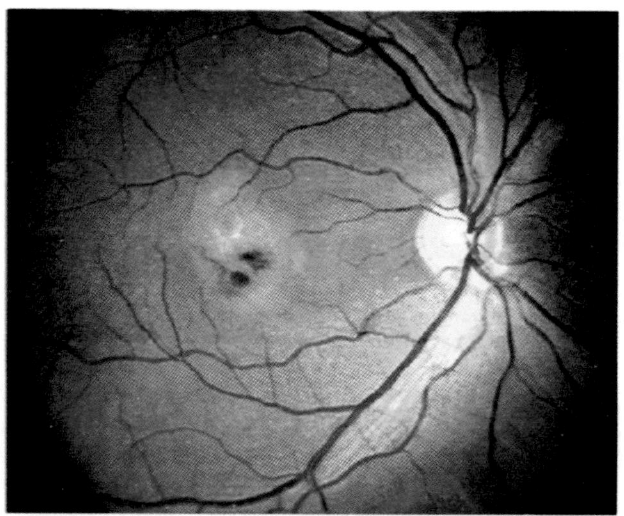

Patients with juxtafoveal telangiectasia (JFT) fall into various subgroups:

Group 1A: Unilateral congenital parafoveal telangiectasis : These patients suffer from a localized mild form of focal telangiectasia with the presence of yellow, lipid-rich exudation at the outer margin of the area of telangiectasis.

Group 1B: Unilateral, idiopathic, focal juxtafoveal telangiectasis : These are middle-aged men having exudation from a minute area of capillary telangiectasis, generally within 2 clock hours or less at the edge of foveal avascular zone.

Group 2A: Bilateral, idiopathic, acquired parafoveal telangiectasis: This is seen in 5th-6th decade of life and involves both the sexes equally. It has 5 stages:

Stage 1: No biomicroscopic abnormality. Fluorescein angiography shows minimal or no capillary dilatation in the early and mild staining in the late phase.

Stage 2: Slight retinal greying with minimal or absent telangiectatic vessels. Fluorescein angiography shows mild capillary telangiectasis.

Stage 3: Clinically shows parafoveolar dilated and blunted retinal venules and refractile deposits. Fluorescein angiography shows capillary dilation with leak in outer retina.

Stage 4: In this stage, the stellate foci of black RPE hypertrophy are seen at the posterior end of retinal venules.

Stage 5: In this stage subretinal neovascularization occurs in the parafoveal area. Cystoid edema and yellow exudates are seen only in subretinal neovascularization.

It is believed that telangiectasia in the capillary wall causes reduced metabolic exchange which in turn causes nutritional deficiencies to the retinal cells including Muller cells. This is seen as diffuse staining of fluorescein into the damaged cells. The changes in the capillary bed may induce altered pattern of venous flow, resulting clinically the formation of right-angled venules. This further leads to degeneration and atrophy of these cells with overlying photoreceptors resembling the lamellar macular hole. This causes RPE cells to migrate along right angles venules and form hyperplastic black plaques. Finally new vessels proliferate in the subretinal space and form type II choroidal neovascular membrane. These new-vessels are believed to be retinal rather than choroidal, thus are also termed as retinal angiomatous proliferation (RAP) (See Chapter 19).

Group 2B: Juvenile occult familial idiopathic JFT.

Group 3A and 3B are rare and thus not discussed here.

OCT IN JFT

The diagnosis of JFT is essentially based on fluorescein angiography that helps in the grouping and staging of the disease. OCT showed the following features in JFT:

1. OCT showed hyporeflective spaces in the inner or outer retina in stage 2 and 3 of group 2A JFT. These spaces probably represent the atrophy of Mullers cells. The retina in many eyes may not show thickening corresponding to the leakage seen on fluorescein angiography that again substantiates the theory that the fluorescein extravascates in the retinal layers due to the atrophy of retinal cells.
2. OCT was helpful in depicting cystoid spaces and neovascular membranes in the retina. The neovascularization in JFT is believed to be due to proliferation of retinal new vessels called Retinal Angiomatous Proliferation (RAP).

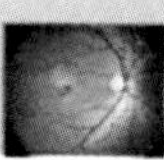

Case 13.1: Group 2A, Bilateral, Idiopathic, Acquired Parafoveal Telangiectasis: Stage 2

Case Summary

A 55-year-old woman was seen with decreased vision in both her eyes of one year duration. Her best corrected visual acuity was 20/50 in the right eye. Fundus showed a greyish-green area temporal to the fovea (A). Fluorescein angiography (B-D) showed telangiectatic vessels temporal to the fovea with staining in the late phase.

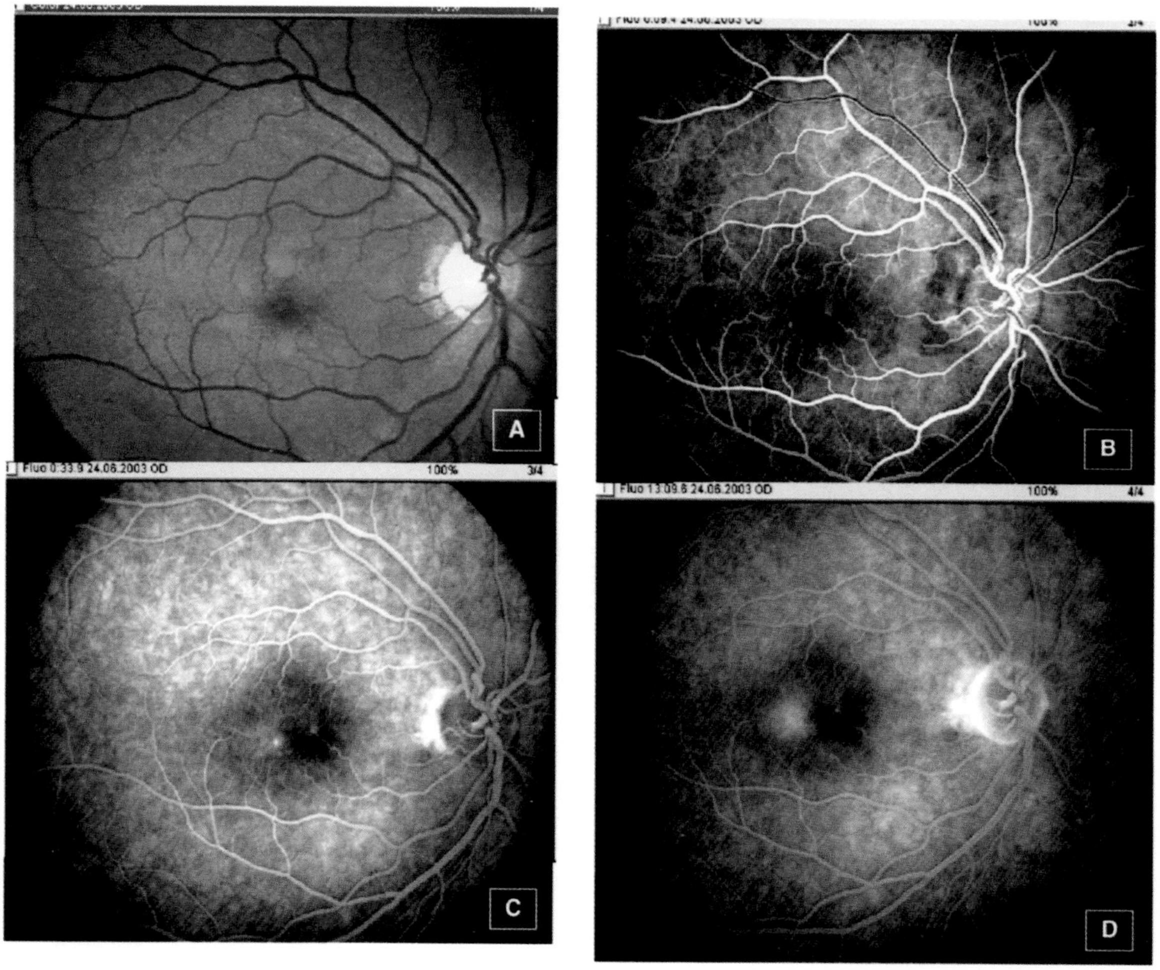

Optical Coherence Tomography

OCT scan through fovea (E) showed a small hyporeflective area at the level of RPE-photoreceptor complex suggesting a localized loss of these layers. **Despite the staining seen on fluorescein angiography, there was no increased thickness on OCT, thus indicating that the diffuse staining on fluorescein angiography that seems to occur at the middle and outer retina is probably the result of diffusion of fluorescein into the damaged retinal cells.**

Fundus and fluorescein angiography of the opposite eye too showed features of juxtafoveal telangiectasia (F).

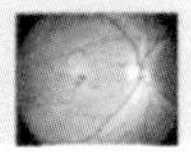

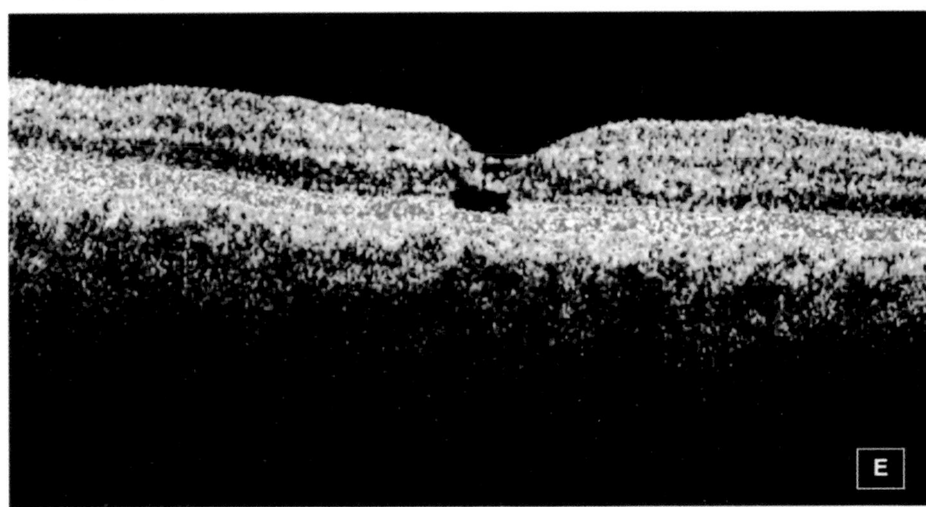
E

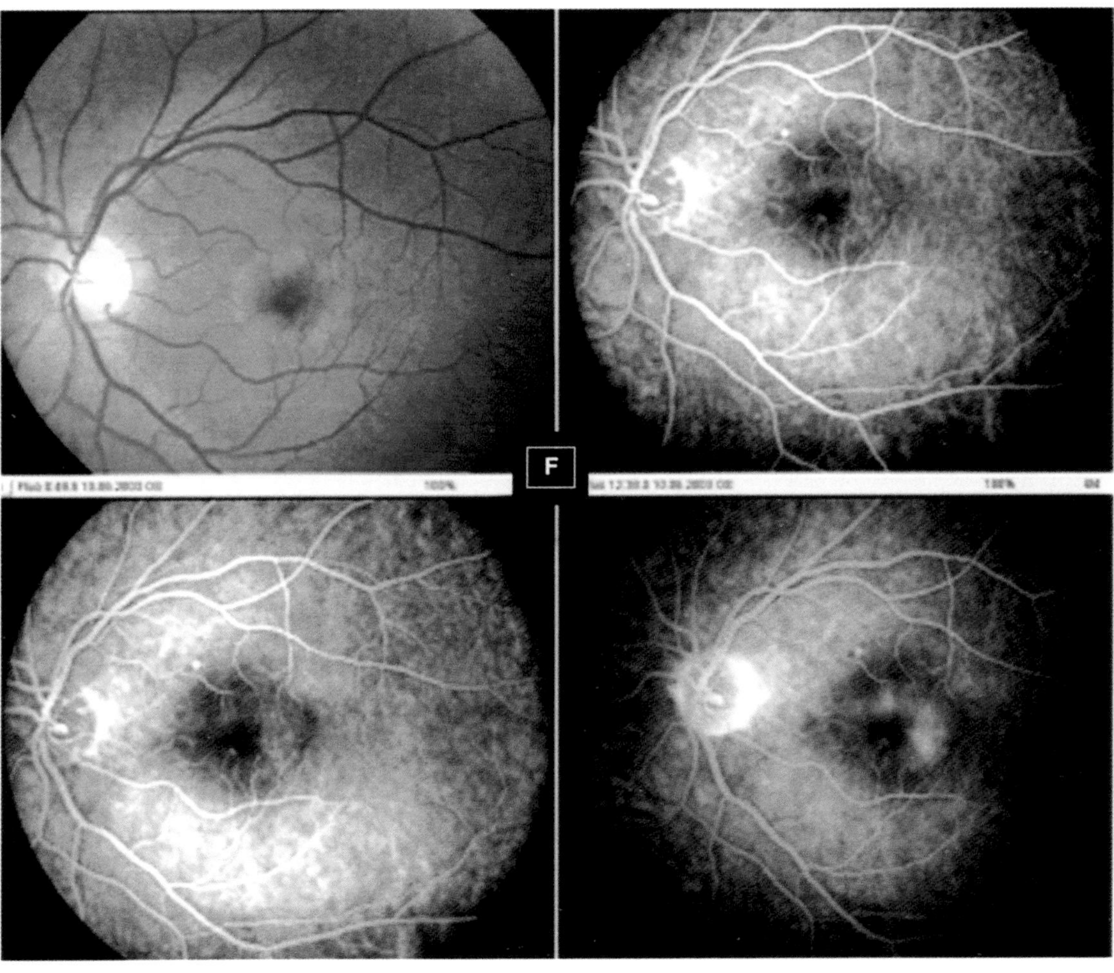
F

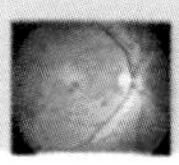

Optical coherence tomography (G) showed the presence of small hyporeflective lesions under the fovea. Also there was thinning and separation of RPE layer from the underlying layer of choriocapillaris, probably representing RPE atrophy. The nasal retina showed a localized area of disrupted RPE-photoreceptor layer. **Despite leakage seen on fluorescein angiography, no increased thickening was seen on OCT suggesting that the dye pooling in juxtafoveal telangiectasia is due to extravasation of the dye and not because of leakage, thus confirming the belief that laser photocoagulation does not have a role.**

The patient was diagnosed as acquired Group 2A juxtafoveal Telangiectasia and no treatment was offered.

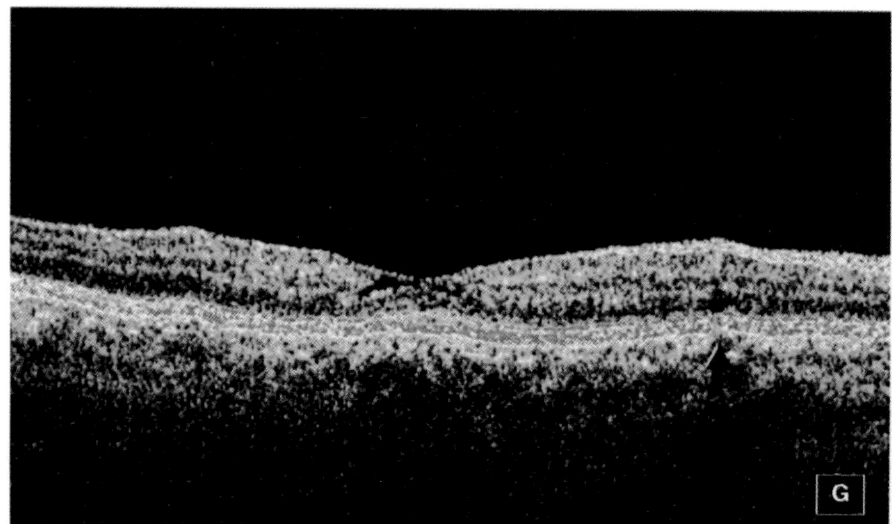

Case 13.2: Group 2A Stage 4 Juxtafoveal Telangiectasia (JFT)

Case Summary

A-45-year-old woman was seen with bilateral, acquired JFT. Her best corrected visual acuity was 20/80 in the right eye. Right eye fundus showed black stellate foci of hyperpigmentation at the end of right angled venules (arrow). The fluorescein angiography showed telangiectasia in the early phase with late staining of the dye (B, C).

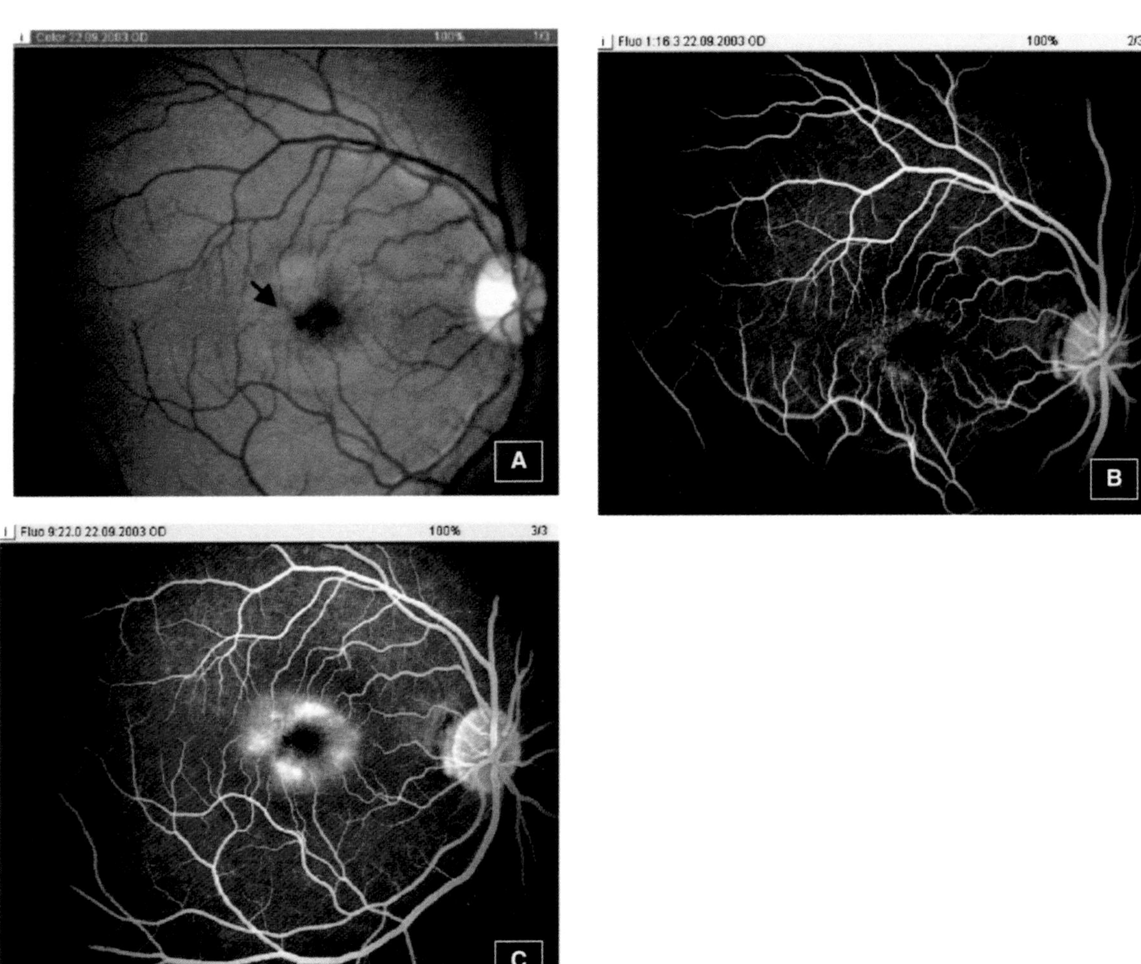

Optical Coherence Tomography

Horizontal line scan through the pigmented scar (D) showed hyperplasia of retinal pigment epithelium (RPE) extending in the inner retinal layers.

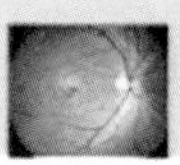

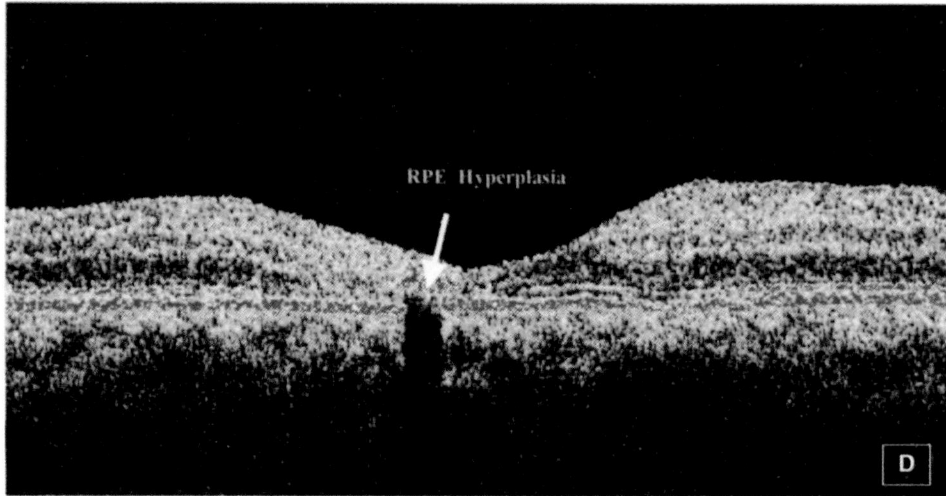

Vertical line scan through the fovea (E) showed multiple red colored hyper-reflective dots suggesting telangiectatic vessels in the inner retinal layers.

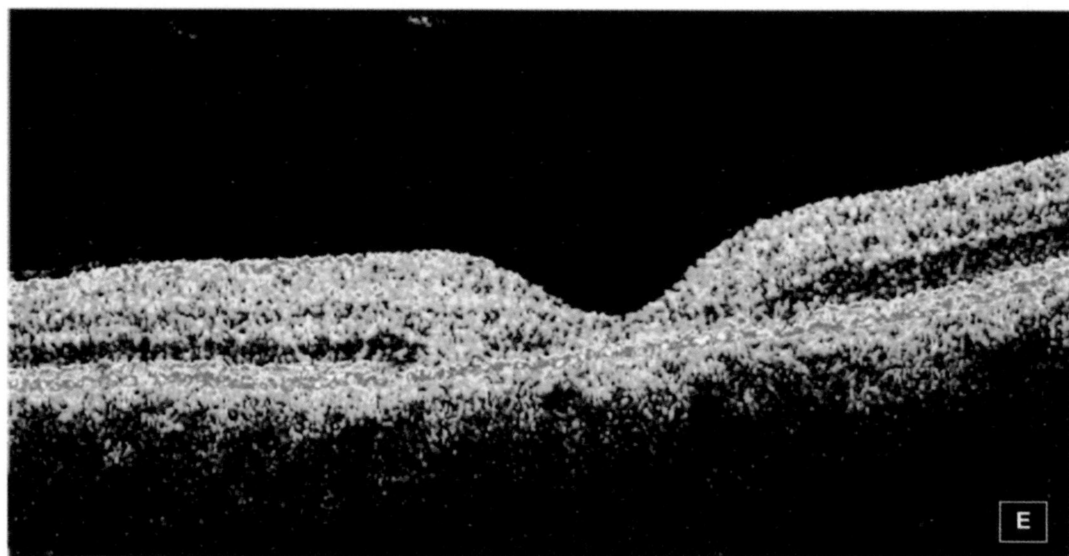

Case 13.3: Group 2A, Stage 5 JFT

Case Summary

A 54-year-old man was seen with blurring of vision caused by bilateral, acquired, perifoveal telangiectasis. His fundus (A) showed right angled venules, pale yellow crystalline deposits with dull foveal reflex. Fluorescein angiography (B-D) showed mottled hyperfluorescence that increased in the late phase suggesting the presence of underlying choroidal neovascular membrane (CNVM).

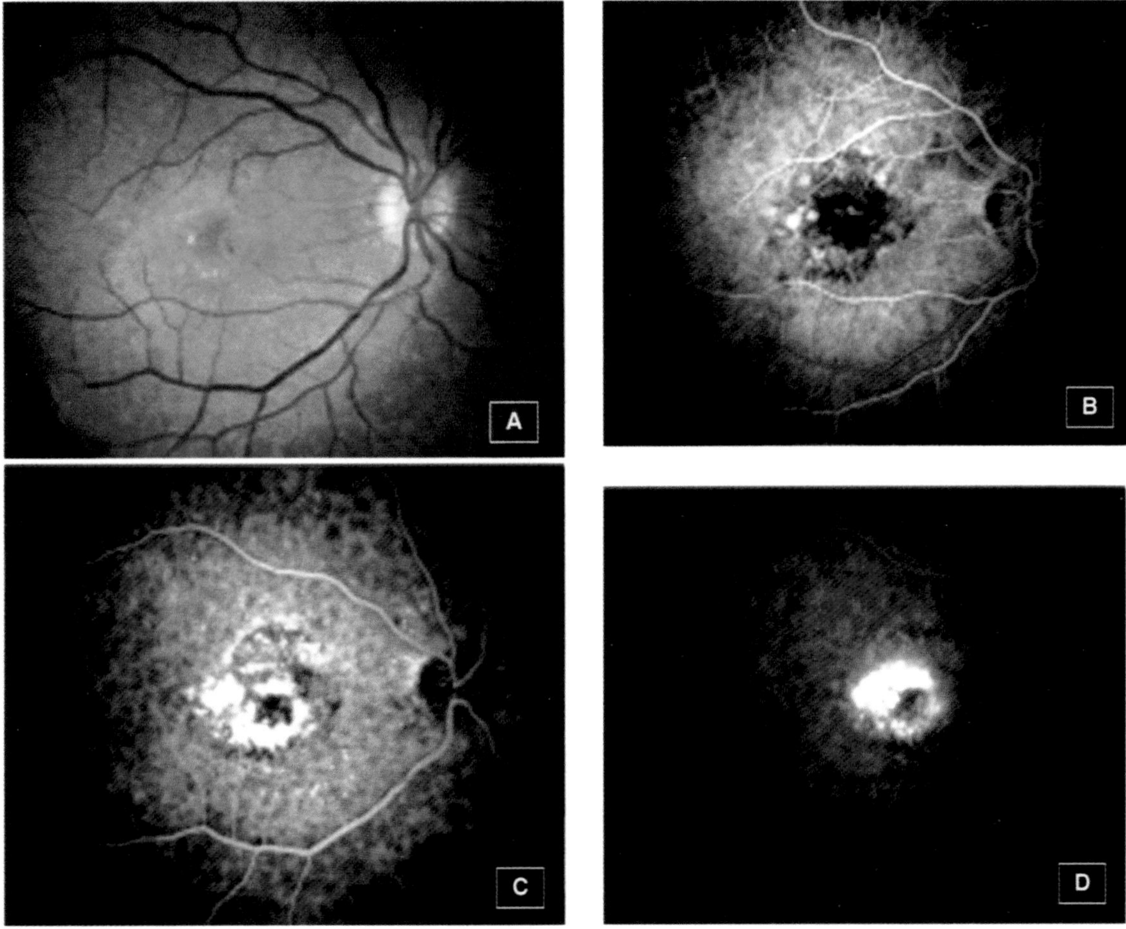

The vertical OCT line scan through the fovea (E) showed increased hyper-reflectivity from the outer retinal layers with overlying cystoid spaces, thus suggesting the presence of a classic choroidal neovascular membrane.

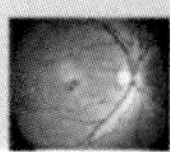

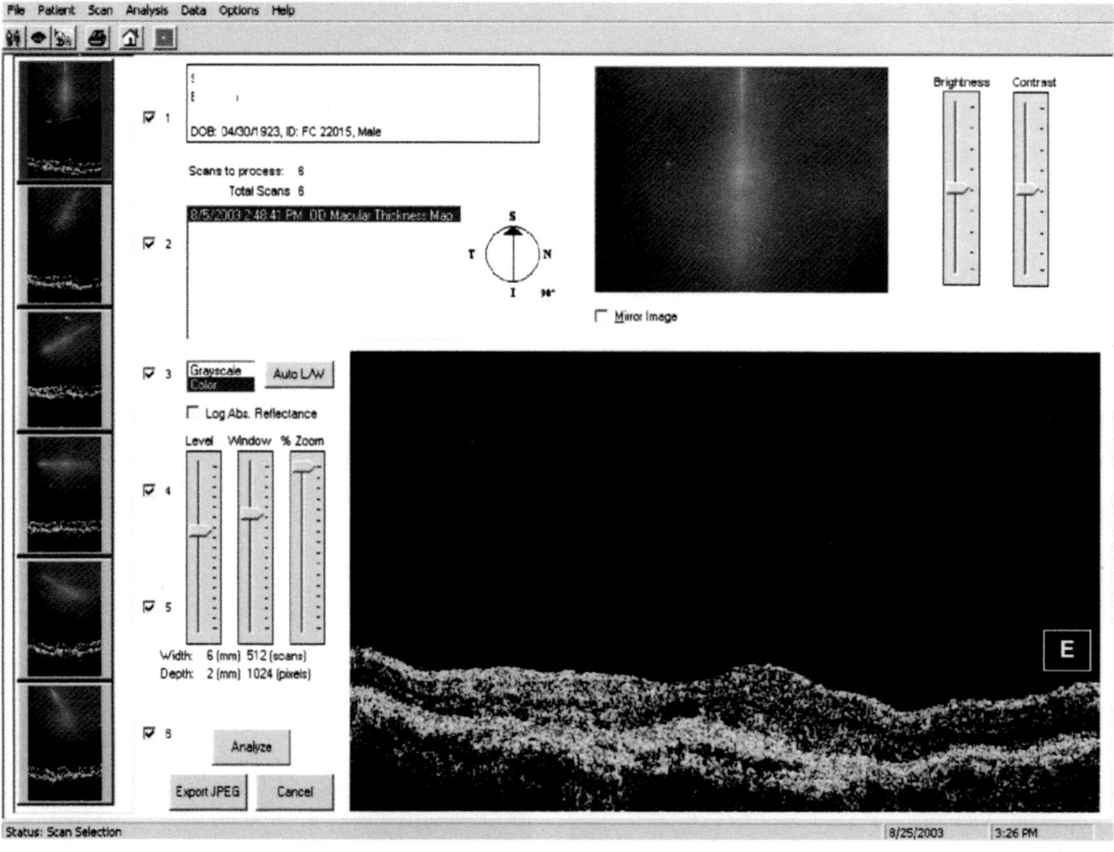
File Patient Scan Analysis Data Options Help
DOB: 04/30/1923, ID: FC 22015, Male
Scans to process: 6
Total Scans 6
8/5/2003 2:48:41 PM OD Macular Thickness Map
S
T
N
I
90°
Mirror Image
Brightness
Contrast
Grayscale
Color
Auto L/W
Log Abs. Reflectance
Level
Window
% Zoom
Width: 6 (mm) 512 (scans)
Depth: 2 (mm) 1024 (pixels)
Analyze
Export JPEG
Cancel
E
Status: Scan Selection
8/25/2003
3:26 PM

Case 13.4: Group 2A Parafoveal Telangiectasia with Choroidal Neovascular Membrane

Case Summary

A 44-year-old man was seen with right eye juxtafoveal telangiectasia and choroidal neovascular membrane diagnosed on fundoscopy and fluorescein angiography (A-D).

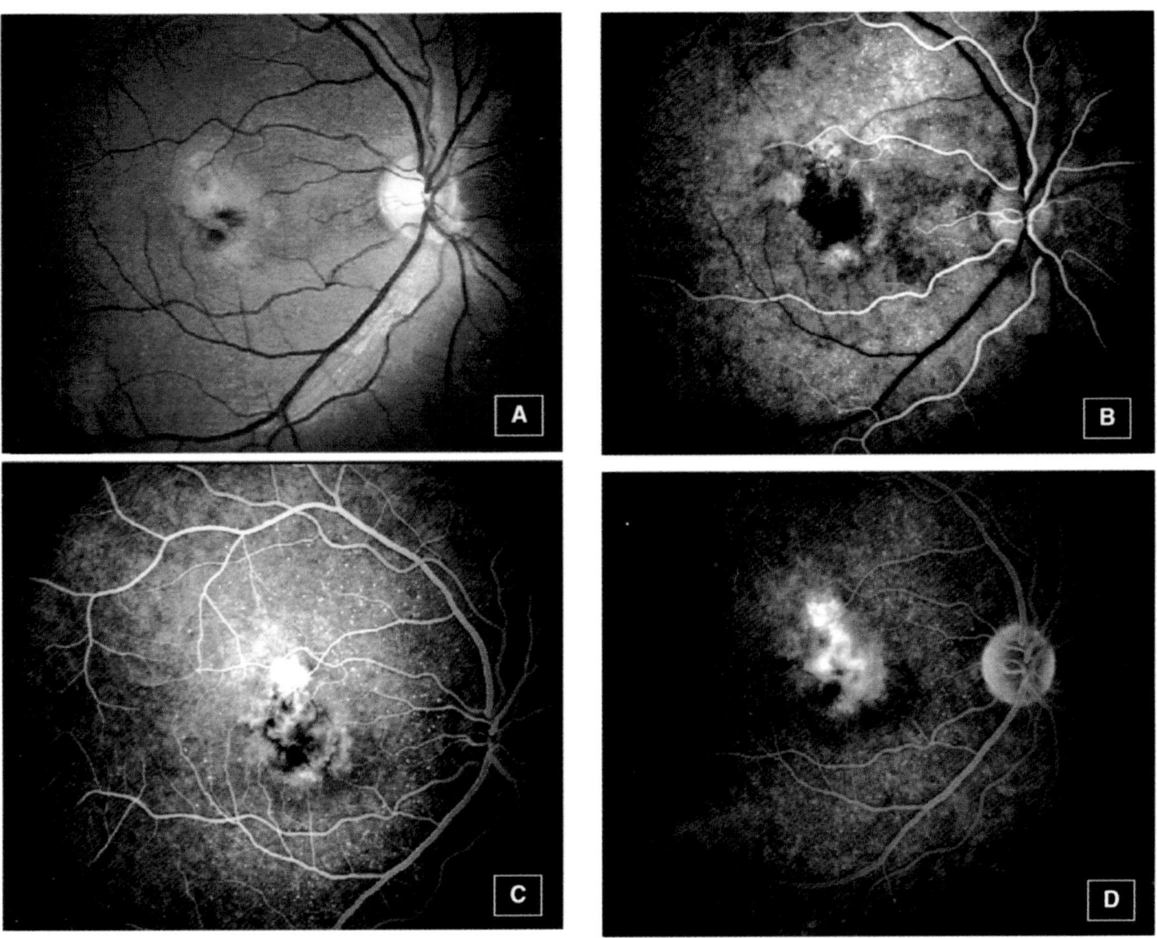

Optical Coherence Tomography

OCT scan of this eye showed an area of hyper-reflectivity in the outer retinal layers under the fovea suggesting subfoveal choroidal neovascular membrane with reduced backscattering from the overlying layers suggesting retinal edema (E). The retinal thickness was increased due to intraretinal fluid accumulation. The patient was advised photodynamic therapy (PDT) but refused for the same.

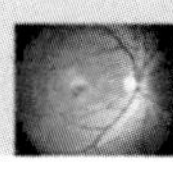

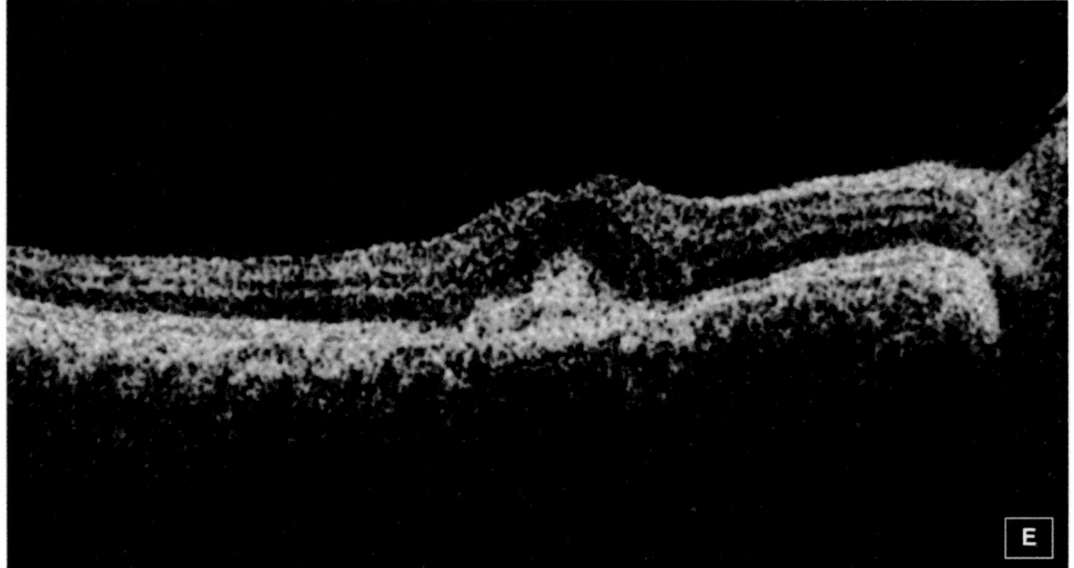
E

Case 13.5: Group 2A, Stage 5 with Hypertrophic Scar of Neovascular Membrane

Case Summary

A 46-year-old man was seen with bilateral juxtafoveal telangiectasis and a choroidal neovascular membrane (A-C). The patient was lost to follow up for one year.

One year later, the patient was seen with hypertrophic scar (D). Vertical OCT scan through the scar (E) showed hyper-reflective layers corresponding to the scar whereas vertical scan through the fovea showed localized defects in RPE with cystic spaces under the fovea (F).

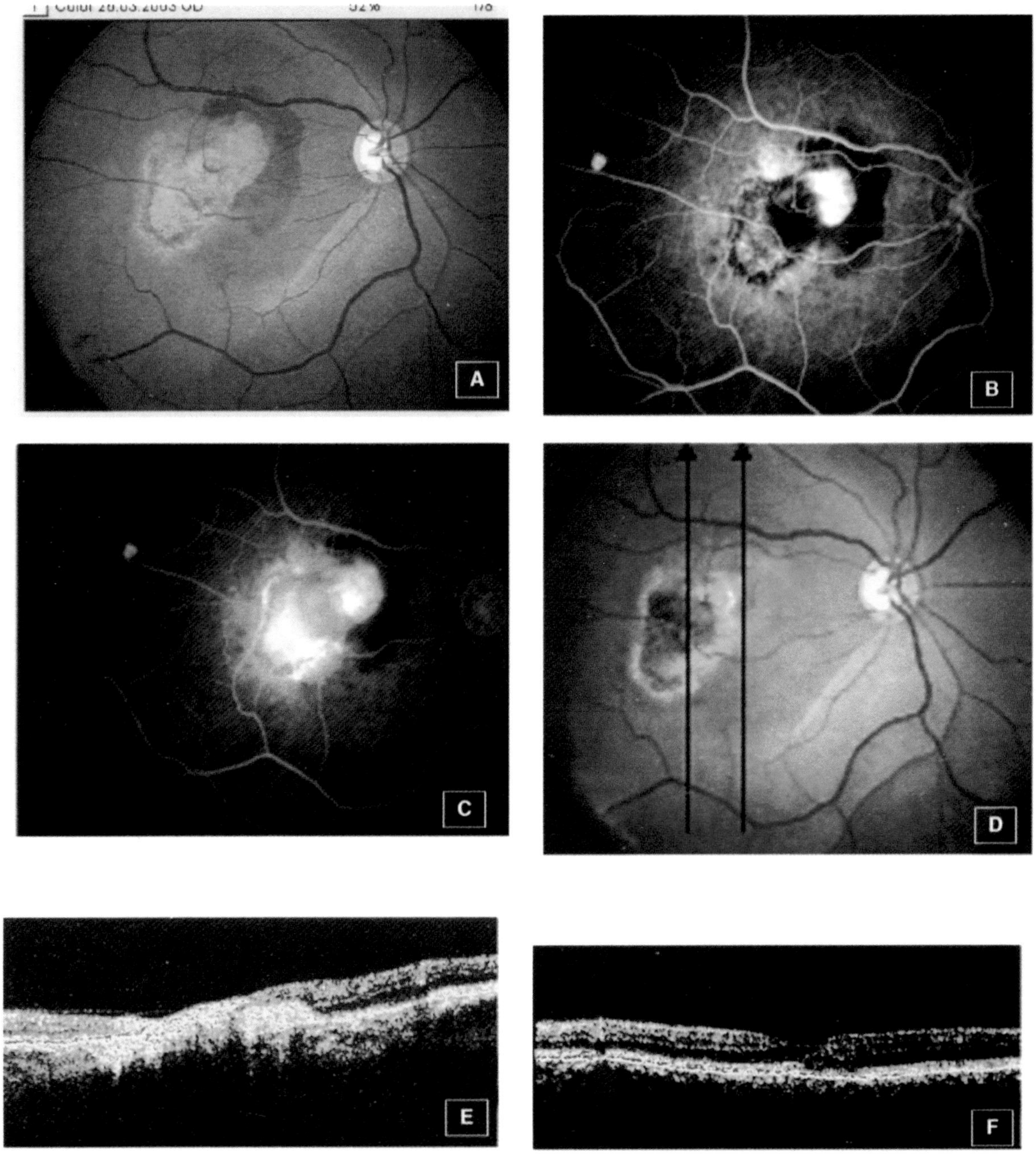

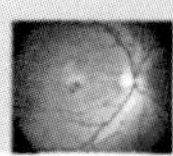

Case 13.6: Intravitreal Triamcinolone Acetonide in Group 2A JFT

Case Summary

A 60-year-old woman was seen with metamorphopsia in her left eye of 2 weeks duration. Her best corrected visual acuity was 20/100. A diagnosis of Juxtafoveal telangiectasia was made based on clinical appearance and fluorescein angiography (A-D).

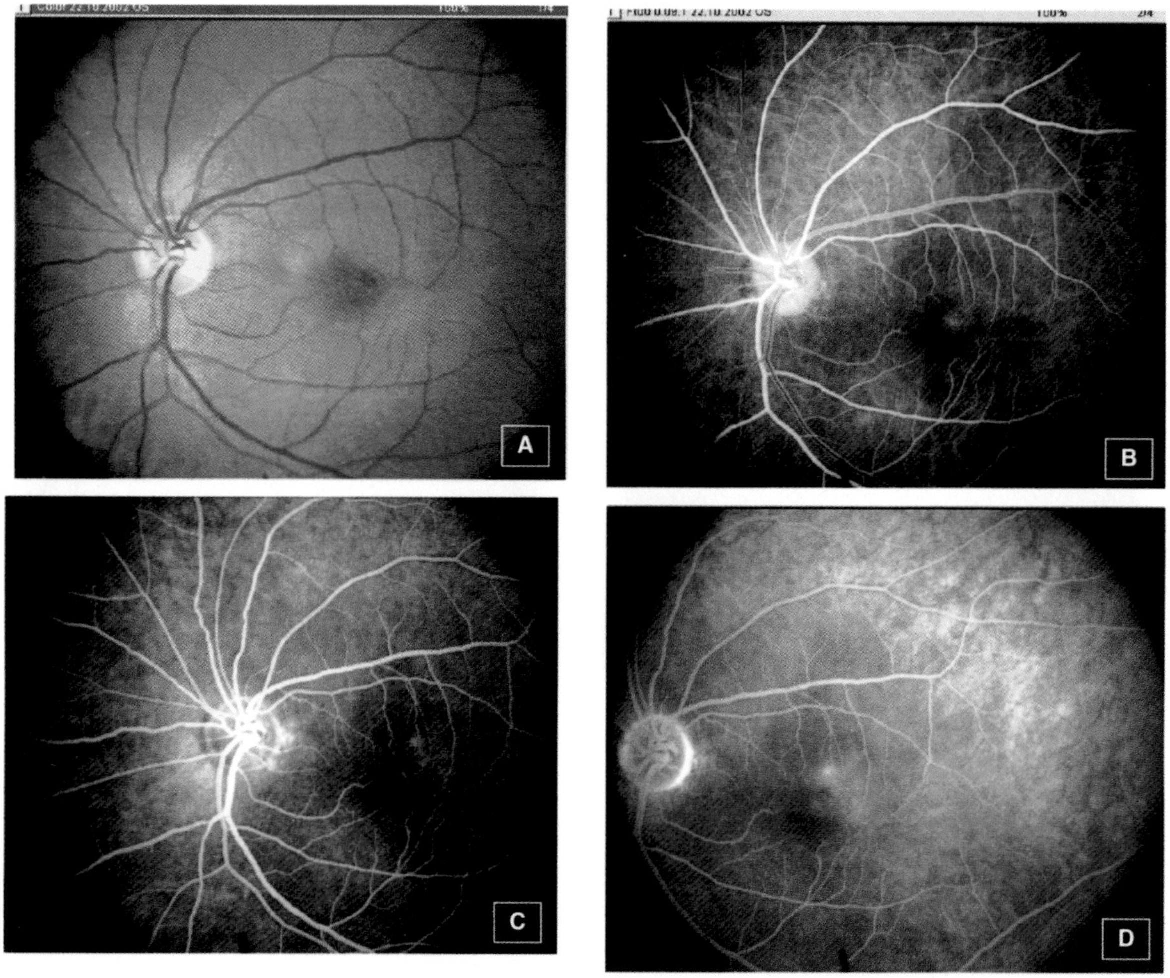

Optical Coherence Tomography

OCT line scans through different angles (E, F) through the fovea showed disruption in the photoreceptor layer under the fovea with the presence of small hyporeflective areas with intervening hyper-reflective septae suggestive of presence of cysts in the inner retina.

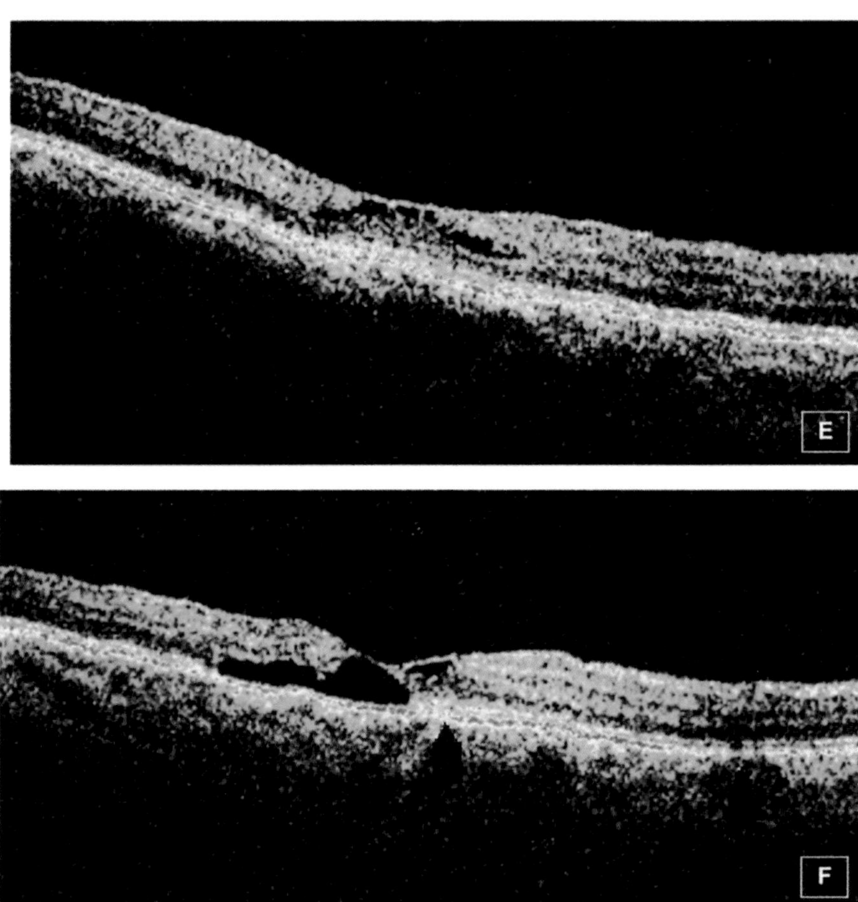

The patient elected to receive intravitreal triamcinolone acetonide injection. Four weeks later, her best corrected visual acuity was 20/80 (G). Repeat fluorescein angiography (G) showed fewer leaks than before.

Repeat OCT scan, done 4 weeks after injection (H, I), showed the persistence of hyporeflective area under the fovea. The vision continued to deteriorate over the next six months.

At six months follow-up, her best corrected visual acuity was 20/90. Repeat OCT showed persistence of hyporeflective lesions in the inner retina (J, K), thus indicating that cases of JFT with primarily atrophic changes probably do not respond to intravitreal triamcinolone acetonide.

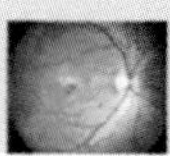

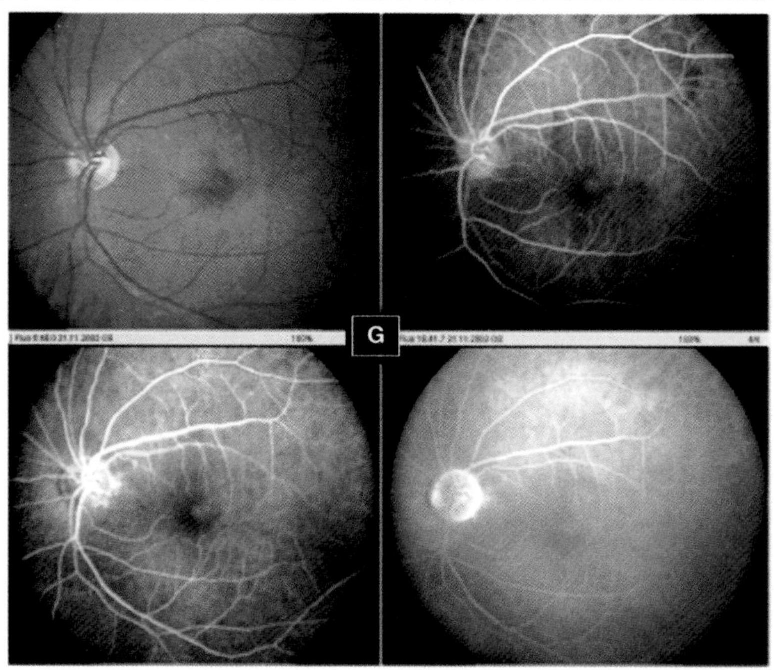
G

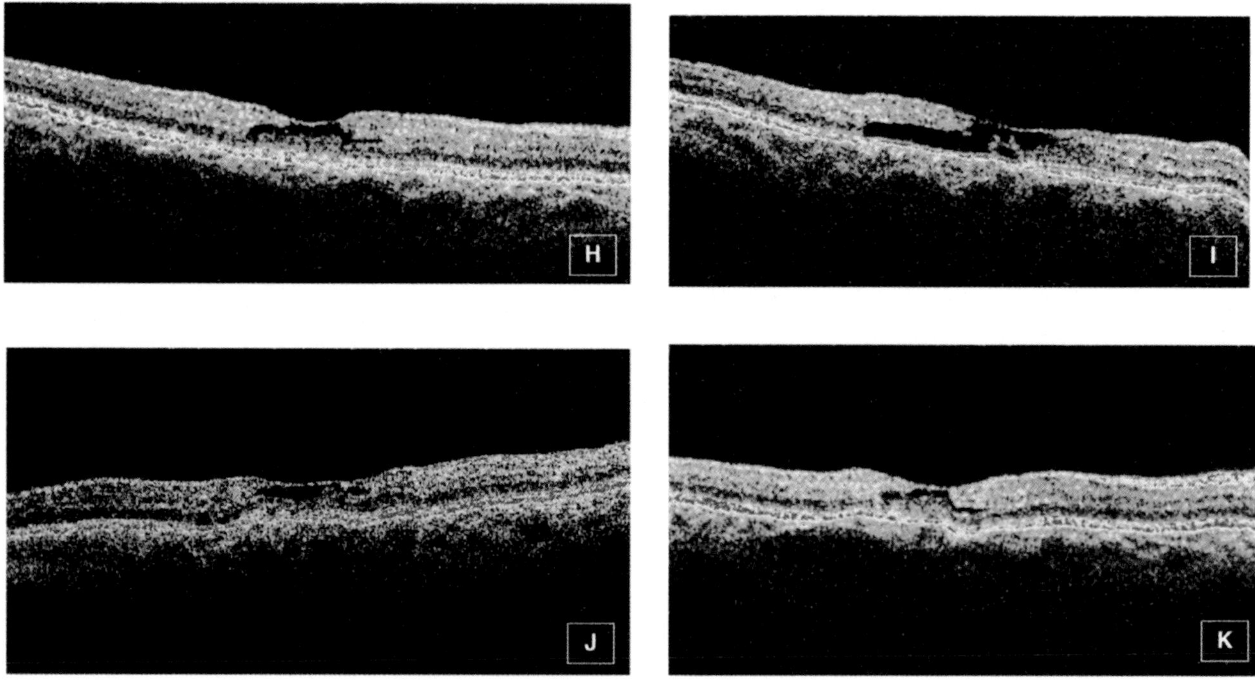
H
I
J
K

Case 13.7: Group 2A Parafoveal Telangiectasia with Cystoid Macular Edema and Serous Retinal Detachment

Case Summary

A 52-year-old man was seen with diminished vision of seven months duration in both his eyes. His best corrected visual acuity was 20/200 in the right eye. Fundoscopy and fluorescein angiography established the diagnosis of Type 2A, i.e. bilateral, idiopathic, acquired, parafoveal telangiectasia with cystoid macular edema (A, B).

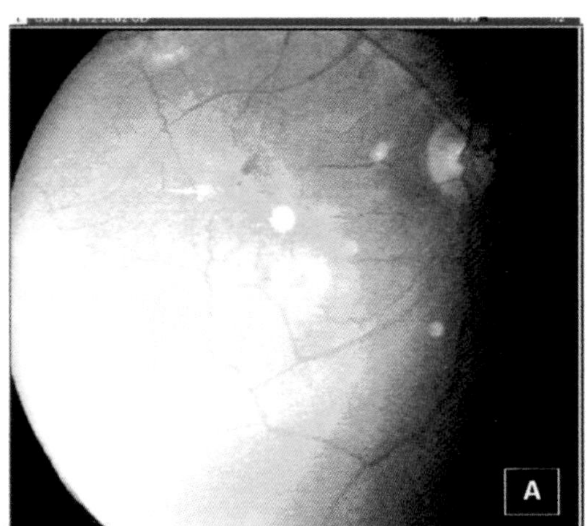
A

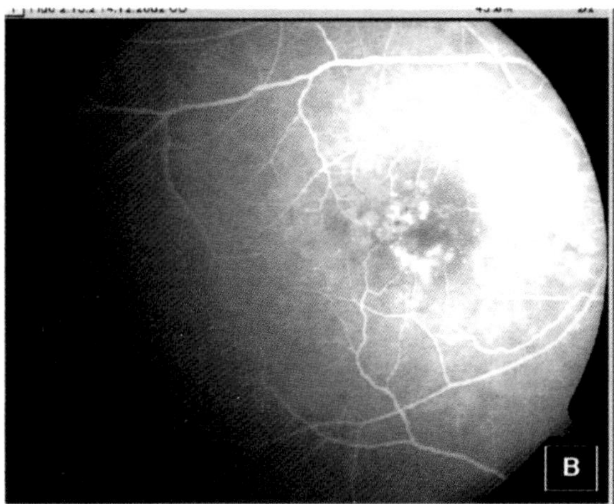
B

Optical Coherence Tomography

Vertical Optical Coherence Tomography line scan of the right eye (C) through the foveal center showed loss of foveal contour, with retinal thickness measuring 460 microns in the foveal center. There was a hyporeflective area in the outer retinal layers under the fovea suggestive of serous retinal detachment. The overlying retina showed multiple hyporeflective areas with intervening hyper-reflective septae arranged in a patelloid fashion suggestive of cystoid macular edema. The temporal retina showed multiple hyper-reflective areas in the neurosensory retina corresponding to the retinal hard exudates. Retinal map analysis of the same showed increased retinal thickness in the central 6 mm retina (D).

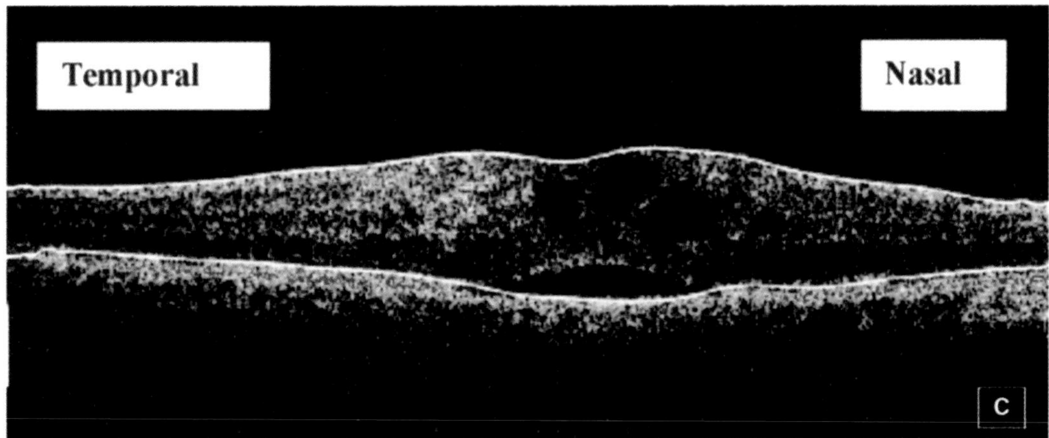

C

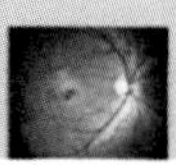

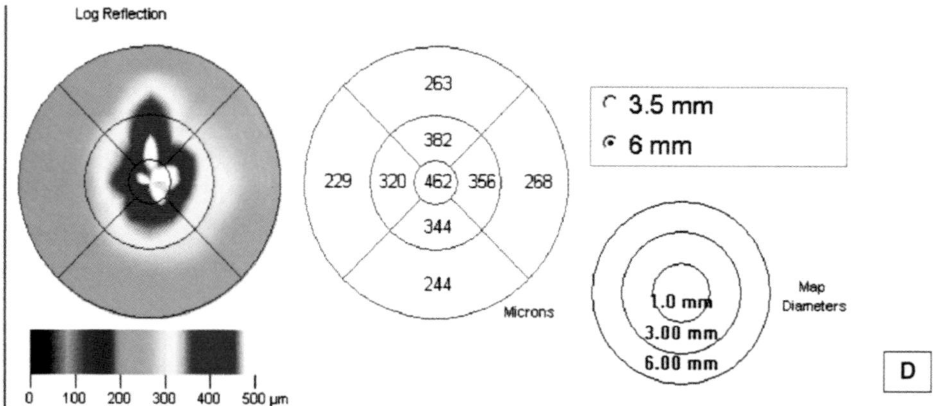

The patient elected to receive intravitreal triamcinolone acetonide 4 mg in this eye. Repeat OCT scan one week later (E & F) showed decrease in retinal thickness with central foveal thickness measuring 389 microns. There was partial resolution in the serous retinal detachment though cystoid spaces persisted

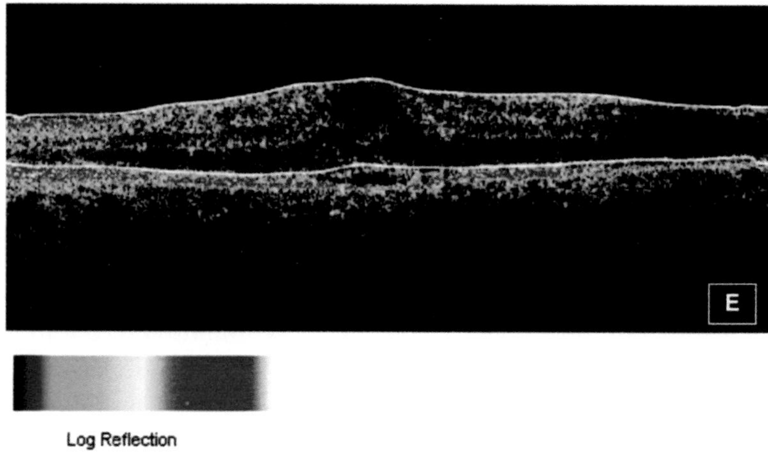

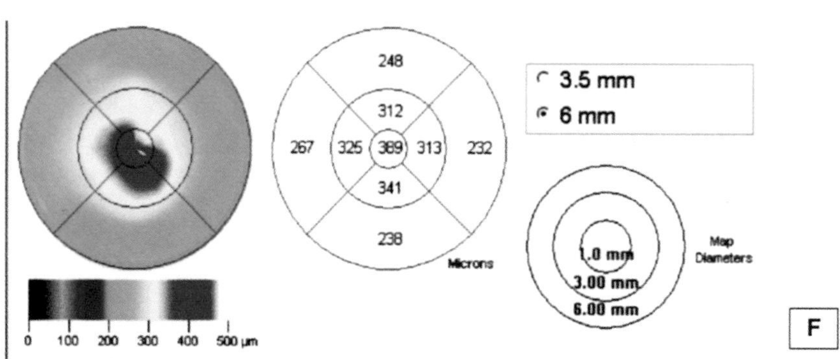

Four weeks later, repeat OCT showed normal foveal contour with resolution of serous retinal detachment as well as cystoid spaces (G). Retinal map showed reduced retinal thickening (H) This case suggests that intravitreal triamcinolone acetonide is effective in patients of JFT with cystoid macular edema

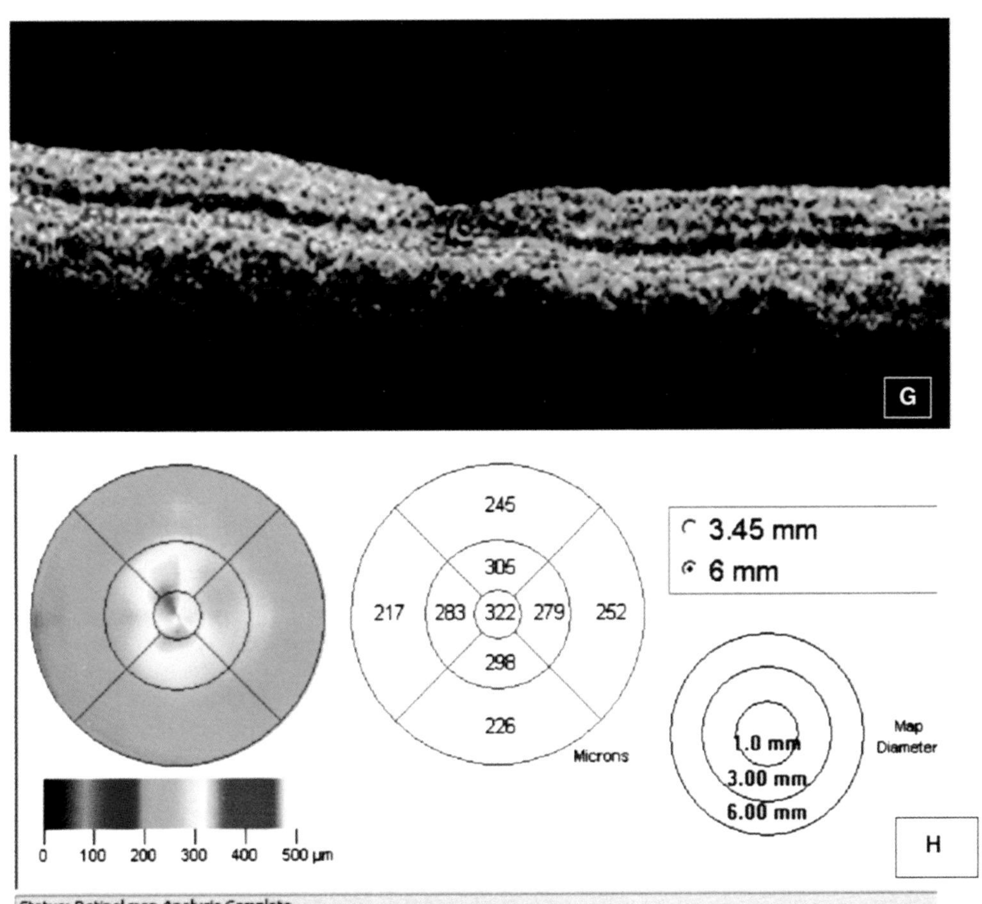

CONCLUSIONS

OCT was found to be a useful tool in differentiating between retinal thickness associated with cystoid retinal spaces and retinal atrophy due to death of retinal cells. This was an important finding where fluorescein angiography may not be able to differentiate between the two due to diffusion of the dye. In our experience, the former variety responded to intravitreal triamcinolone acetonide while the latter did not.

SUGGESTED READING

1. Gass JDM. Congenital and acquired idiopathic juxtafoveolar retinal telangiectasis. In Stereoscopic Atlas of Macular Diseases Diagnosis and Treatment. Mosby-Year Book Inc. 1997 ; 504-12.

Chapter 14

Heredodystrophic Disorders

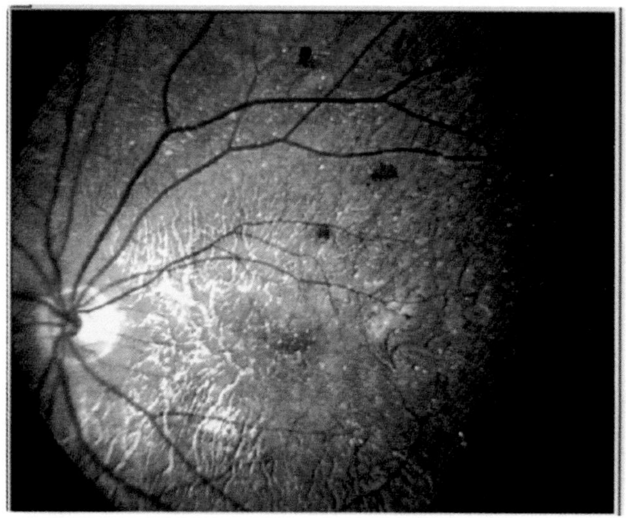

OCT IN HEREDODYSTROPHIC DISORDERS

Macula could get involved in a number of heredodystrophic disorders. OCT is helpful in more than one ways in these disorders.

1. Retinal edema and cystoid spaces: In our experience, we found OCT to be a very useful tool in diagnosing cystoid macular edema even in situations where the cystoid macular edema was non-staining on fluorescein angiography.
2. Retinal Atrophy: Many of these disorders eventually show atrophy of the neurosensory retina with reduced central foveal thickness, that can be measured precisely on OCT.
3. OCT has been found to be useful in differentiating Adult-onset vitelliform dystrophy from Best disease as the former shows a well defined thickness of retinal pigment epithelium while the latter tends to show central serous retinal detachment more often.
4. Prognostication of disease: In cases with atrophy of neurosensory retina, OCT is able to measure the thickness of neurosensory retina with precision. This may help in determining the disease progression over long-term period that would indicate whether the disease is progressive or not.

OCT in Retinitis Pigmentosa

OCT showed two patterns in retinitis pigmentosa:

1. Cystoid macular edema: OCT was very useful in depicting the cystoid spaces in retinitis pigmentosa even when the cystoid macular edema was non-staining on fluorescein angiography. This might be an indication to prescribe oral acetazolamide.
2. Retinal Atrophy: characterized by reduced retinal thickness where no intervention is required.

Case 14.1: Cystoid Macular Edema in Retinitis Pigmentosa

Case Summary

An eleven-year-old girl child was seen with bilateral retinitis pigmentosa. Her visual acuity in the right eye was 20/40 (A). Fluorescein angiography did not show any macular edema (B)

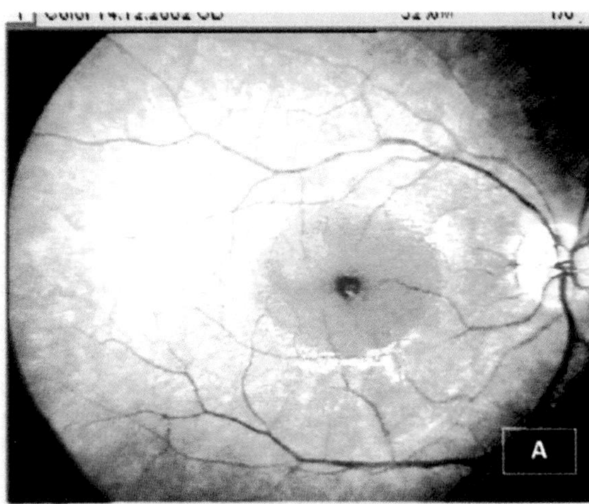
A

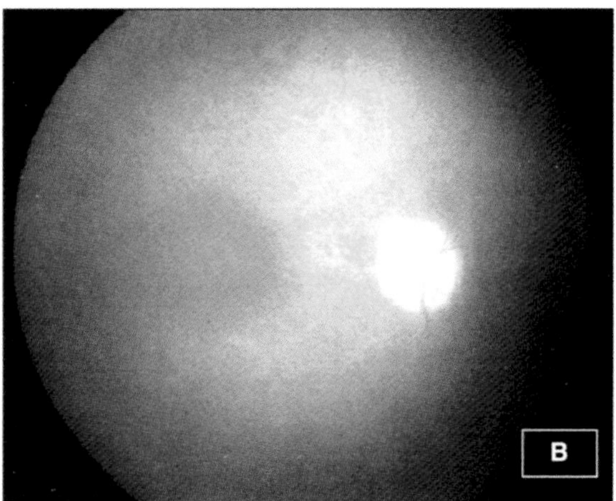
B

Optical Coherence Tomography

OCT scan through the fovea (C) showed loss of foveal contour, increased foveal thickness measuring 449 microns, hyporeflective spaces under the fovea with intervening hyper-reflective walls arranged in the patelloid pattern suggestive of cystoid macular edema. Retinal thickness analysis map showed increased retinal thickness. **OCT was able to depict non-staining cystoid macular edema.**

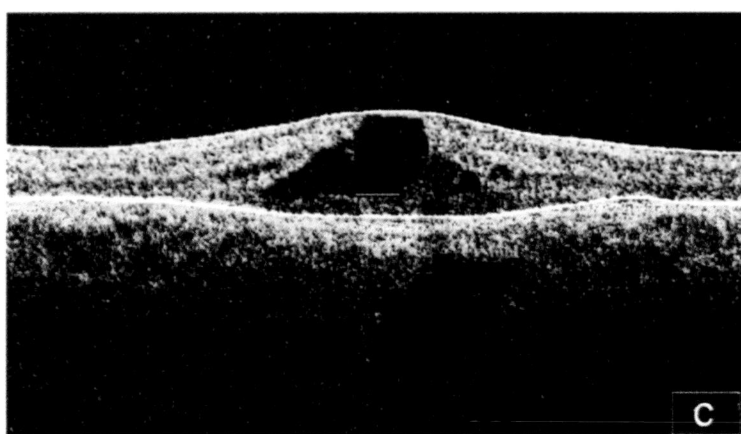
C

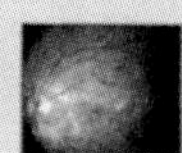

The patient received oral acetazolamide for cystoid macular edema. Eight weeks later, repeat OCT scan showed central retinal thickness measuring 363 microns with persistence of cystoid spaces (D, E).

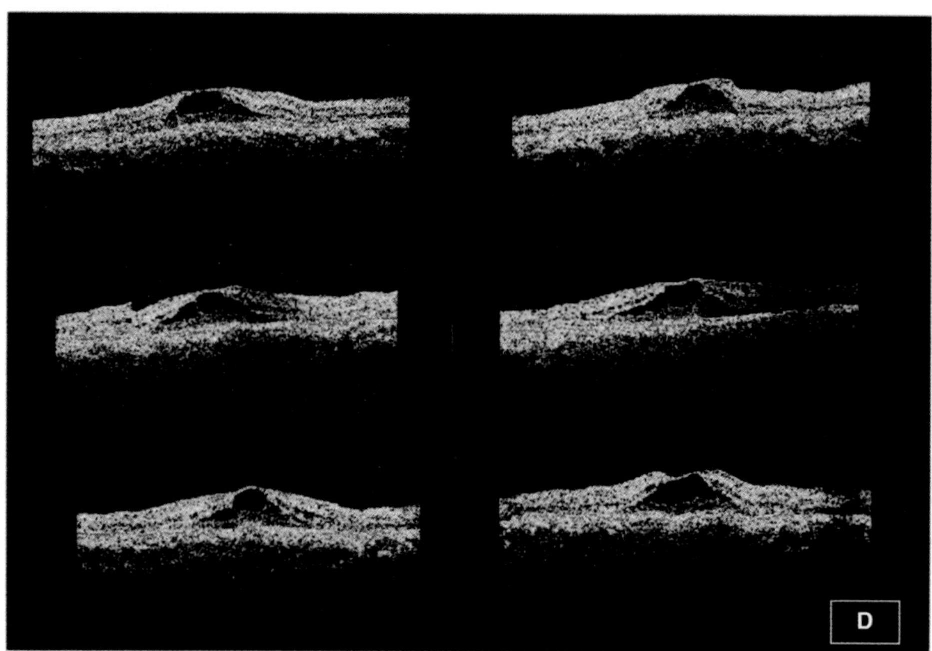

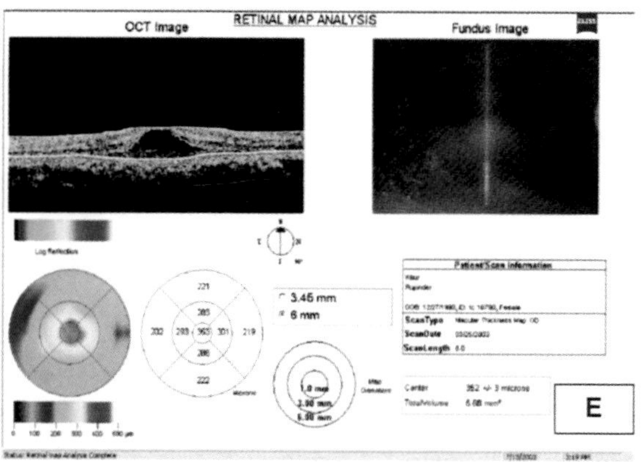

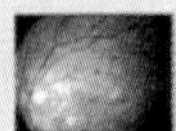

Three months later, her visual acuity in this eye was 20/30. Repeat OCT scan (F, G) showed persistence of macular edema with no response to oral acetazolamide. Oral acetazolamide was discontinued at this stage.

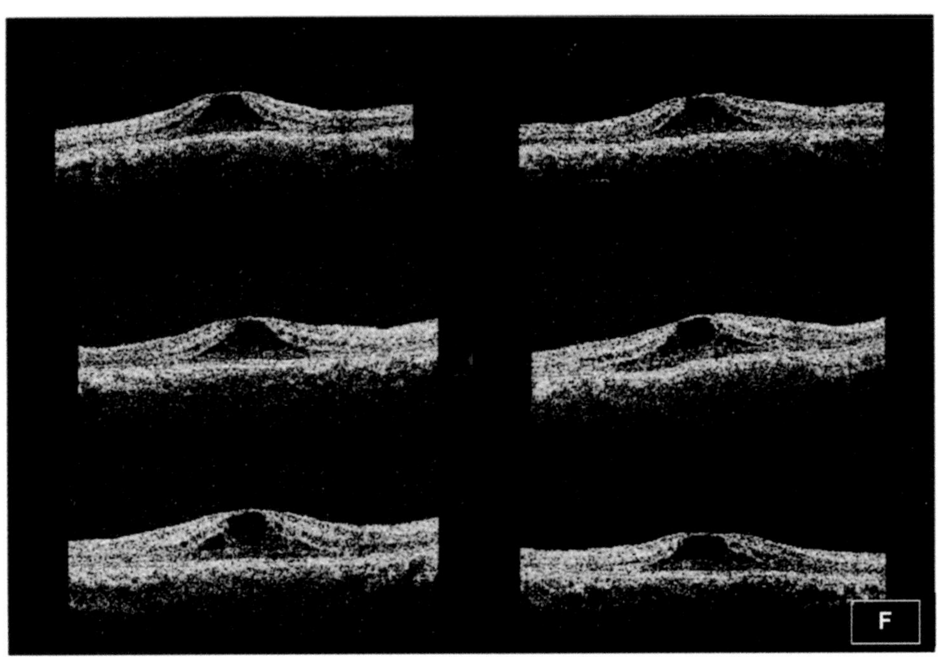

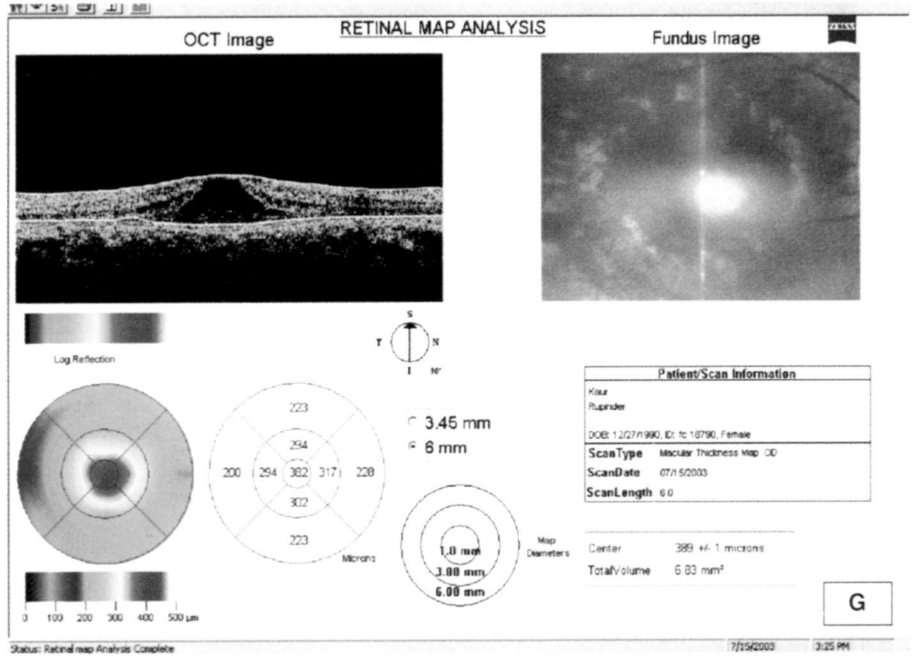

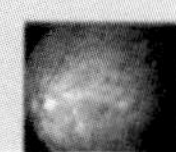

The left eye too showed similar features (H-K). The visual acuity in this eye was 20/30.The patient received oral acetazolamide.

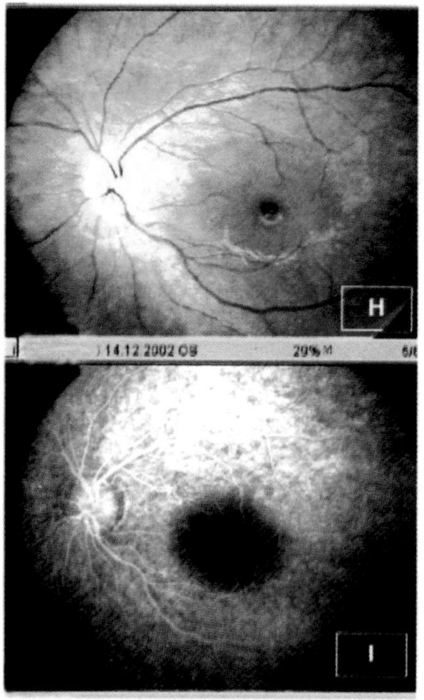

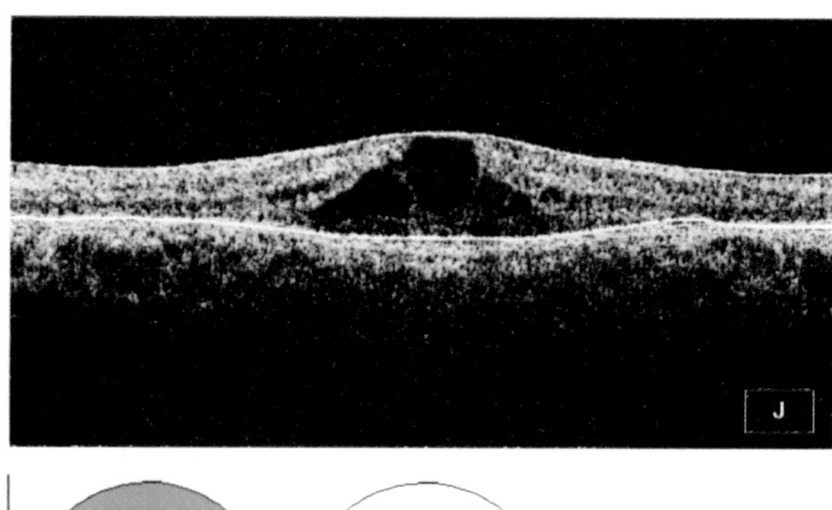

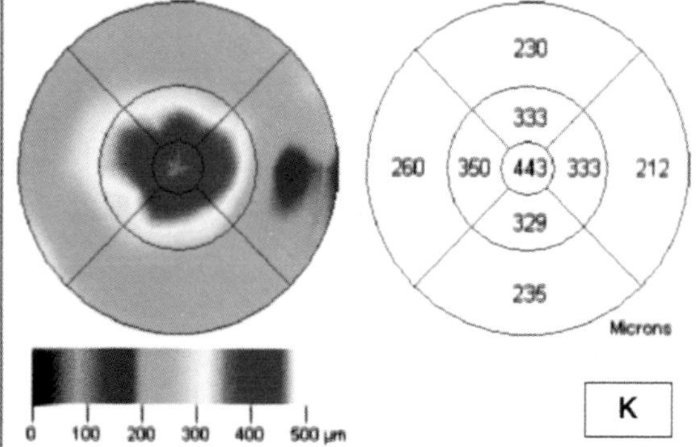

Repeat OCT scan of the left eye six weeks later showed persistence of cystoid spaces with retinal thickness measuring 402 microns in the foveal center (L, M).

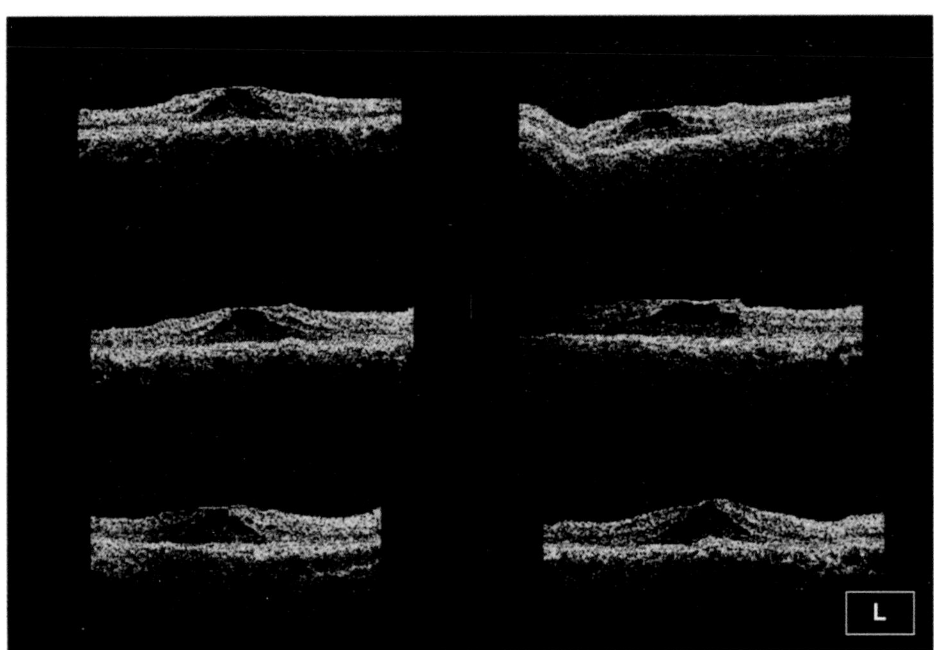

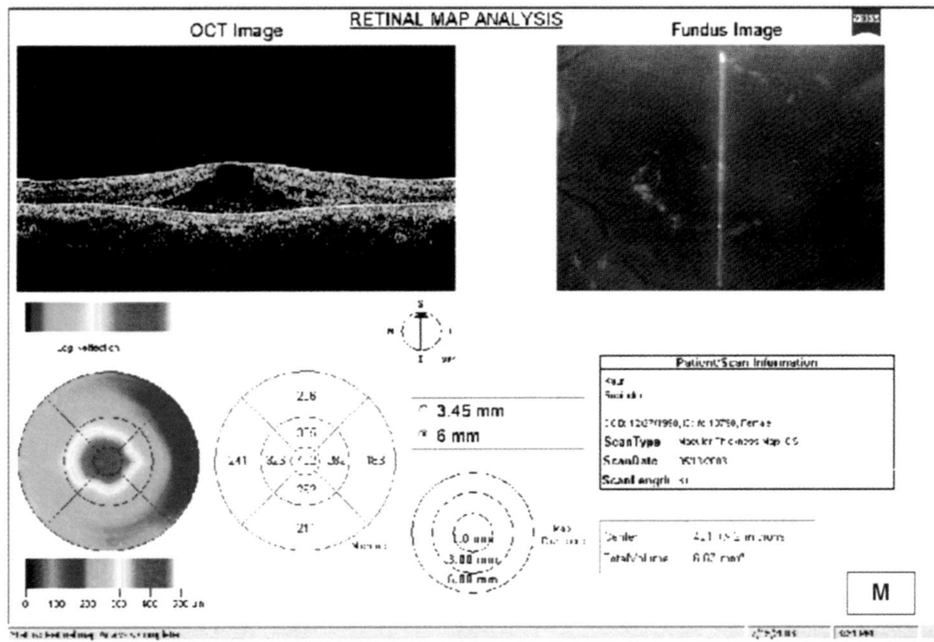

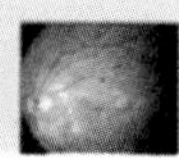

The patient still continued to receive oral acetazolamide. Three months later, her best-corrected visual acuity was 20/30. Repeat OCT scan still showed the persistence of cystoid spaces with central foveal thickness measuring 350 microns (N, O) following which oral acetazolamide was discontinued.

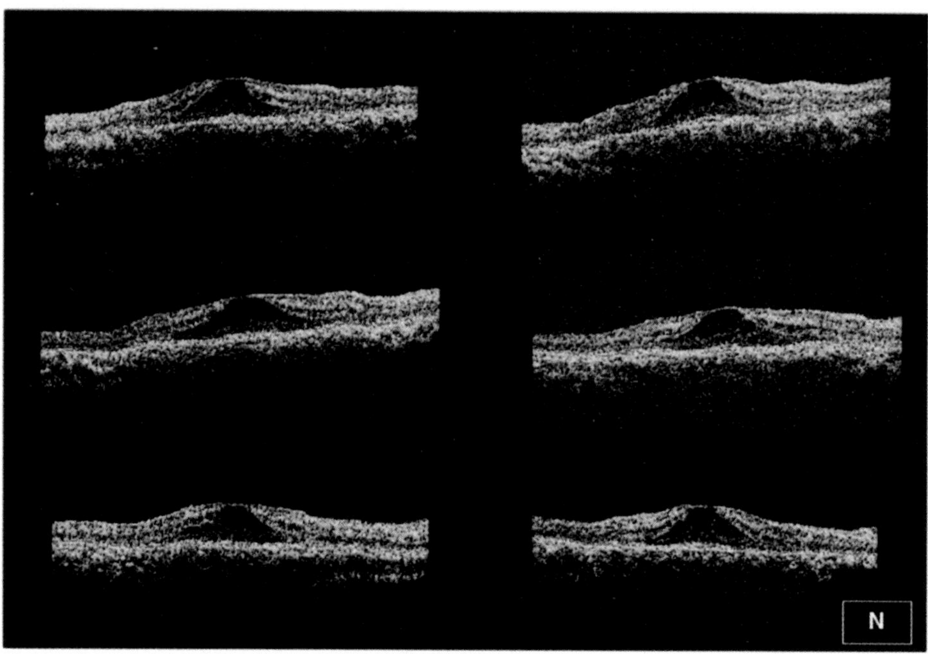

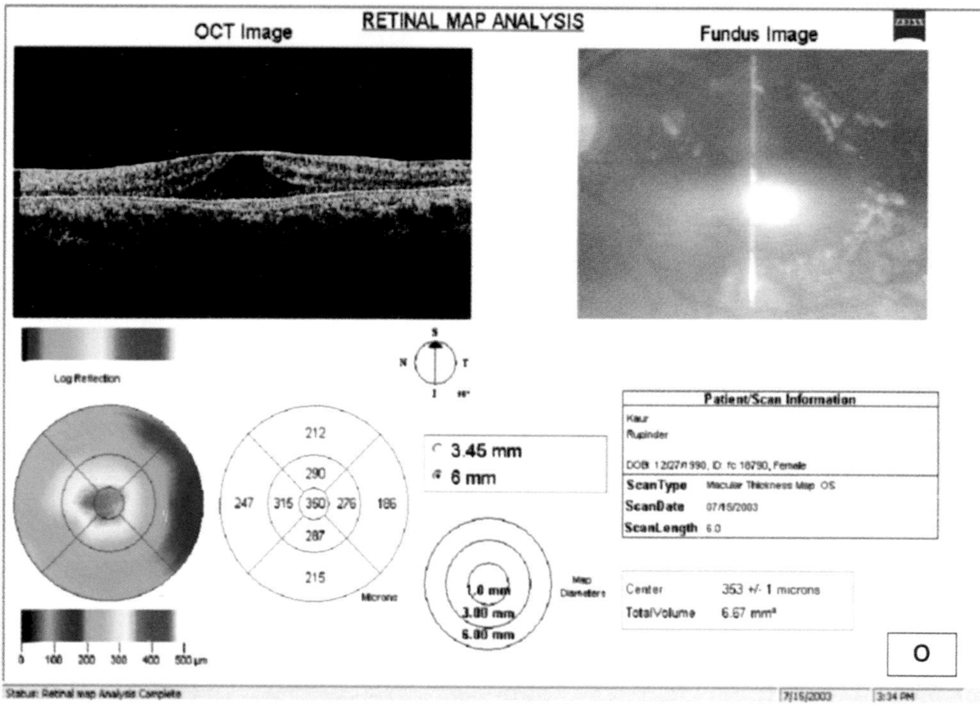

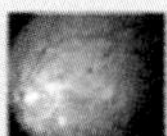

Case 14.2: Retinitis Pigmentosa with RPE Atrophy

Case Summary

A 18-year-old girl was suffering from retinitis pigmentosa (A, B). Her best corrected visual acuity was 4/ 60 in the right eye.

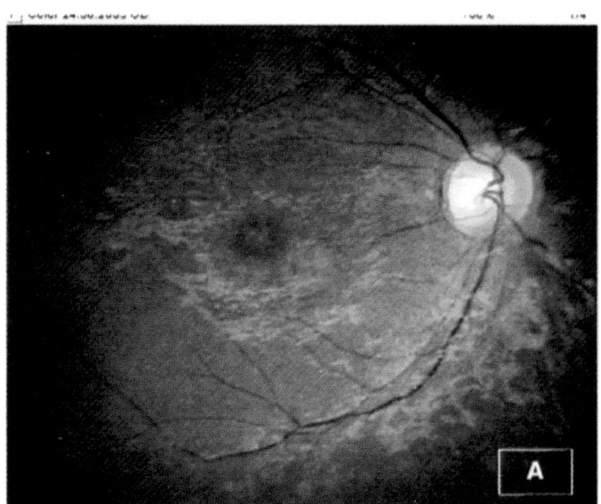

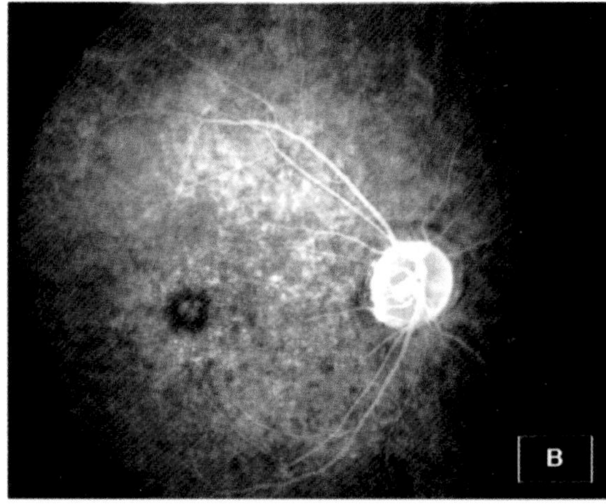

Optical Coherence Tomography

Optical coherence tomography line scan of the right eye (C) showed atrophy of neurosensory retina with central foveal thickness measuring 87 microns. There were no cystoid spaces in this, eye.

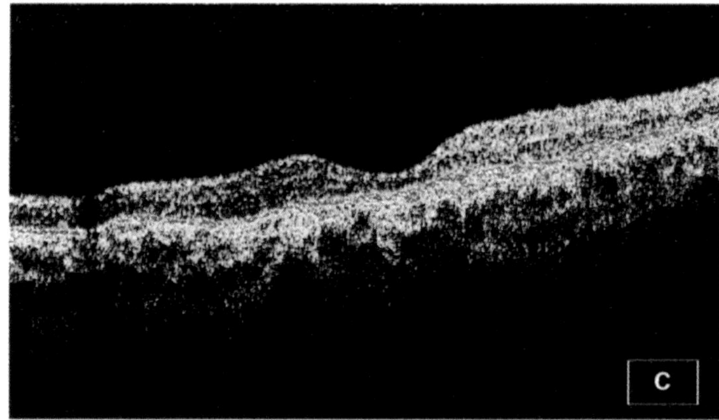

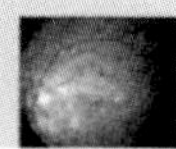

She had similar features in the opposite eye as well (D, E). The OCT in this eye too showed features of retinal atrophy with central foveal thickness measuring 83 microns (F). This patient showed atrophy of retinal layers on OCT. Thus no intervention was planned for this patient.

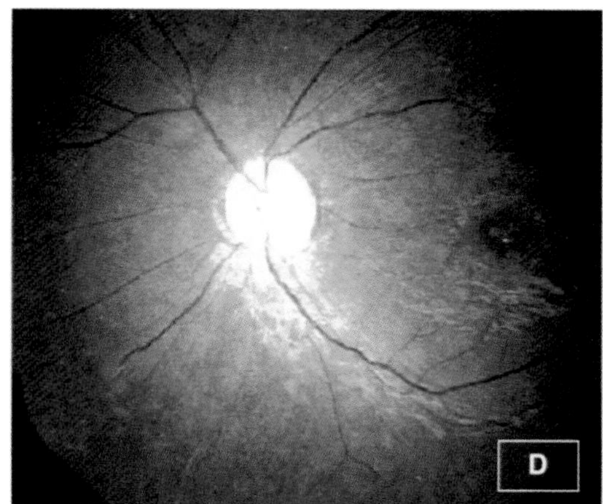

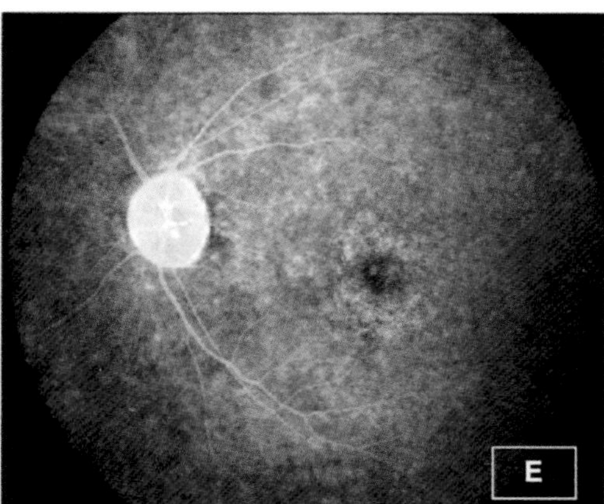

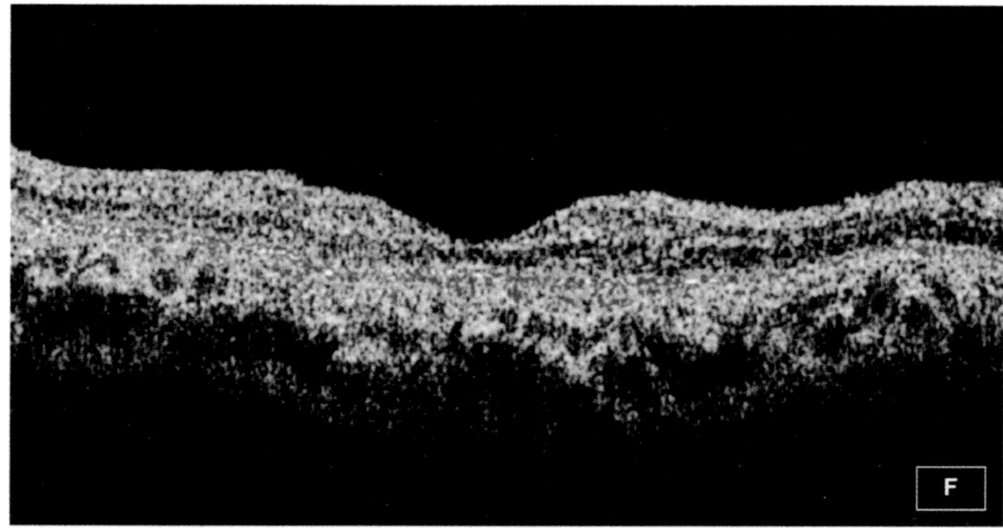

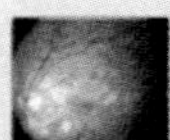

Case 14.3: Cone Dystrophy

Case Summary

A 12-year-old boy was diagnosed as a case of bilateral cone dystrophy based on clinical and electrophysiologic features that showed subnormal cone responses with normal rod response. His best corrected visual acuity was 20/80 in the right eye (A). Fluorescein angiography of this eye showed hyperfluorescence in the fovea (B).

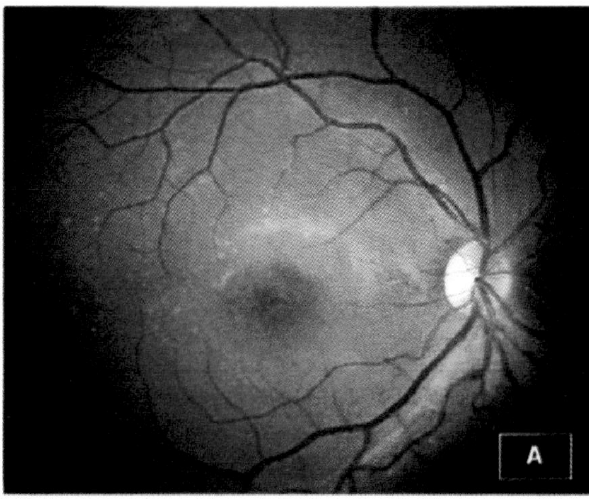

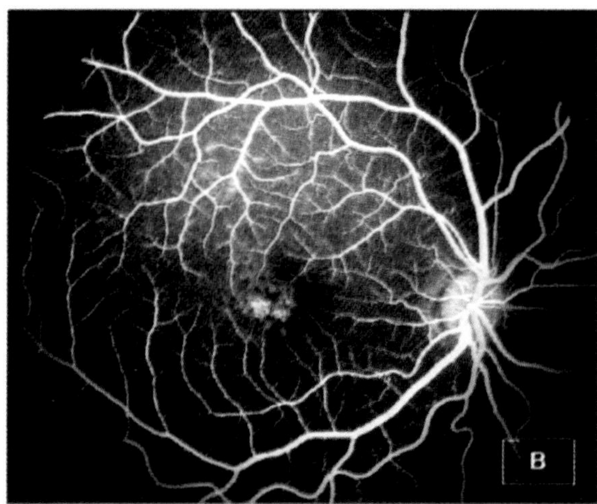

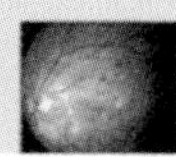

The OCT scan through the fovea (C) and at different angles (D-I) showed irregular retinal pigment epithelial layer, central foveal atrophy with foveal thickness measuring 87 microns in the foveal center. The left eye of the patient showed identical changes (not shown). In view of atrophic changes, no active intervention was planned for this patient.

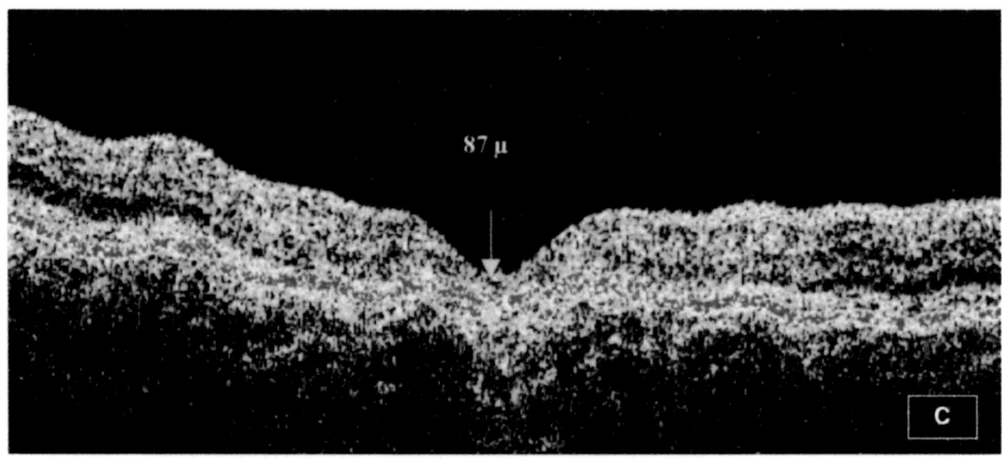

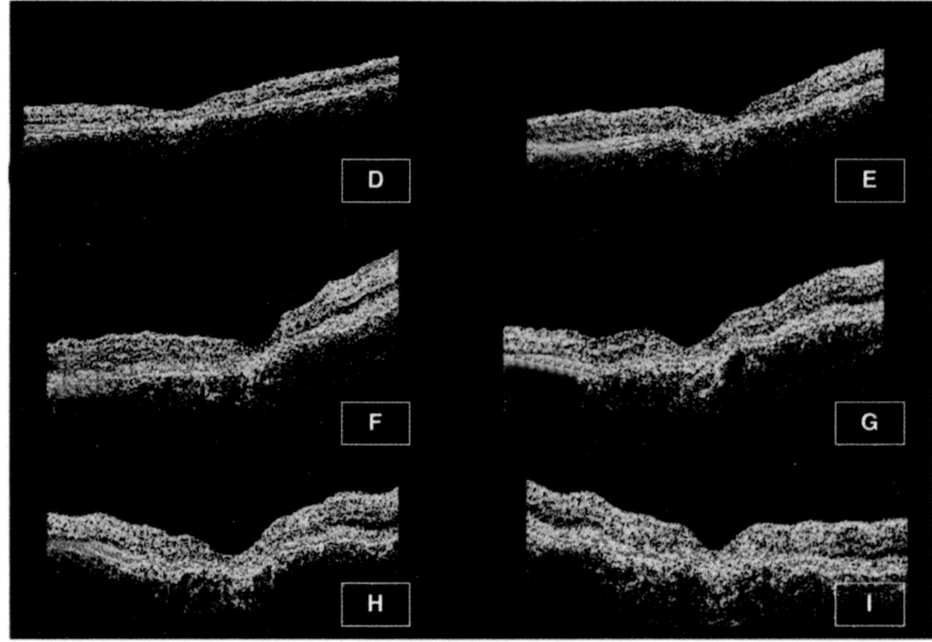

STARGARDT'S DISEASE/ FUNDUS FLAVIMACULATUS

14.4: Atrophic Maculopathy without Flecks

Case Summary

A 23-year-old woman was seen with mild red-green dyschromatopsia. Her best corrected visual acuity was 20/30 in the right eye (A). Fluorescein angiography (B) showed bull's eye pattern of RPE atrophy with ring shaped area of mottled hyperfluorescence. The electroretinogram was normal while electrooculogram was subnormal.

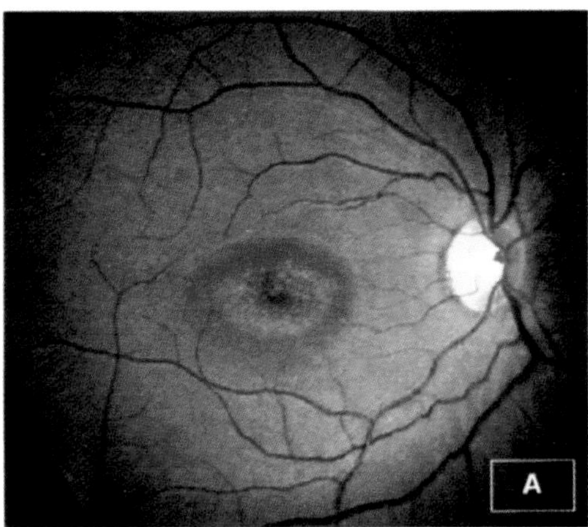

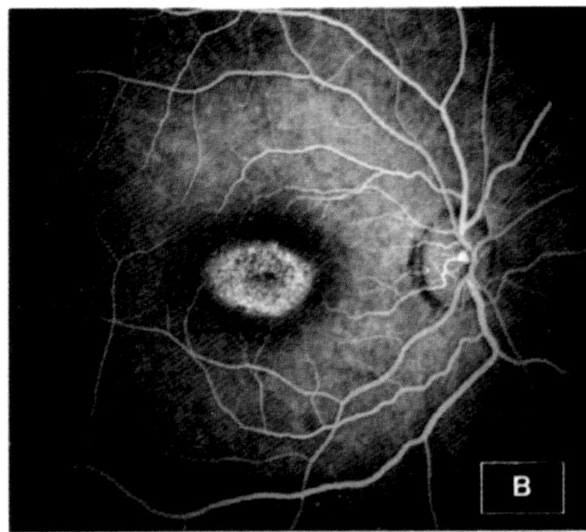

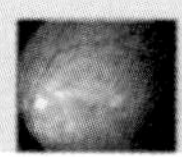

Optical Coherence Tomography

OCT scan of the right eye (C, D) showed atrophy of neurosensory retina in the foveal center with central foveal thickness measuring 65 microns. The underlying RPE –choroid complex showed hyper-reflectivity.

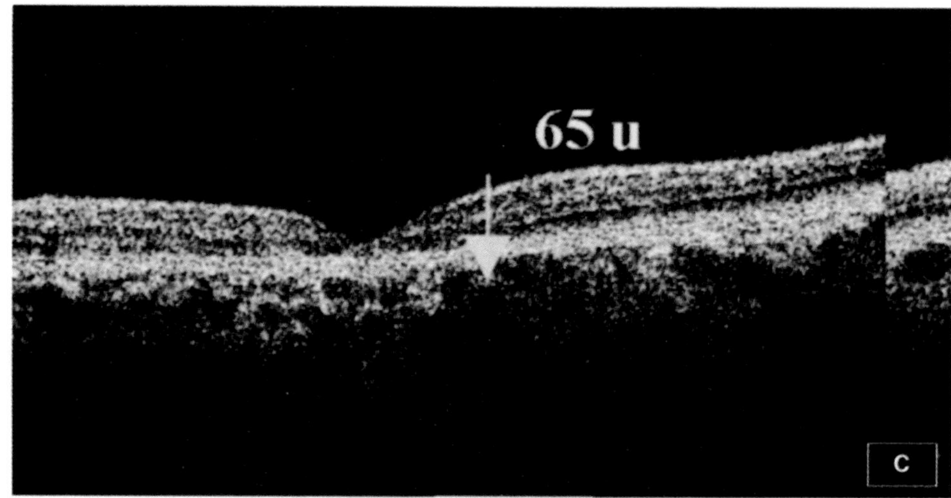

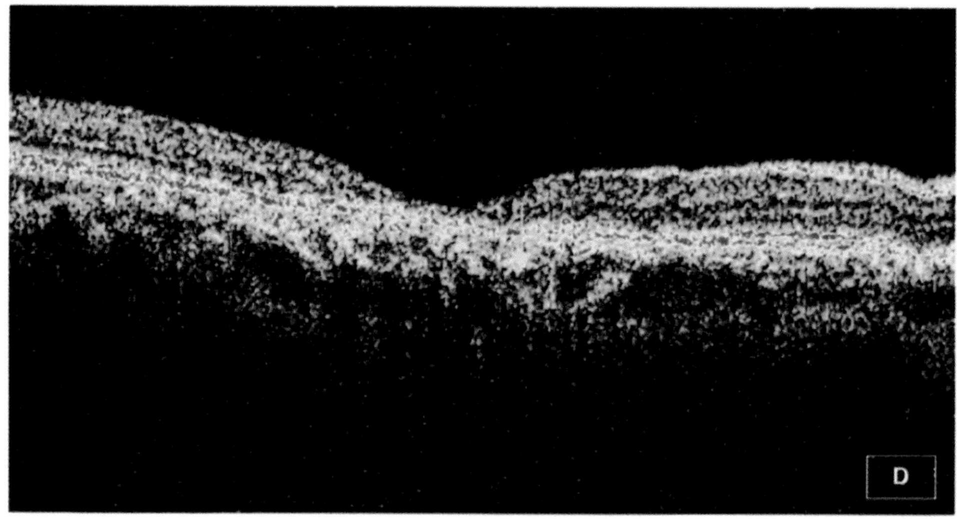

Case 14.5: Atrophic maculopathy with flecks

Case Summary

A 20-year-old man was seen with progressive decrease in vision in both his eyes of three years duration. His best corrected visual acuity in the right eye was 20/200. The fundus showed a central area of a beaten metal appearance with flecks in the posterior pole (A). Fluorescein angiography (B) showed "dark " choroid with central atrophy resembling "bulls eye lesion" while flecks showed irregular pattern of fluorescence.The electro-oculogram was subnormal.

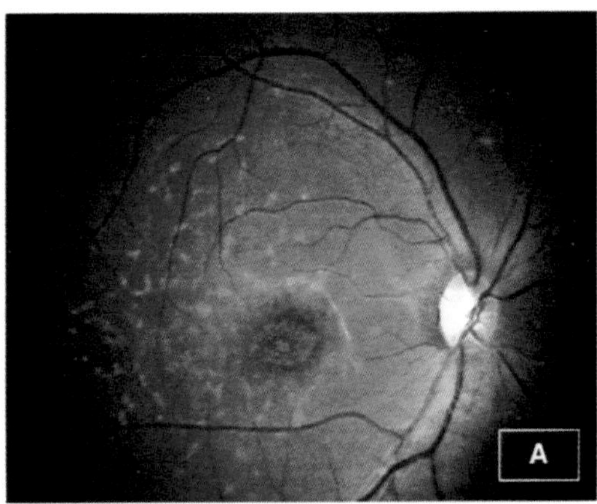

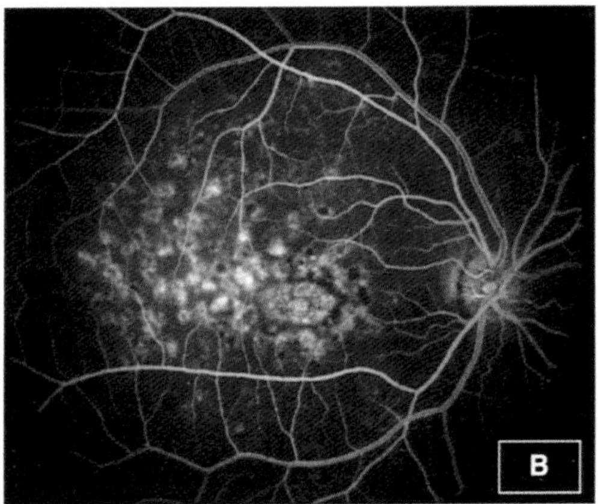

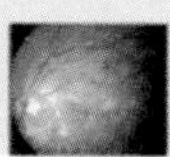

Optical Coherence Tomography

OCT scan (C, D) of the right eye showed atrophy in the foveal center with central foveal thickness measuring 58 microns. The flecks have been shown histopathologically as RPE cells that are enlarged and densely packed with PAS-positive substance. On OCT, these were seen as hyper-reflective areas with irregular RPE (arrows).

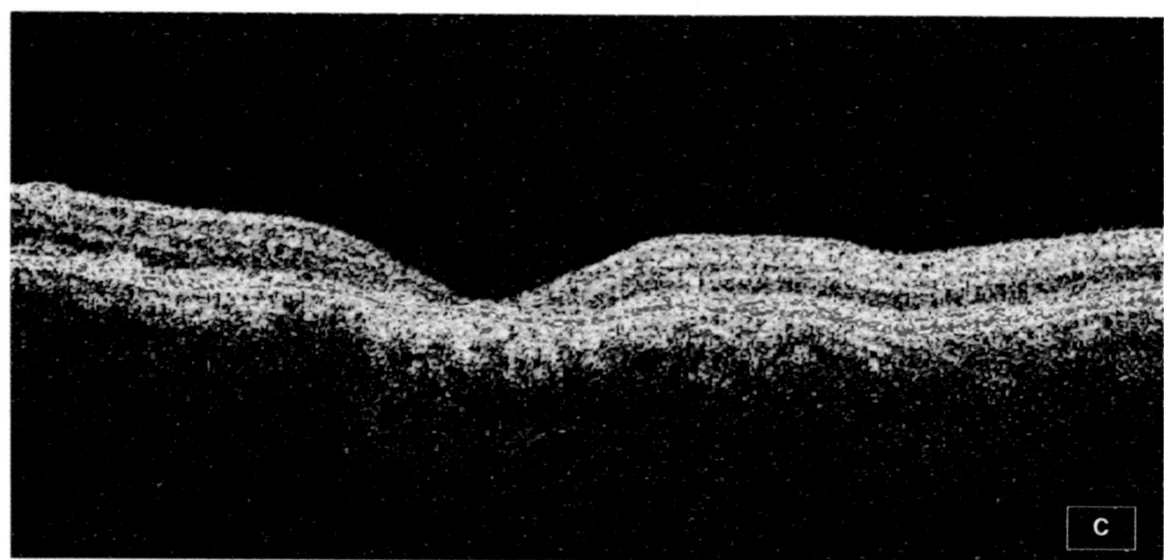

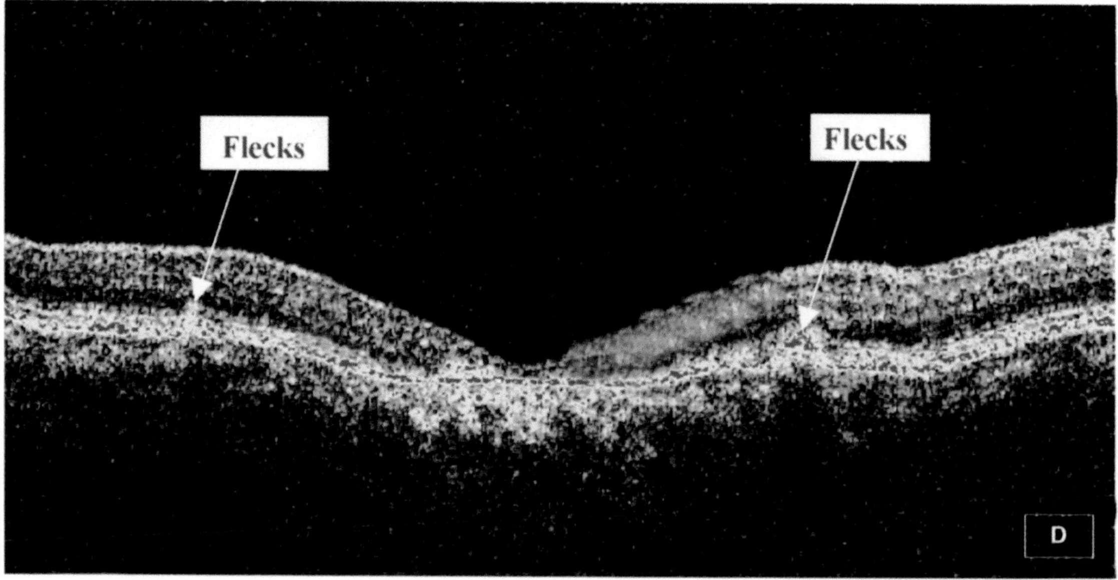

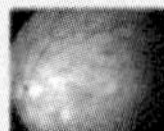

Case 14.6: Bietti's Crystalline Tapetoretinal Dystrophy

Case Summary

A 34-year-old man was seen with complaints of paracentral scotoma in both the eyes. His best corrected visual acuity was 20/30 in the right eye. The fundus in this eye showed glittering crystals seen throughout the posterior pole with central geographic atrophy (A). Fluorescein angiography (B) revealed choriocapillary atrophy corresponding to RPE atrophy.

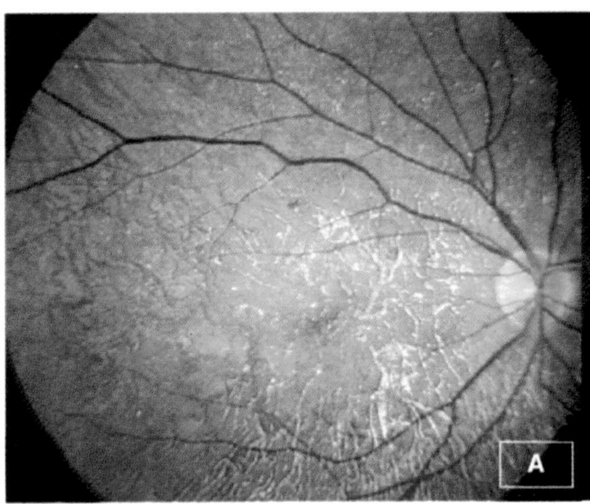

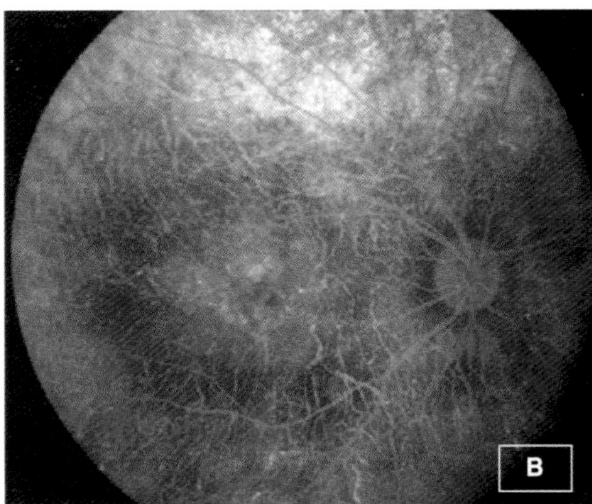

Optical Coherence Tomography

OCT scan of this eye (C, D) showed increased backscattering from neurosensory retina under the fovea suggestive of some intraretinal fluid accumulation with few cystoid spaces (arrow). The underlying RPE-choroid complex showed increased hyper-reflectivity probably due to overlying thinning of the retina. The crystals were seen as multiple pin point hyper-reflective dots located in inner as well as outer retinal layers.

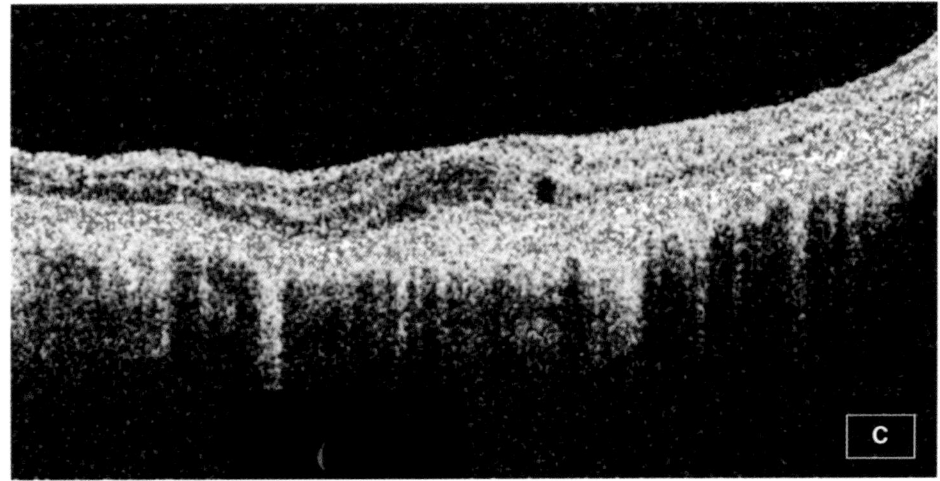

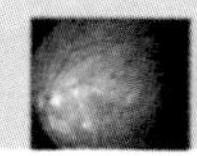

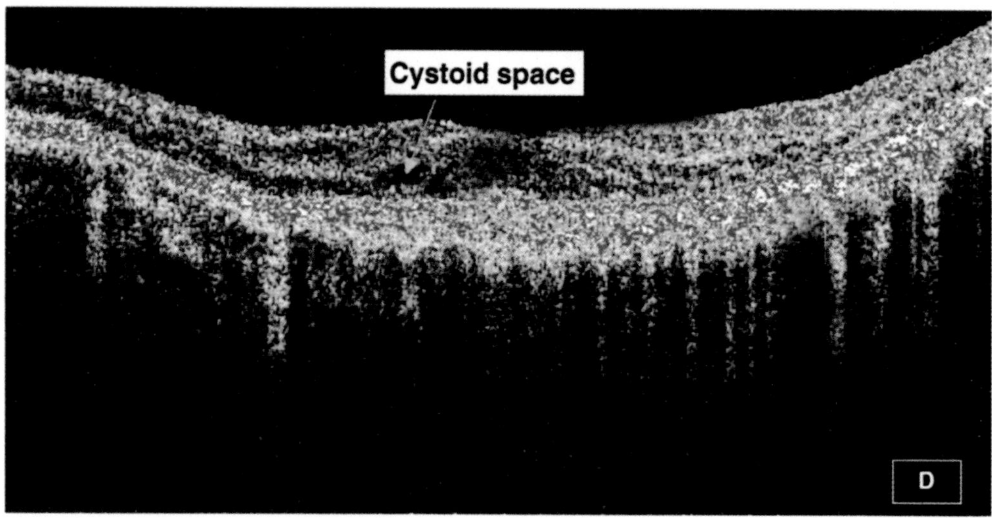

The fundus in the left eye too showed glittering crystals seen throughout the posterior pole with central geographic atrophy (E). Fluorescein angiography (F) revealed choriocapillary atrophy corresponding to RPE atrophy.

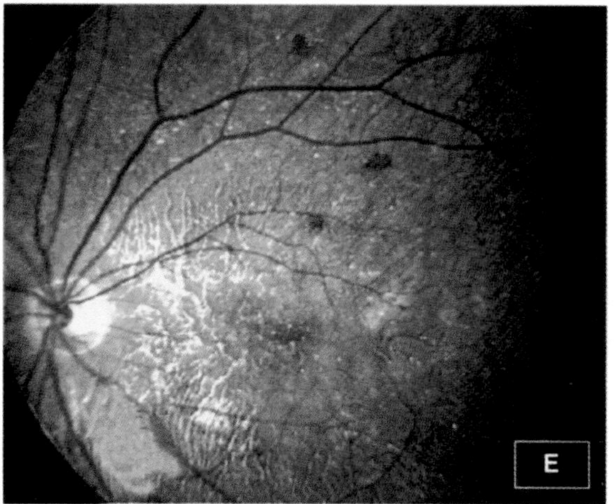

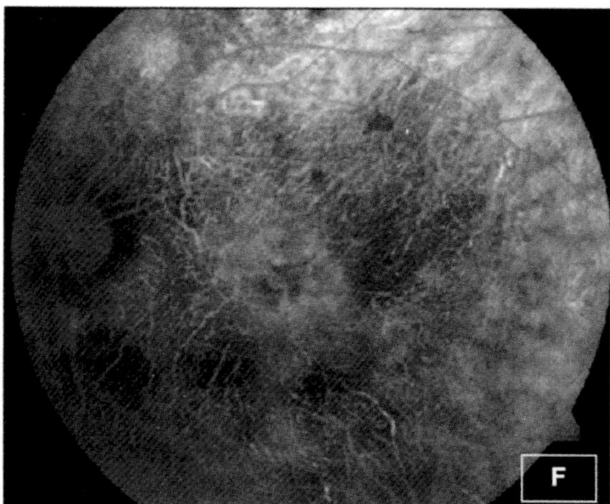

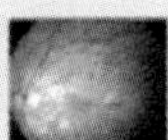

Optical Coherence Tomography

OCT scan of this eye (G, H) showed the presence of small cystic spaces (arrow) in the neurosensory retina nasal to the fovea. The underlying RPE-choroid complex showed increased hyper-reflectivity probably due to overlying thinning of the retina.

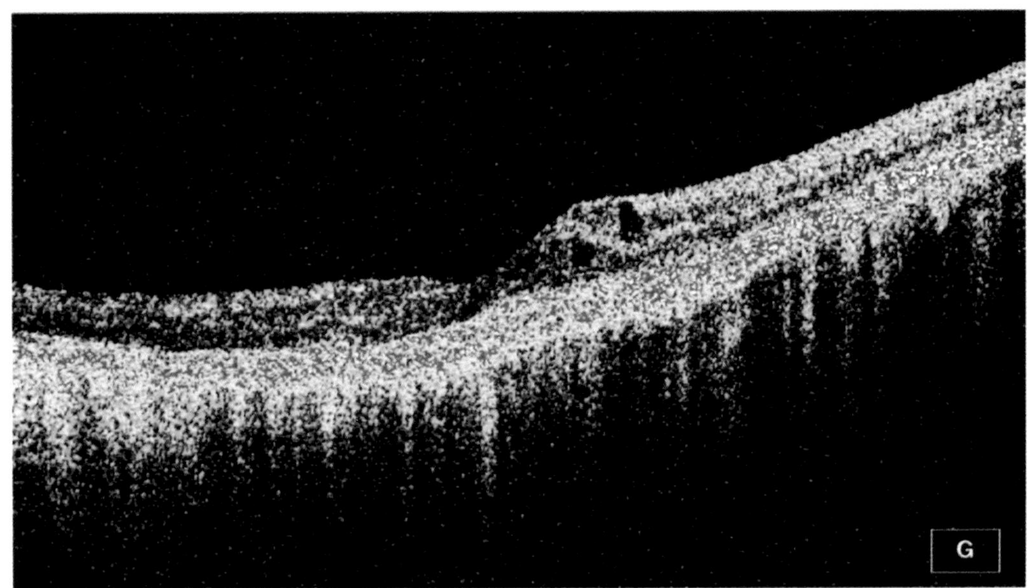

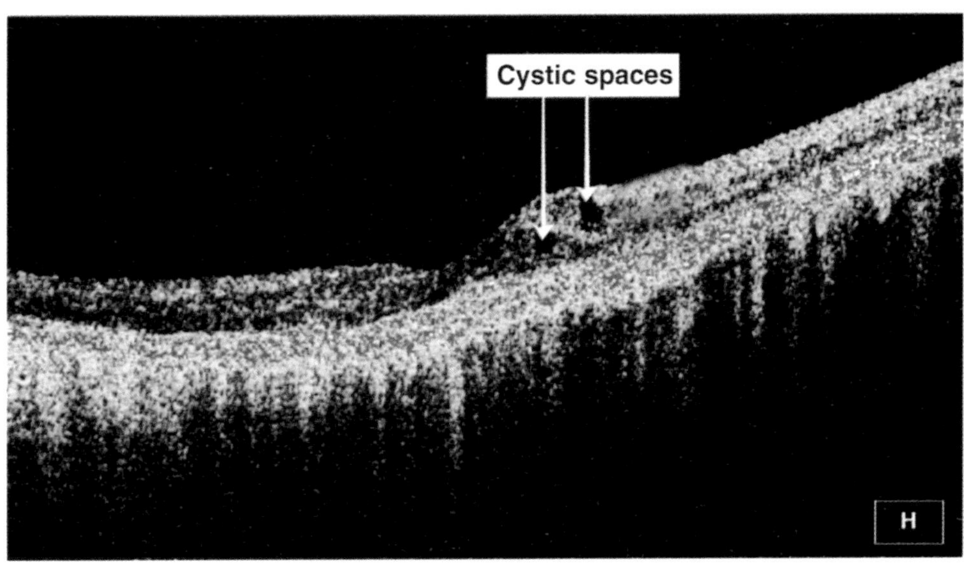

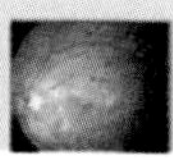

In view of cystic spaces seen on OCT alone, patient was offered a trial of oral acetazolamide. Six weeks later, repeat OCT of both right and left eye respectively (I, J) showed no change. Oral acetazolamide was discontinued.

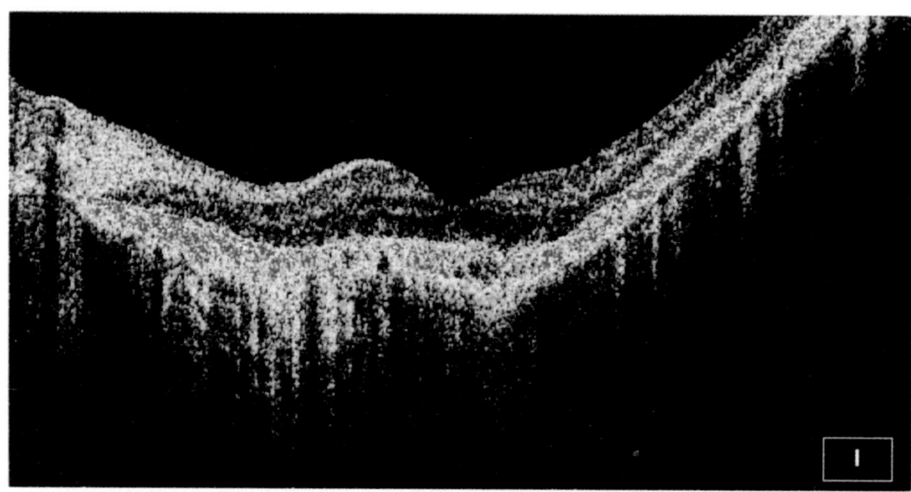

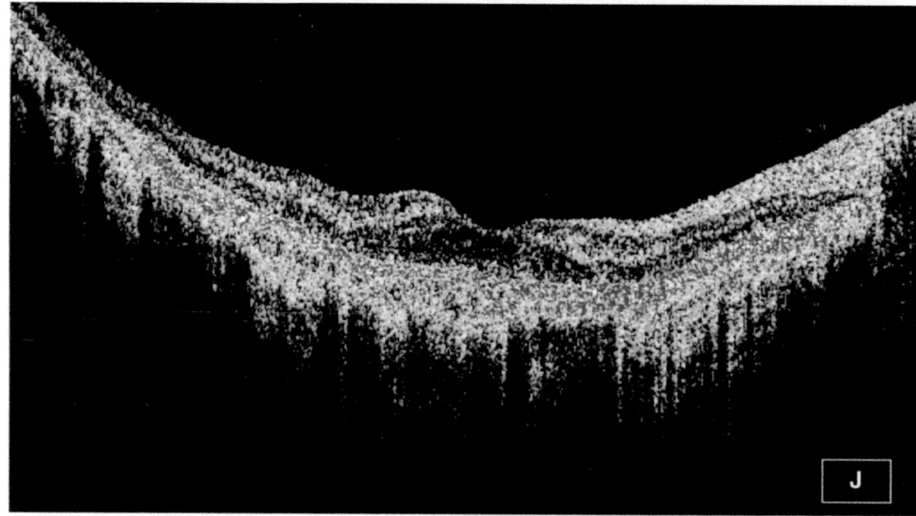

CENTRAL AREOLAR CHOROIDAL DYSTROPHY

Case 14.7: CACD

Case Summary

A 64-year-old man was seen with complaints of paracentral scotoma in both the eyes. His best corrected visual acuity was 20/80 in the right eye. The fundus in this eye showed advanced atrophy of the central retina (A). Fluorescein angiography revealed choriocapillary atrophy corresponding to RPE atrophy.

Optical Coherence Tomography

OCT scan of this eye (B, C) showed increased backscattering from neurosensory retina under the fovea with loss of normal retinal architecture. The underlying RPE-choroid complex showed increased hyper-reflectivity probably due to overlying thinning of the retina.

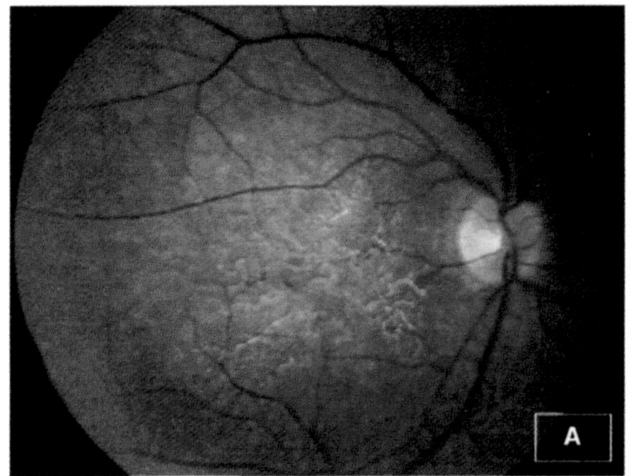
A

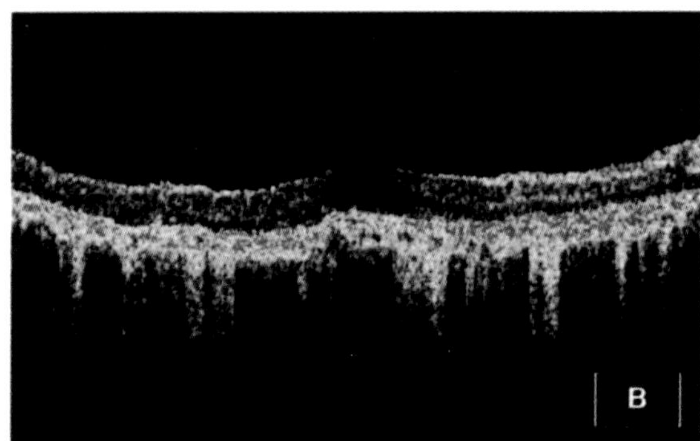
B

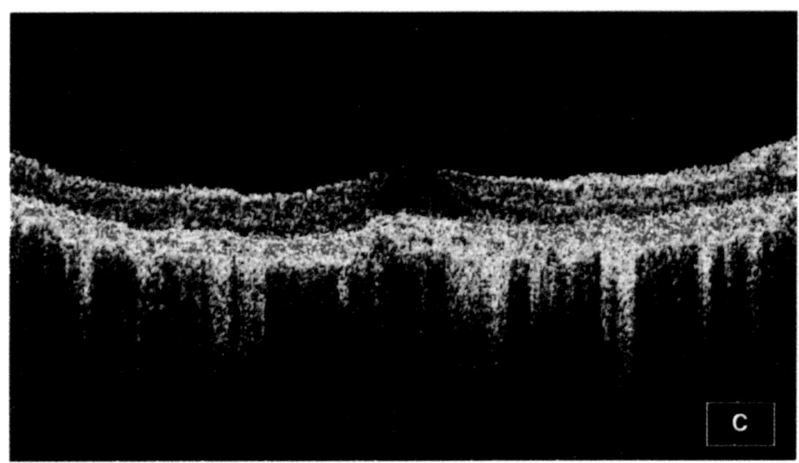
C

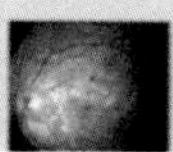

ADULT –ONSET FOVEOMACULAR VITELLIFORM DYSTROPHY

(*Courtesy* of Dr. Monique Leys, West Virginia University Eye Institute, Morgantown, USA)

Case 14.8: Adult-Onset Foveomacular Vitelliform Dystrophy

Case Summary

A 56-year-old glaucoma patient had visual acuity of 20/50 in the right eye with yellow lesion in the fovea (A, B).

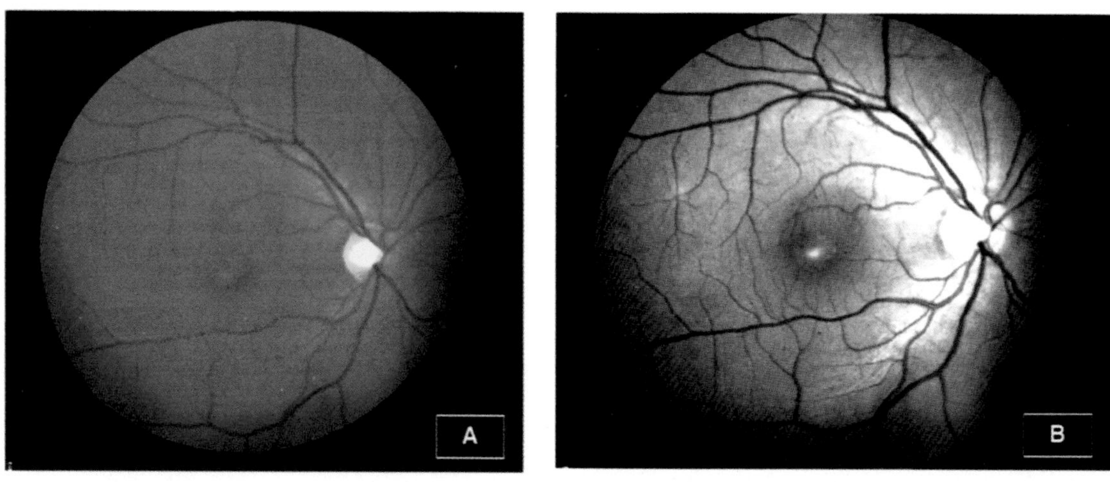

The horizontal OCT line scan showed a central, hyper-reflective area of thickening corresponding to retinal pigment epithelial thickening. This has resuted in the altered foveal contour with displacement of photoreceptors.

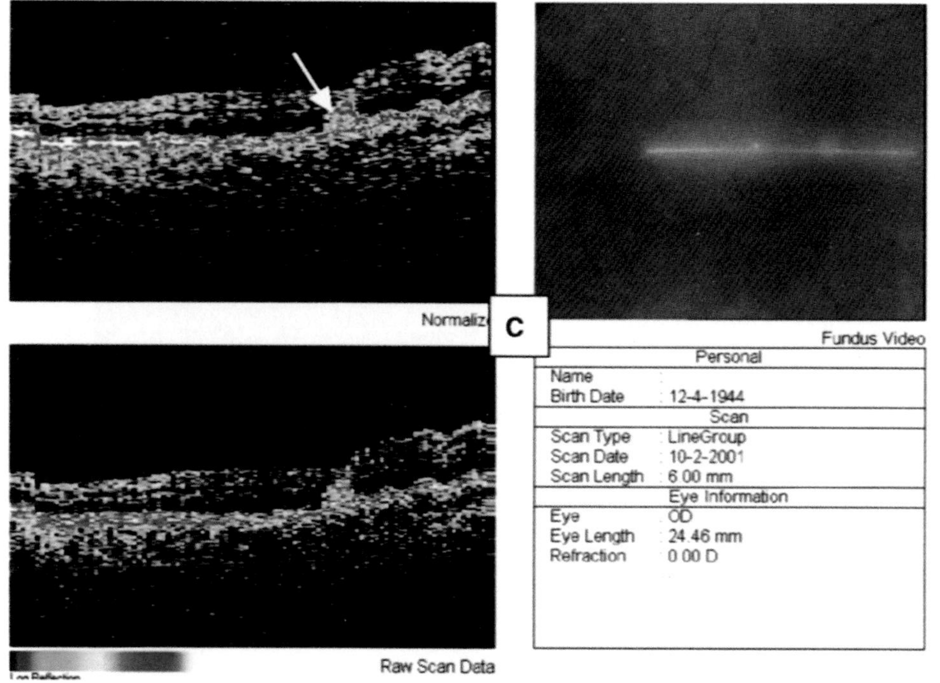

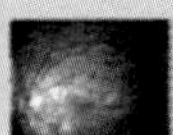

Case 14.9: Best Disease with Choroidal Neovascular Membrane

(*Courtesy* of Dr. Monique Leys West Virginia University Eye Institute, Morgantown, USA)

Case Summary

This 12-year-old patient has a mother and sister with Best disease. The mother has a flat EOG. In 2000, this patient had visual acuity of 20/20 OD and 20/30 OS. He had atrophy and subretinal fibrosis OU (not shown). The patient returned an year later with complaints of reduced visual acuity in the left eye following minor injury. The visual acuity in the left eye was reduced to 20/200. Fundus showed subretinal fibrosis and subretinal hemorrhage (A). Fluorescein angiography of the left eye (B) indicated subretinal hemorrhage associated with CNV.

Optical Coherence Tomography

The OCT of the left eye (C) shows thin atrophic retina with an area of hyper-reflectivity in the retina suggesting subretinal fibrosis. There was hyporeflective area on either side indicating the fluid accumulation.

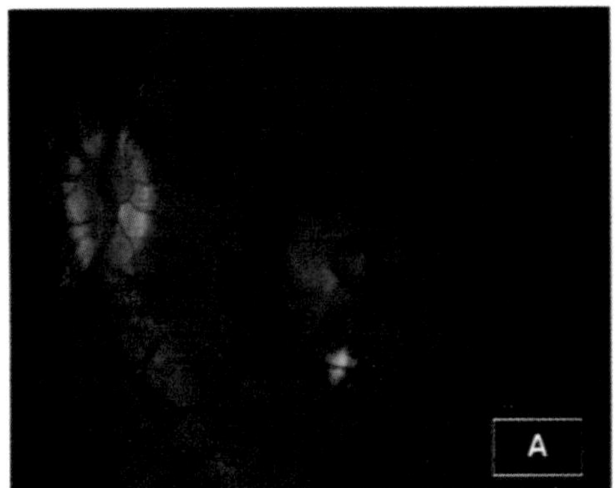

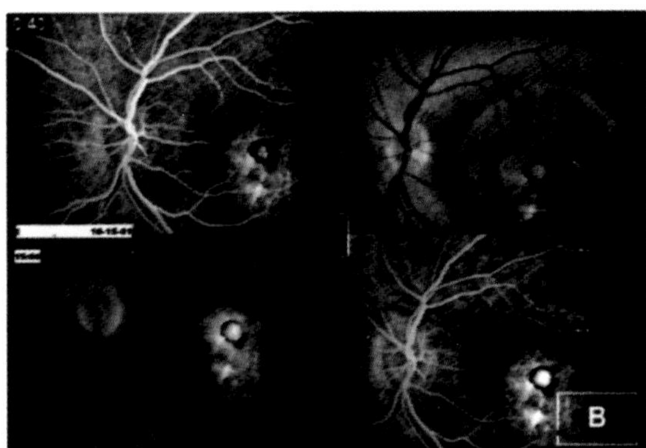

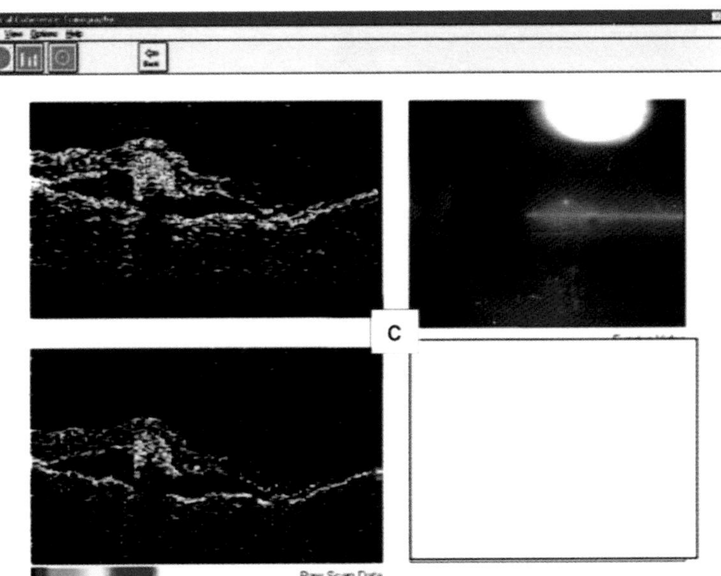

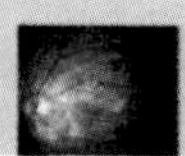

The fundus in the right eye (D) showed subretinal fibrosis with retinal atrophy. The OCT scan of this eye (E) showed hyper-reflectivity within the retinal layers with serous detachment on either side.

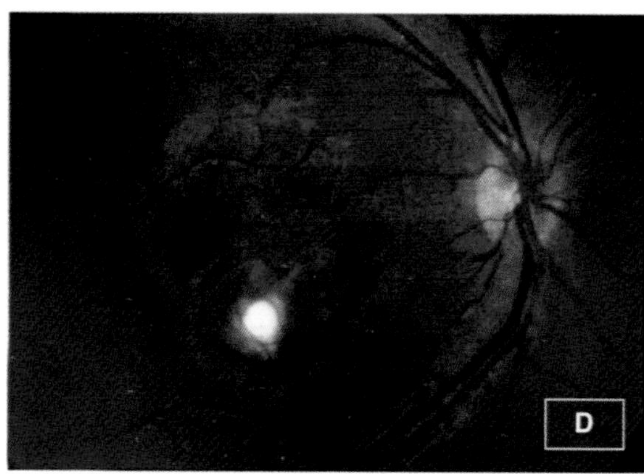

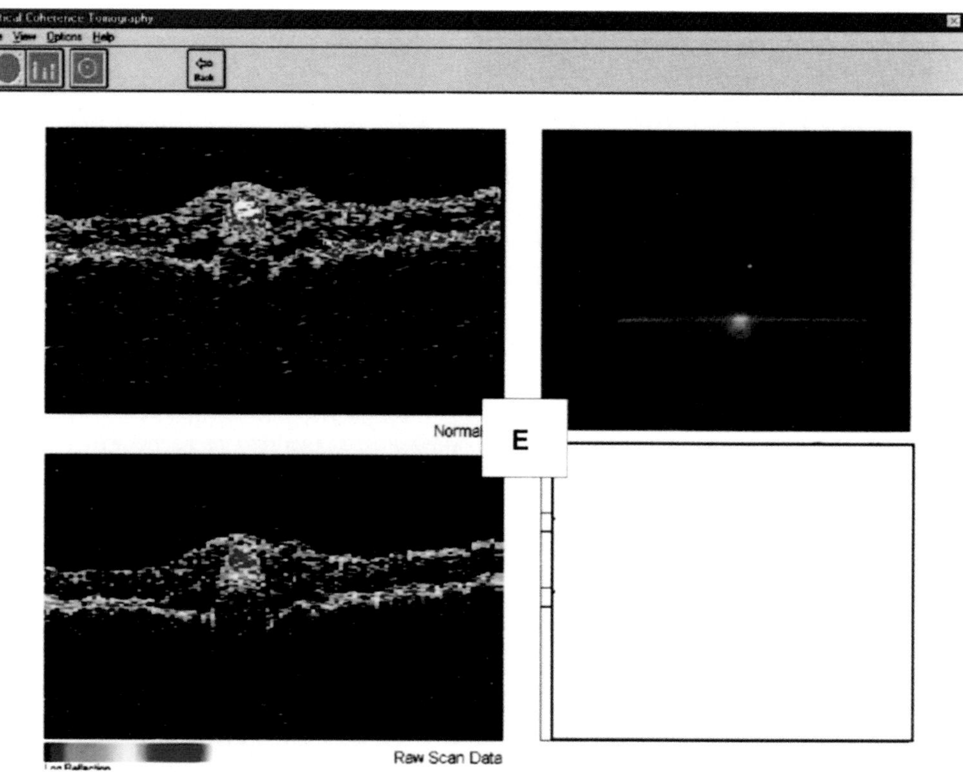

CONCLUSIONS

1. OCT provides useful information regarding the morphology of these disorders. It helps in better understanding of the disease process in these disorders.
2. It demonstrates the foveal thinning that can probably help in predicting the progressive visual loss and monitor the disease progression.
3. As demonstrated in the cases, OCT was helpful in measuring retinal thickness and document cystoid macular edema where fluorescein angiography showed none. Such cases might be the candidates for medical management and again OCT could be used to monitor the response to the intervention.
4. Recent report has suggested that OCT was useful in diagnosing a taut posterior hyaloid membrane in retinitis pigmentosa that responded to surgical intervention. Though we have no personal experience of pars plana vitrectomy in retinitis pigmentosa as yet, it seems a promising strategy.

SUGGESTED READINGS

1. Heredodystrophic Disorders affecting the Retinal Pigment Epithelium and Retina. Chap 5.In Gass JDM (ed) Stereoscopic Atlas of Macular Diseases Diagnosis and Treatment. 1997, Mosby- Year Book, Inc.303-436.
2. Gracia Aruni J, Martinez V, Sararols L, Corcostegui B. Vitreoretinal surgery for cystoid macular edema associated with retinitis pigmentosa. Ophthalmology 2003;110:1164-69.
3. Benhamou N, Souied EH, Zolf R et al. Adult-onset foveomacular vitelliform dystrophy: A study by optical coherence tomography. Am J Ophthalmol. 2003;135: 362-67.
4. Pianta MJ, Aleman TS, Cideciyan AV et al. In vivo micropathology of Best macular dystrophy with optical coherence tomography. Exp Eye Res 2003;76:203-11.
5. Pierro L, Introini U, Calori G, Brancato R. Optical coherence tomography findings in adult-onset foveomacular vitelliform dystrophy. Am J Ophthalmol; 2002;134:675-80.

Chapter 15

Foveal Hemorrhage

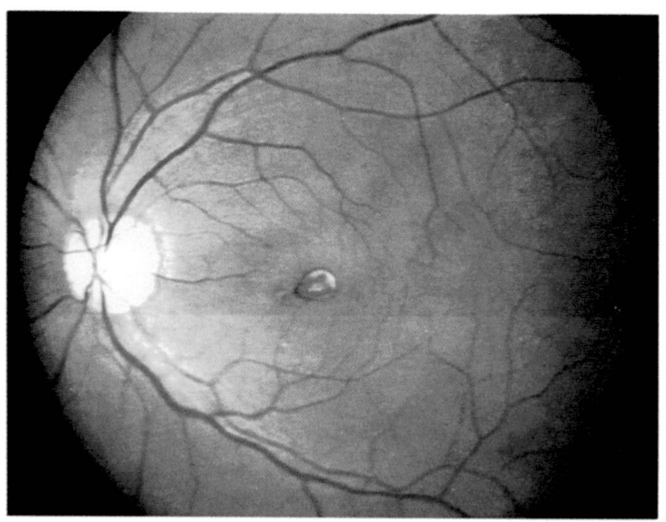

FOVEAL/SUBFOVEAL HEMORRHAGE

Case 15.1: Sub-internal Limiting Membrane Hemorrhage

Case Summary

A 45- year-old woman was seen with complaints of reduced vision in the left eye of 5 days duration. Her best corrected visual acuity was 20/60. Fundus showed the presence of bright red spot in the fovea (A). Fluorescein angiography did not show any hyperfluorescence (B).

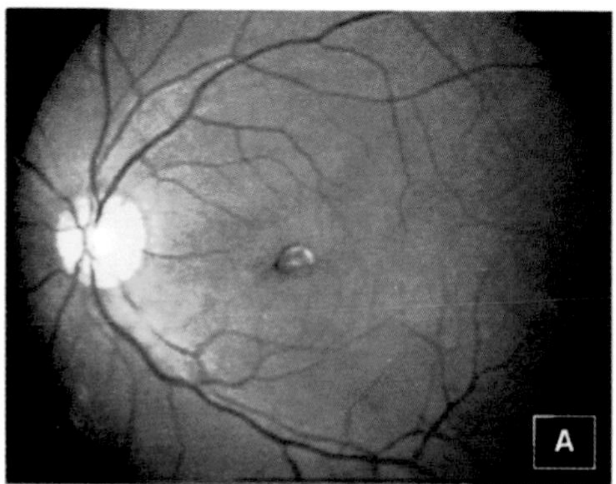

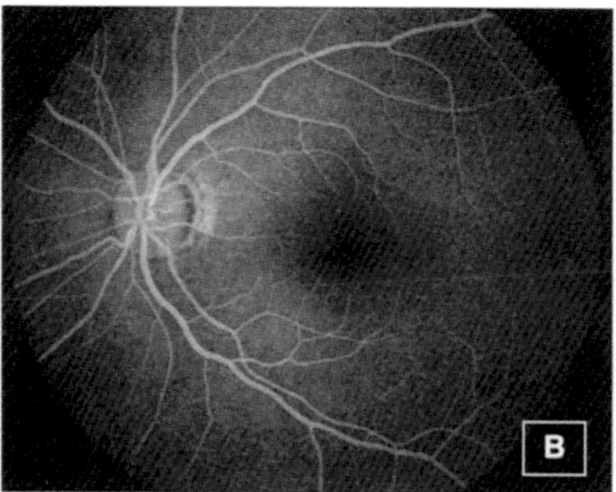

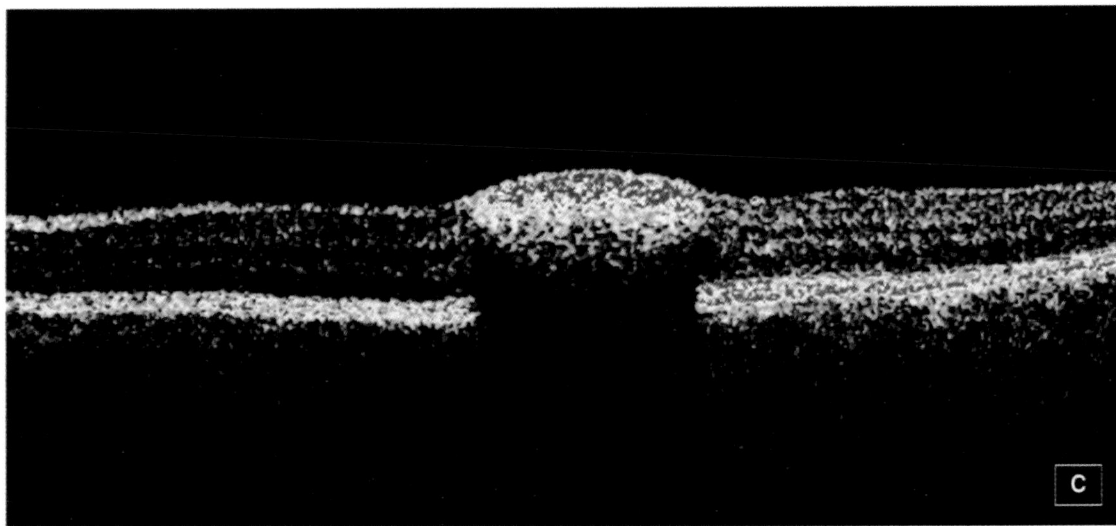

Optical Coherence Tomography

Horizontal OCT line scan (C) through the foveal center showed the presence of focal area of enhanced backscatter underlying the reflection from internal limiting membrane, corresponding to the area of blood seen clinically, that blocked all the reflections from the underlying retina and choroid.

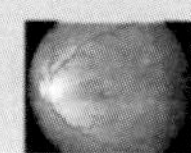

Case 15.2: Sub-hyloid Foveal Hemorrhage

Case summary

A 34-year-old woman (A) with a diagnosis of epidemic dropsy and anemia was seen with bilateral retinal hemorrhage. Her best-corrected visual acuity was 20/80 in the left eye.

Optical Coherence Tomography

OCT scan (B) showed the presence of focal area of blocked reflections. Also there was a hyper-reflective membrane seen anterior to this indicating subhyloid nature of the hemorrhage (arrow).

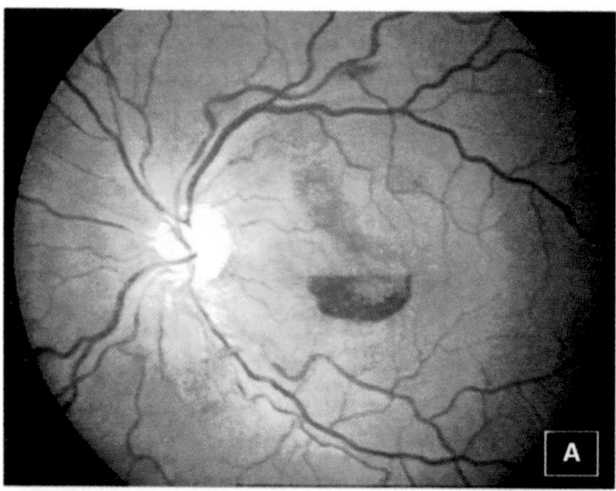

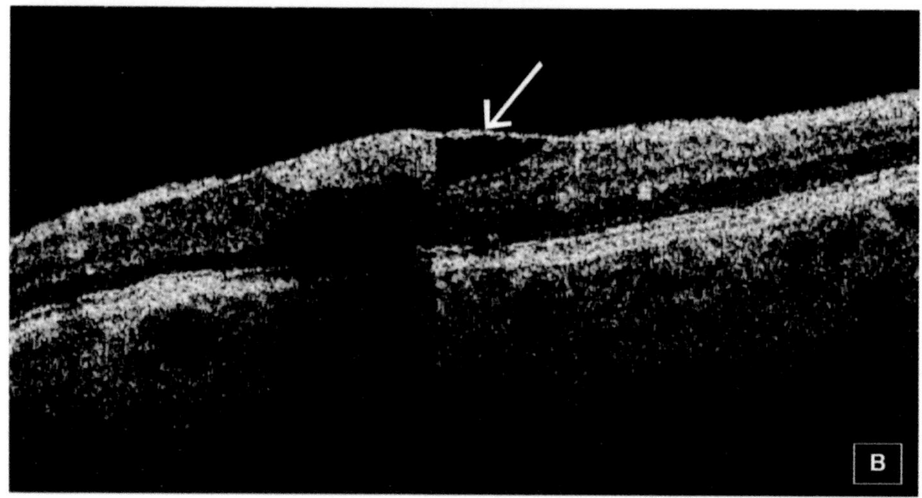

CONCLUSIONS

In patients with foveal hemorrhage, OCT helps in delineating the precise location of the blood. In cases where bleed is small, it may be able to depict underlying choroidal neovascular membrane, if any. However, in cases of large bleeds, the OCT beam is unable to penetrate, resulting in shadowing behind, thus not allowing the visualization of underlying structures.

Chapter 16

Photic Maculopathy

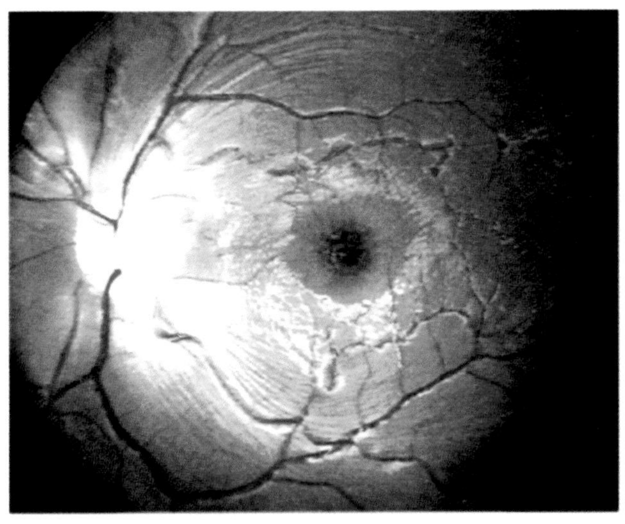

Case 16.1: Solar Retinopathy following Eclipse Viewing

Case Summary

A 34-year-old man was seen with complaints of decreased vision in both his eyes of one year duration following viewing of an eclipse. His best corrected visual acuity was 20/70 in both the eyes. The fundus examination showed a small reddish spot in the center in both eyes (A, B). Fluorescein angiography (C, D) didn't show any abnormality during early or late phase of the disease in either eye.

Optical Coherence Tomography

Horizontal OCT line scans through the foveal center of the right and left eye respectively (E, F) showed normal foveal contour with intact inner layers and disruption in the RPE complex under the fovea suggesting an outer lamellar hole (arrow). **OCT was able to diagnose lamellar macular hole that could not be diagnosed on fundoscopy or fluorescein angiography.**

A
B
C
D
Outer lamellar hole
E
Outer lamellar hole
F

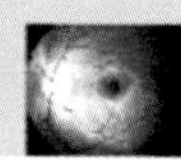

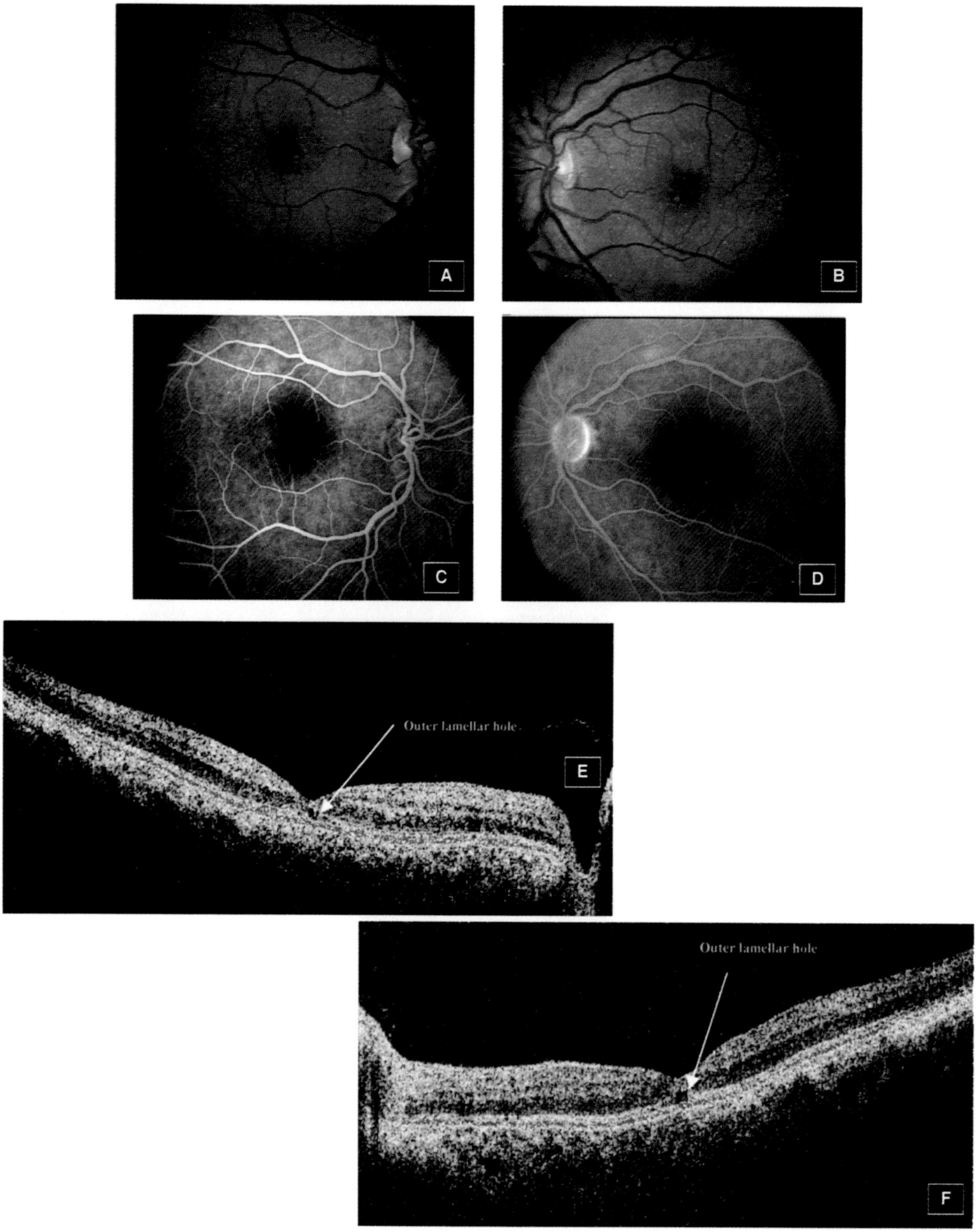

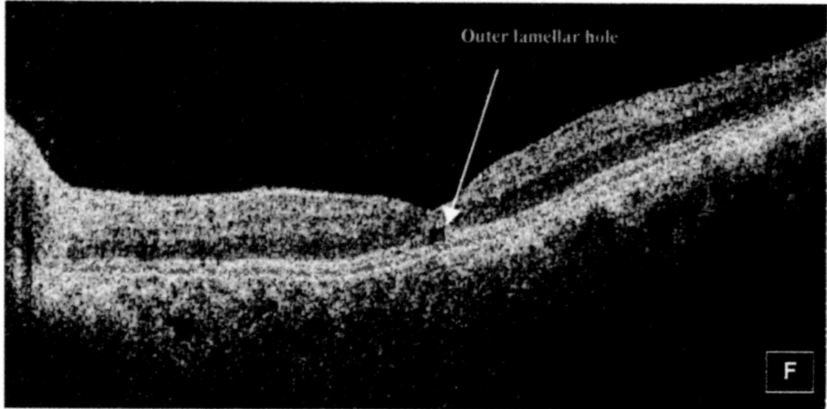

Case 16.2: Welding Arc Maculopathy

Case Summary

An 18-year-old boy was seen with complaints of persistent visual loss following exposure to welding arc 3 months ago. He gave history of developing keratoconjuctivitis following welding arc exposure that resolved a week later but the visual loss persisted. The fundus was unremarkable (A, B)

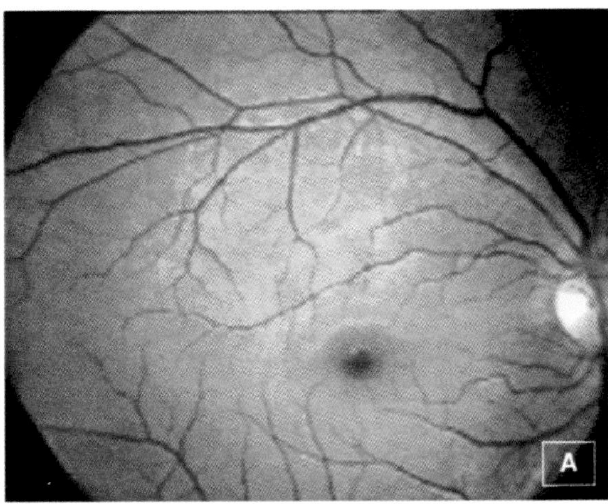
A

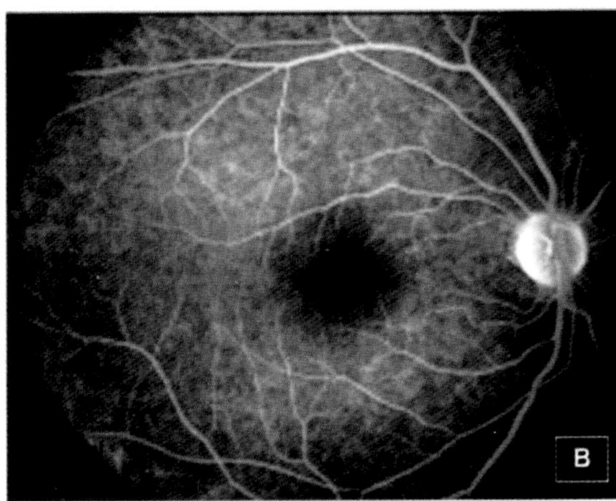
B

Optical Coherence Tomography

Horizontal OCT line scans through the foveal center (C) showed normal foveal contour with intact inner layers and disruption in the RPE complex under the fovea. **OCT was able to depict subtle changes at the ultrastructural level that could not be seen either on fundus examination or fluorescein angiography.**

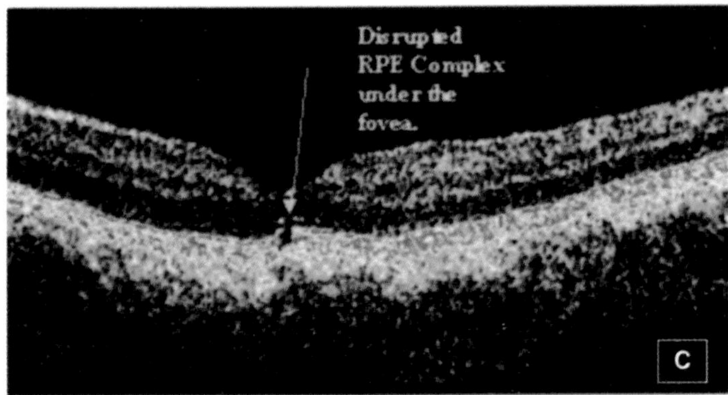

C

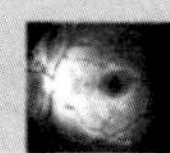

Case 16.3: Lightening Maculopathy

Case Summary

A 19-year old Indian male was exposed to lightening when it struck his house 2 years back, following which he had progressive decrease in vision in both eyes. At the time of presentation, his best-corrected visual acuity was 20/300 in both eyes. Slit lamp bimicroscopy revealed bilateral posterior subcapsular cataract. He underwent phacoemulsification with posterior chamber intraocular lens implantation in the left eye. One-week postoperatively, his best-corrected visual acuity was 20/200 in the left eye. Fundus examination showed prominent retinal striae with linear and circumlinear, granular, hypopigmented bands and granular pigmentation in the foveal center (A). Fundus fluorescein angiography (FFA) was non-contributory (B).

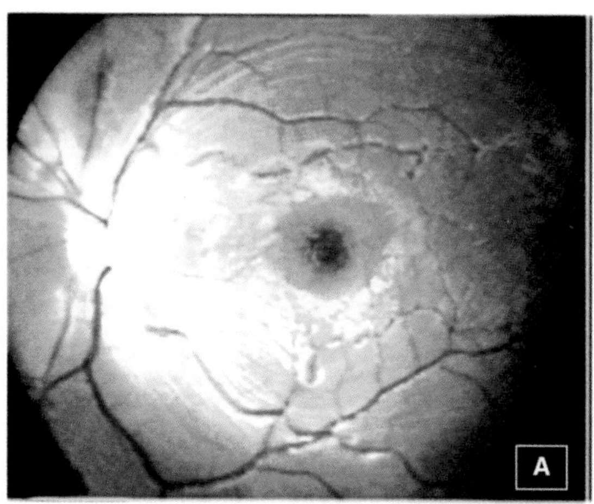

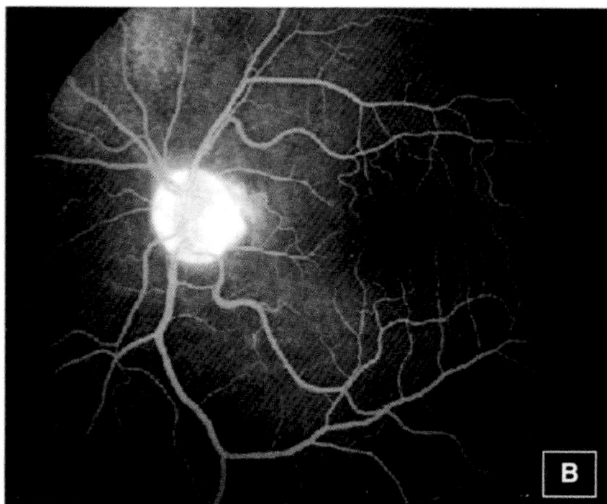

Optical Coherence Tomography

OCT scan of the left eye through the fovea showed a hypo-reflective area between the inner and outer reflective bands with few bridging septae seen in-between. There was a loss of foveal contour with thinning of overlying retina and the presence of cystic spaces in the inner retinal layers (C). OCT scan of the right eye too showed similar changes though a good quality scan could not be obtained due to the cataract. **The intraretinal fluid accumulation that was seen on OCT was not seen on fundoscopy or fluorescein angiography.**

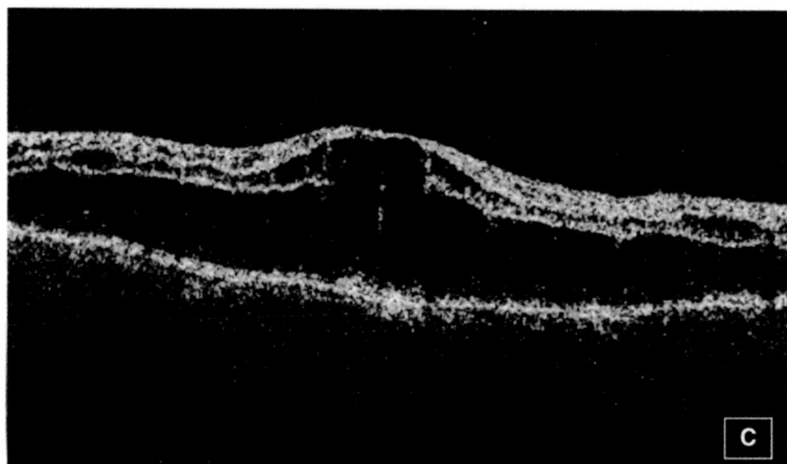

The diagnosis of lightening maculopathy was made and the patient received oral acetazolamide 125 mg thrice a day. Three weeks later his vision in the left eye improved to 20/80 and fundus showed disappearance of retinal striae, though cystic changes persisted. Repeat OCT scan showed foveal contour returning to normal, both inner and outer reflective bands could be demarcated and the bridging septae became better delineated (D).

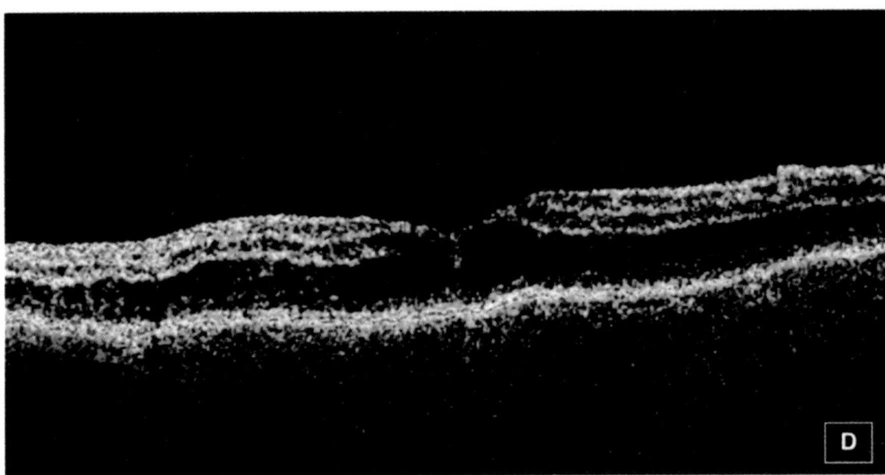

The patient discontinued oral acetazolamide four weeks later following which his vision in the left eye dropped to 5/60 with repeat scan showing loss of foveal contour and both inner and outer reflective bands were separated with hypo-reflective band in-between (E).

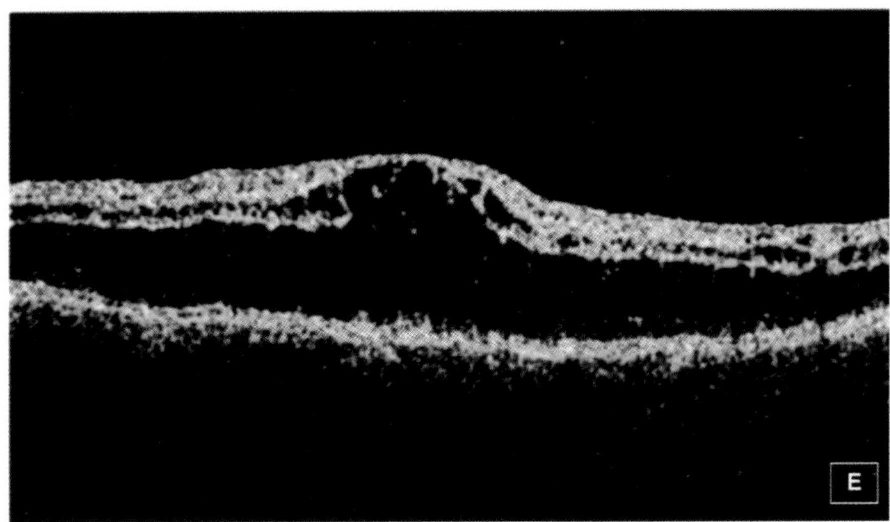

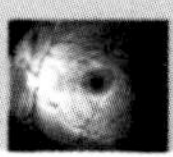

Oral acetazolamide 125 mg t.i.d was restarted. Repeat OCT scan, 6 weeks later (F), again showed good response to oral acetazolamide with vision improving to 6/24 in the left eye; with normal foveal contour and retinal structure though few cystic spaces were still persistent in the inner retinal layers. The patient continued to receive oral acetazolamide.

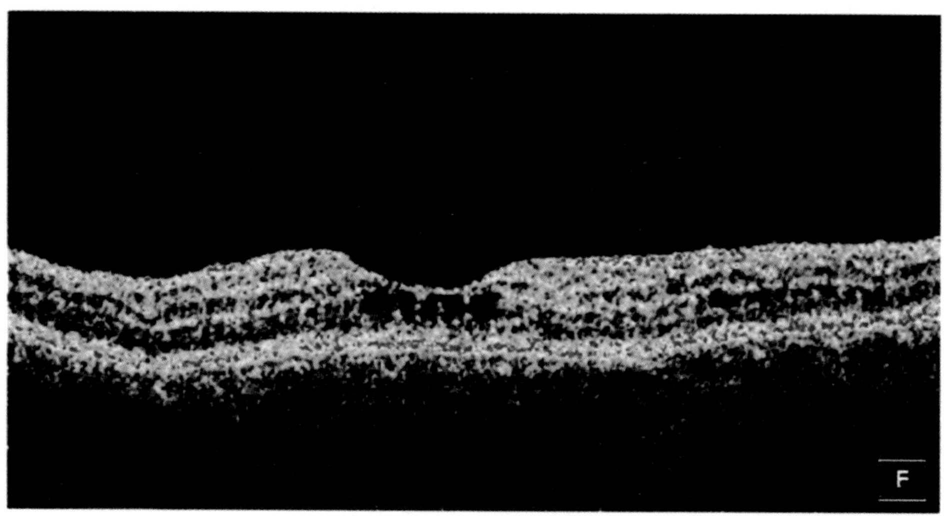

CONCLUSIONS

Photic maculopathy might produce many subtle changes in the RPE-photoreceptor complex or in the neurosensory retina. OCT was useful in depicting these changes, where conventional imaging techniques including fundus photography and fluorescein angiography failed. In lightening induced maculopathy, OCT was found to be helpful in depicting macular edema that responded to oral acetazolamide.

SUGGESTED READING

1. Gass JDM. Photic maculopathy. In Gass JDM (Ed). Steroscopic Atlas of Macular Diseases 1997, Mosby-Year Book Inc.1997, 760-69.

Chapter 17

Optic Disc Pit

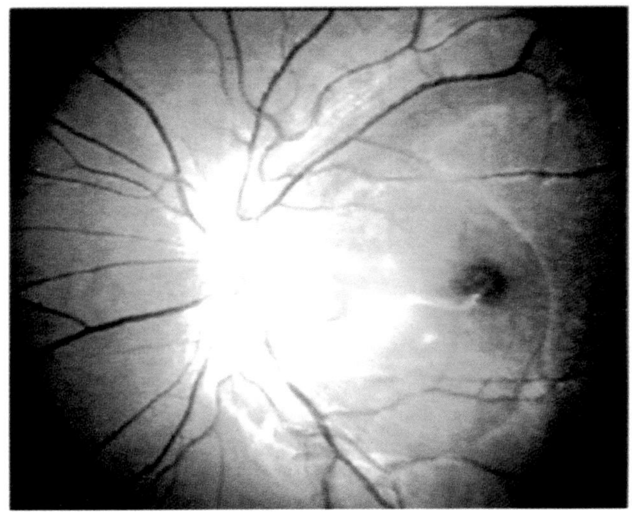

Congenital pits of the optic nerve head develop serous detachment of macula usually between 20 to 40 years of age in 25 to 75 percent of the patients. The pathogenesis of the detachment is believed to be the passage of fluid from the area of pit into the subretinal space. The origin of this fluid is unclear, though it is believed to be probably originating from the vitreous cavity, vessels at the base of the pit or cerebrospinal fluid from subarachnoid space.

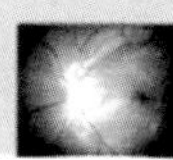

Case 17.1: Optic Disc Pit with no Clinical Macular Detachment

Case Summary

A 24-year-old boy was diagnosed to have an optic nerve head pit in his right eye on routine checkup. His best-corrected visual acuity was 20/20 in this eye. Fundoscopy (A) revealed a small, round; optic nerve head pit inferotemporally (arrow). The macula did not show any changes.

Optical Coherence Tomography

Horizontal OCT line scan through the optic disc pit (B, C) showed a deep pit in the temporal aspect of the cup (arrow). The peripapillary retina and fovea were normal on OCT.

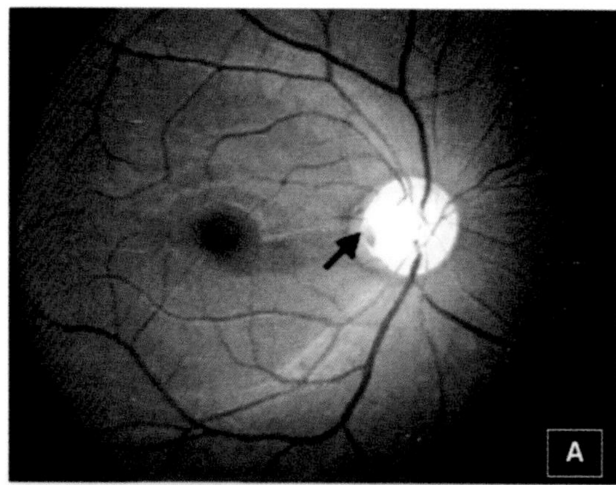

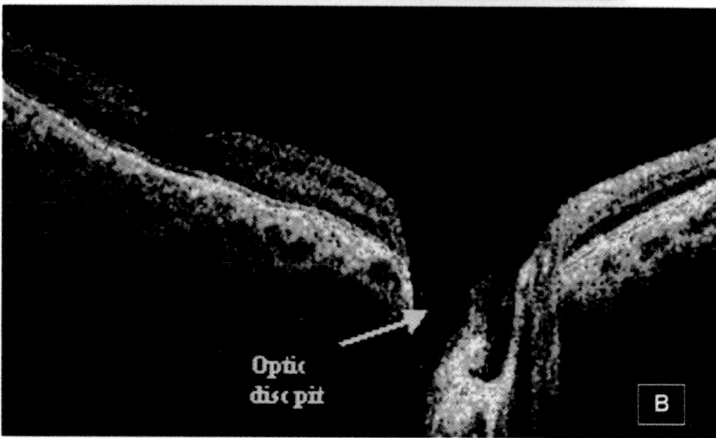

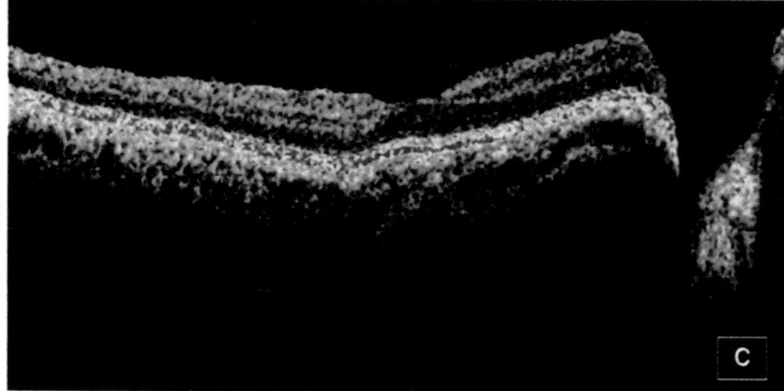

Case 17.2: Optic Disc Pit with Serous Macular Detachment

Case Summary

A 22- year-old man presented with blurred vision that fluctuated in the left eye of 3 months duration. His best-corrected visual acuity was 20/200. There was serous detachment of the macula that extended to the margin of the optic disc pit (arrow) (A). Fluorescein angiography showed the staining in the area of optic disc pit and absence of dye in the subretinal fluid (B). The lack of fluorescein dye indicated probably the presence of cerebrospinal fluid.

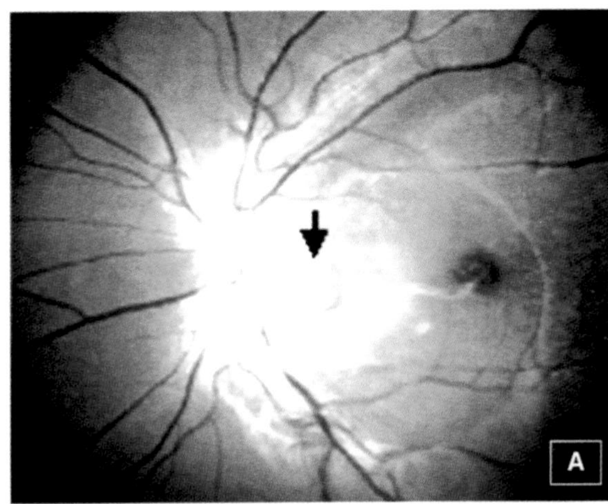

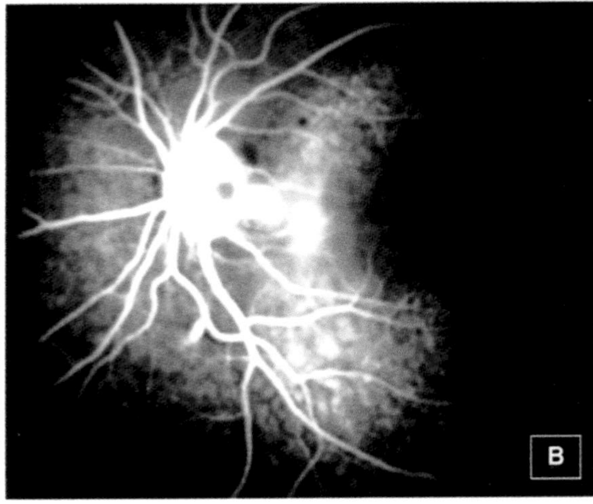

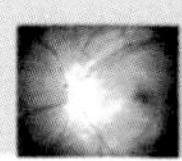

Optical Coherence Tomography

Optical coherence tomography of the left eye through different levels (C, D) showed cystoid changes and schisis cavity formation in the peripapillary retina. The retinoschisis in the peripapillary area seemed to continue into a neurosensory retinal detachment under the fovea. This detachment seemed to communicate with the optic nerve head. The retina showed small cystic spaces.

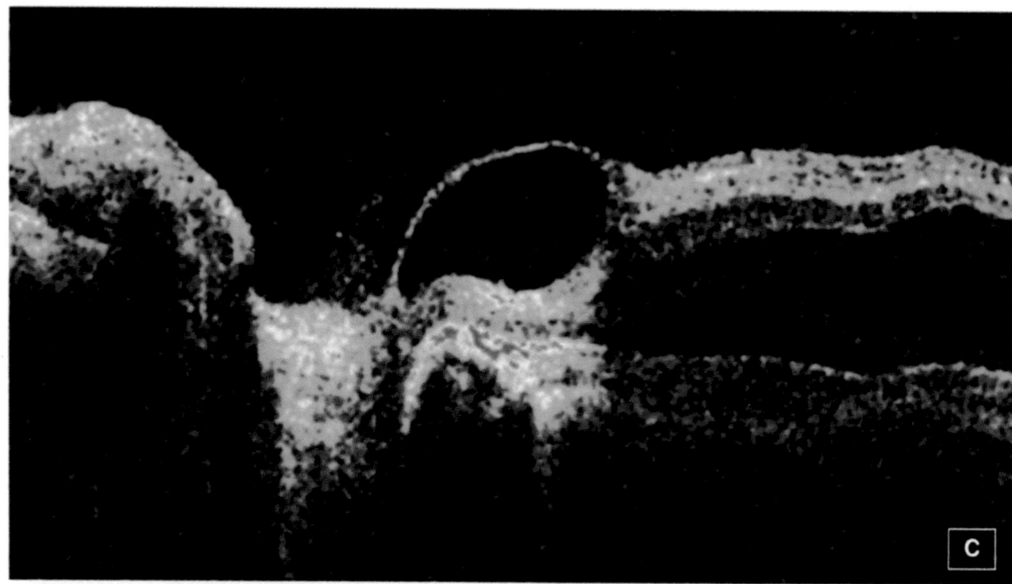

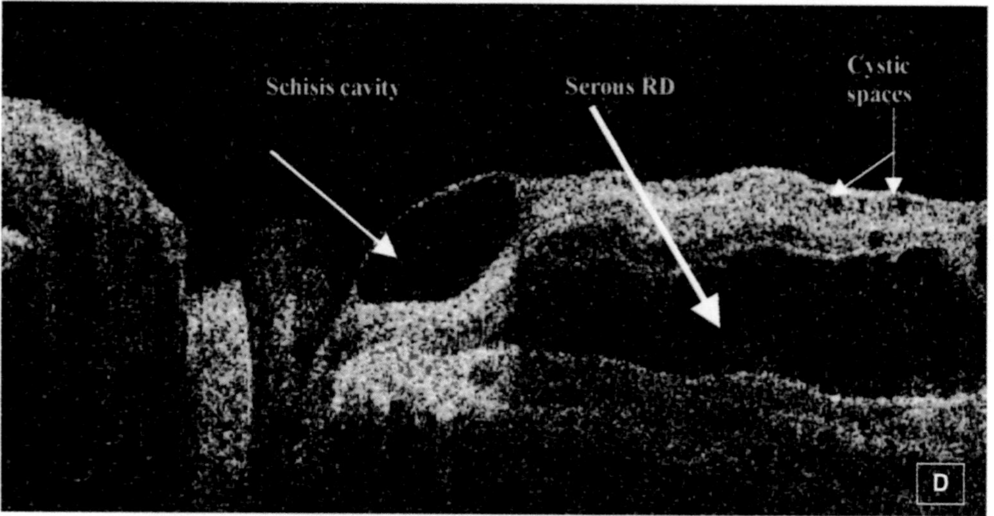

Case 17.3: PPV for Optic Disc Pit and Serous Macular Detachment

Case Summary

A 30-year-old woman was seen with visual loss in her right eye of two years duration. Her best-corrected visual acuity in this eye was 20/100. Fundoscopy (A) revealed an optic nerve head pit with associated macular detachment.

Optical Coherence Tomography

A horizontal OCT line scan through the macula (B) showed inner retinoschisis cavity with retinal tissue bridging the two layers suggesting schisis cavities and cystoid spaces. This inner cavity communicated with a space that dissected through the temporal aspect of the optic nerve suggesting a probable communication between this cavity and optic nerve head. In addition, there was another cavity below the inner cavity seen under the fovea that did not seem to communicate with the inner cavity.

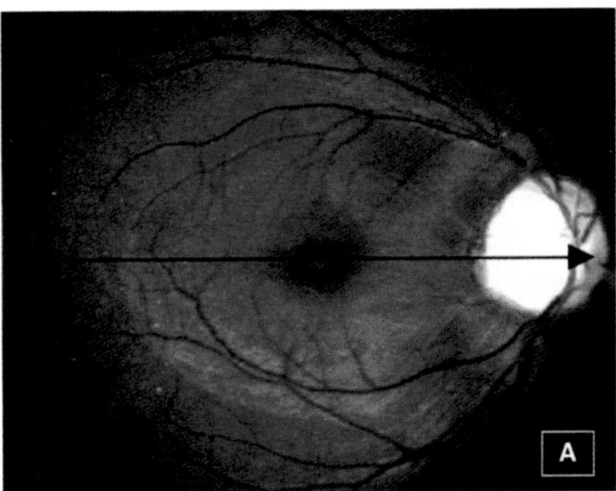

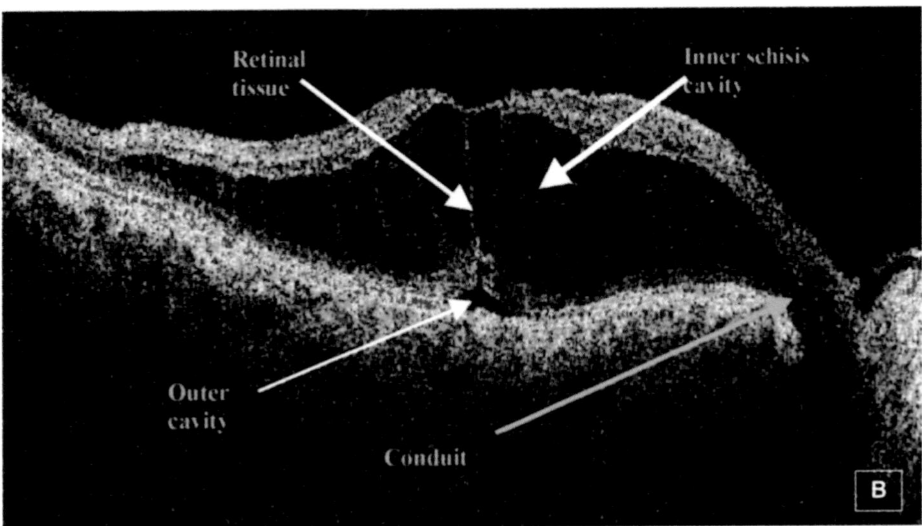

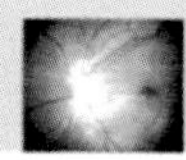

Two months later, the repeat OCT scan (C) showed an increase in the outer schisis cavity with the development of a hole in the outer lamella of retinoschisis. The inner retina temporal to the disc showed cystoid stages. In view of progression of the disease, the patient was offered pars plana vitrectomy.

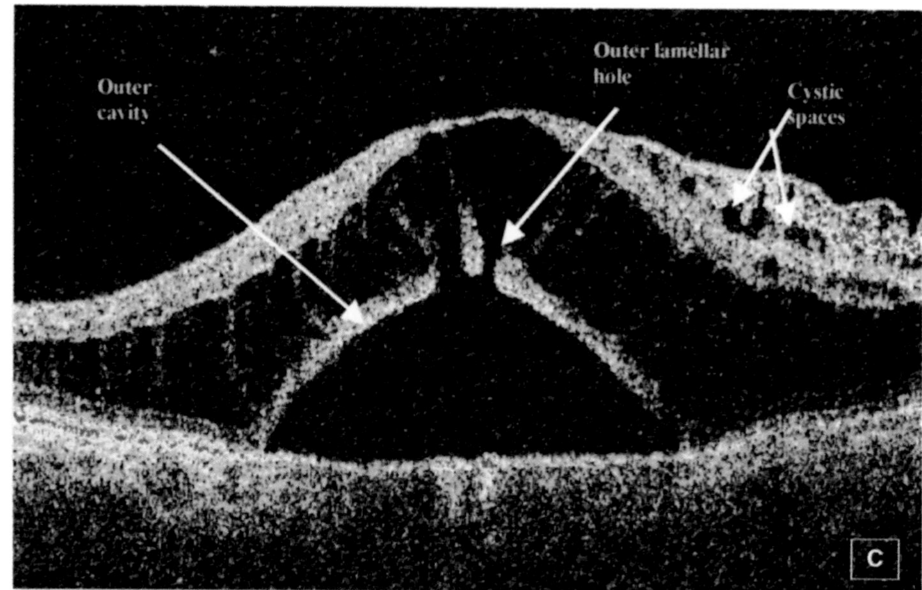

The patient underwent pars plana vitrectomy with separation of posterior hyloid, drainage of fluid through optic disc pit, $C_3 F_8$ gas temponade and laser photocoagulation around the tract. The fluid drained through the pit was sent for biochemical analysis and was found to be cerebrospinal fluid. One week following surgery, fundus showed approximately 30 percent gas fill with central macular detachment (D).

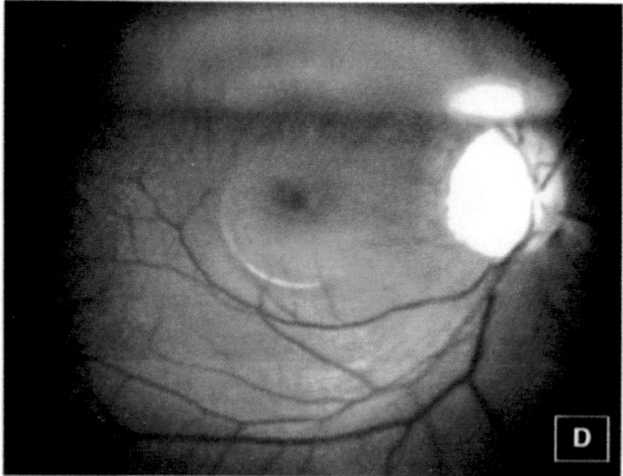

Repeat OCT scan(E, F) through the pit showed closure of track communicating between the optic disc pit and retina. The temporal edge of the retinoschisis cavity started getting attached to the overlying neurosensory retina and collapse of inner retinoschisis cavitiy was seen temporally.

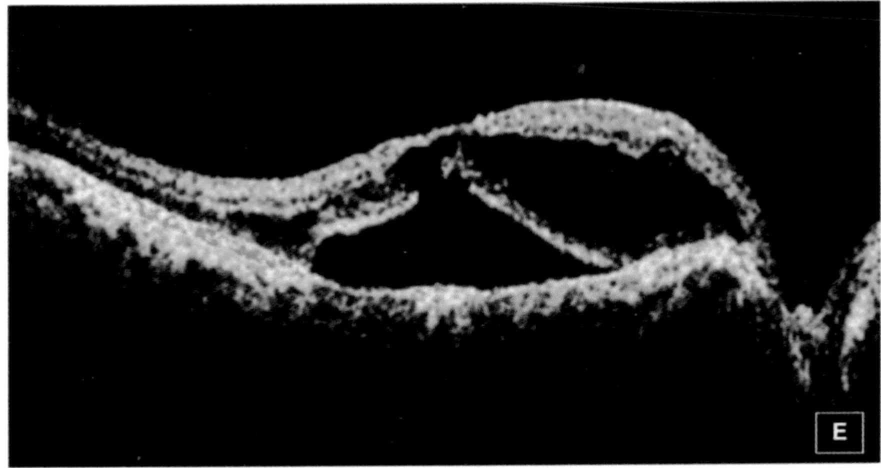

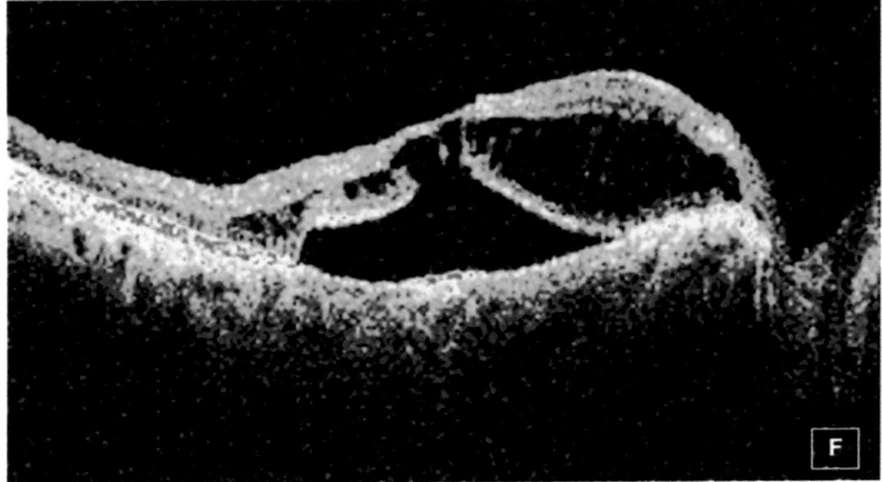

CONCLUSIONS

OCT confirms the original belief that schisis formation is crucial in the development of serous retinal detachment in optic disc pits. This also confirms the theory that the optic disc pit is infact a conduit that allows the flow of cerebrospinal fluid between the subarachnoid and subretinal space.

SUGGESTED READINGS

1. Lincoff H, Lopez R, Kreissig I et al. Retinoschisis associated with optic nerve pits. Arch Ophthalmol 1988;106:61-67.
2. Krivoy D, Gentile R, Geffery M et al. Imaging congenital optic disc pits and associated maculopathy using optical coherence tomography. Arch Ophthalmol 1996;114:165-70.

Chapter 18

Inflammatory Diseases of Retina-choroid

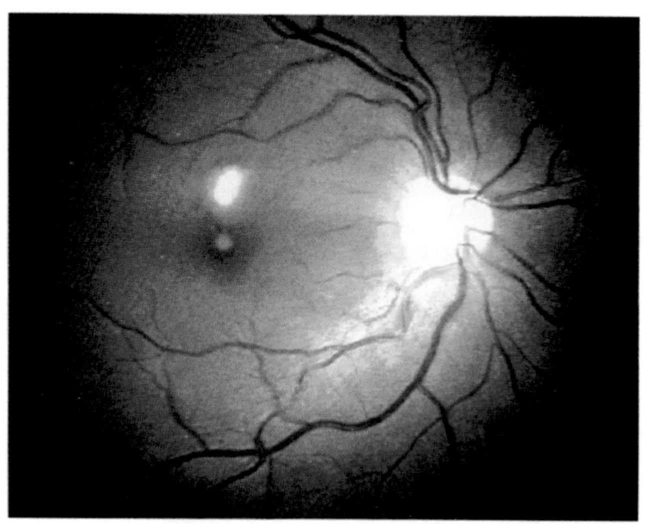

OCT IN CHORIORETINAL INFLAMMATIONS

OCT has been found to be useful in the management of intraocular inflammations in the following ways:

1. OCT is able to define the extent, depth and thickness of the inflammatory lesion. It helps to localize the layer of retina-choroid harboring the lesion. This localization is helpful in not only diagnosing the disease but also in monitoring the response to treatment.
2. OCT is helpful in depicting the associated secondary changes like cystoid macular edema, choroidal neovascular membrane, epiretinal membrane, subretinal fluid and subretinal fibrosis.

TOXOPLASMIC RETINOCHOROIDITIS

Toxoplasma gondii, an intracellular parasite can get transmitted to the fetus either *in utero,* i.e. congenital, or, less commonly, retina gets involved in acquired variety due to ingestion of the organism. In congenital toxoplasmosis, the retinal involvement is a part of generalized infection and is characterized by the presence of a large, atrophic, excavated scar in the macula or elsewhere. Acquired form is characterized by the presence of focal necrotizing retinitis with involvement of inner retinal layers and overlying vitritis. These active lesions may be seen adjacent to the old chorioretinal scar. Another variant is the development of punctuate outer or deep retinal lesions. Choroidal neovascular membrane may develop in some of these patients.

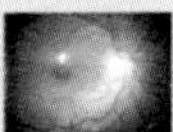

Case 18.1: Congenital Toxoplasmic Scar

Case Summary

A 20-year-old boy was seen with bilateral congenital toxoplasmic scar (A). The scar showed three zones

1. Outer white zone,
2. Intermediate zone with pigmentary hyperplasia
3. Inner dark zone of atrophy.

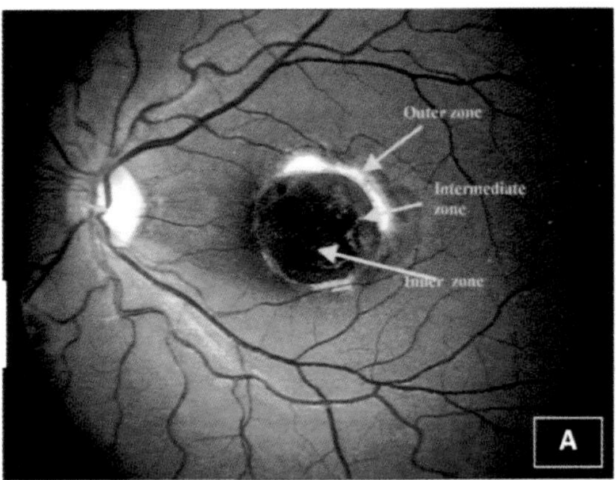

OCT line scan through the superior margin of the scar (B) showed increased hyper-reflectivity from the underlying Retinal Pigment Epithelium (RPE) and choroid with intact overlying neurosensory retina. The scan line through the outer whitish band showed hyper-reflectivity suggesting the presence of a fibrous scar (arrow).

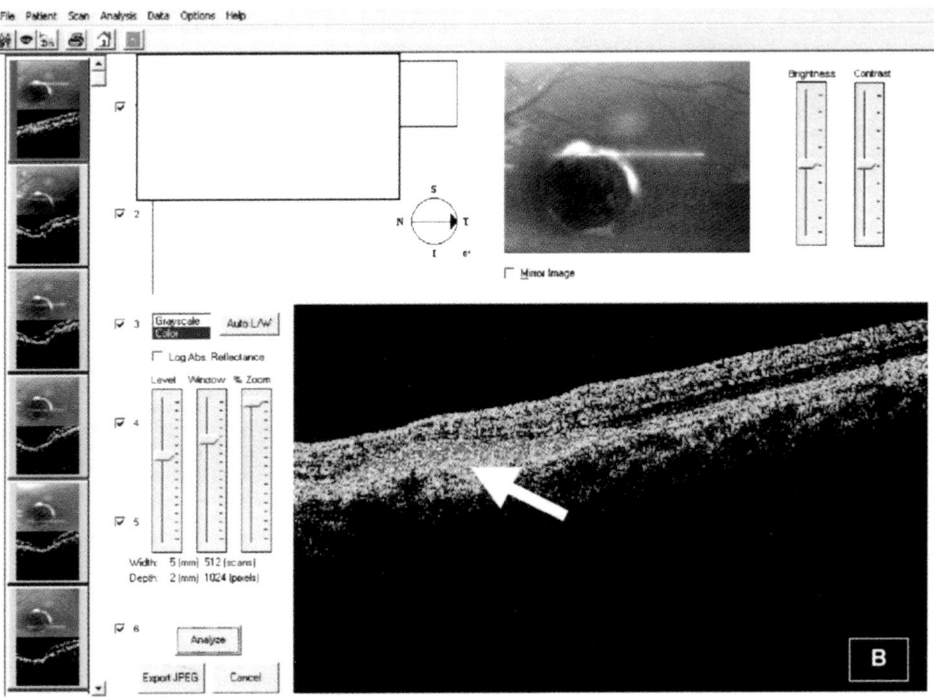

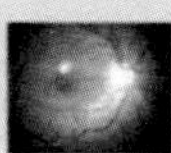

Optical Coherence Tomography

The line scan passing through the intermediate zone (C) showed atrophy of neurosensory retina though some redundant tissue was still persistent.

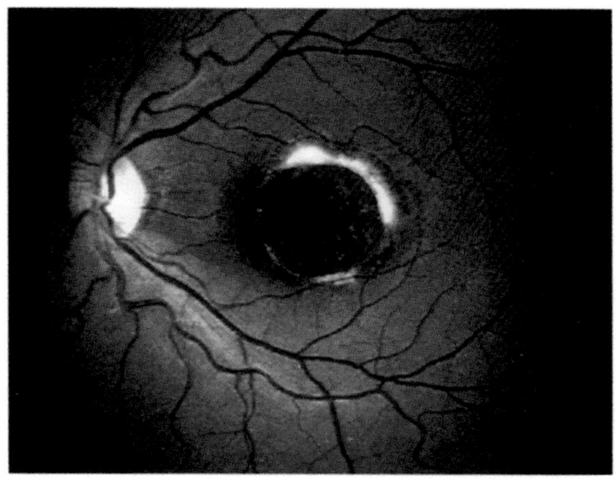

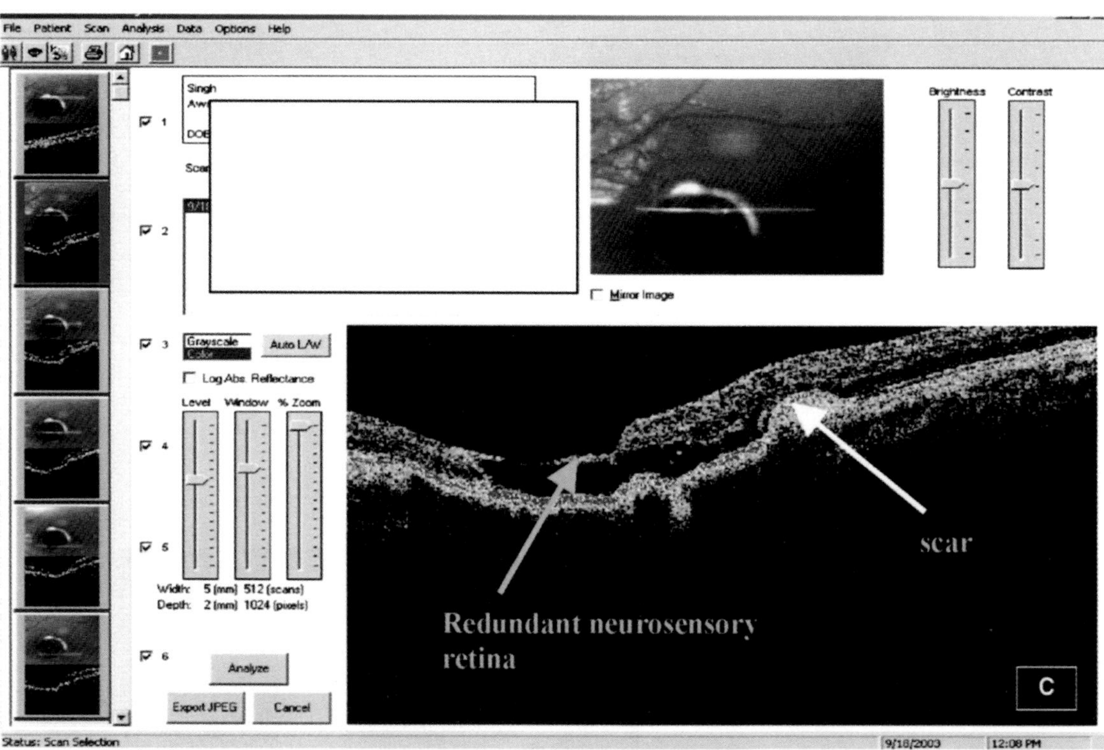

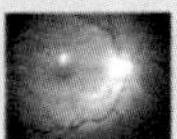

Optical Coherence Tomography

The OCT line scan through the central zone (D) showed total absence of neurosensory retina over the central area. **Note the absence of RPE-choroid hypertrophy indicating that the congenital toxoplasmosis scar has the central area of retinal atrophy**.

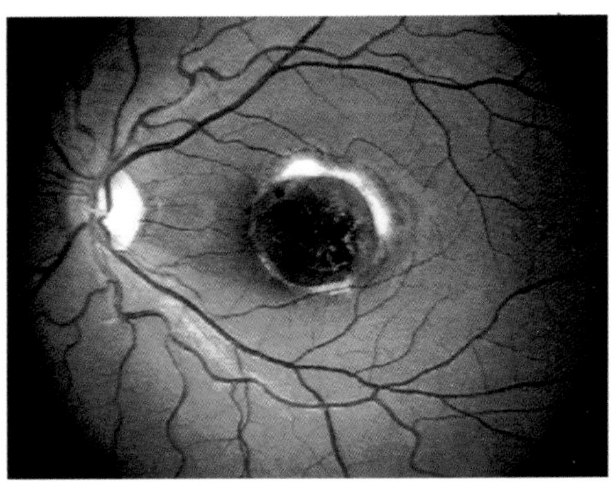

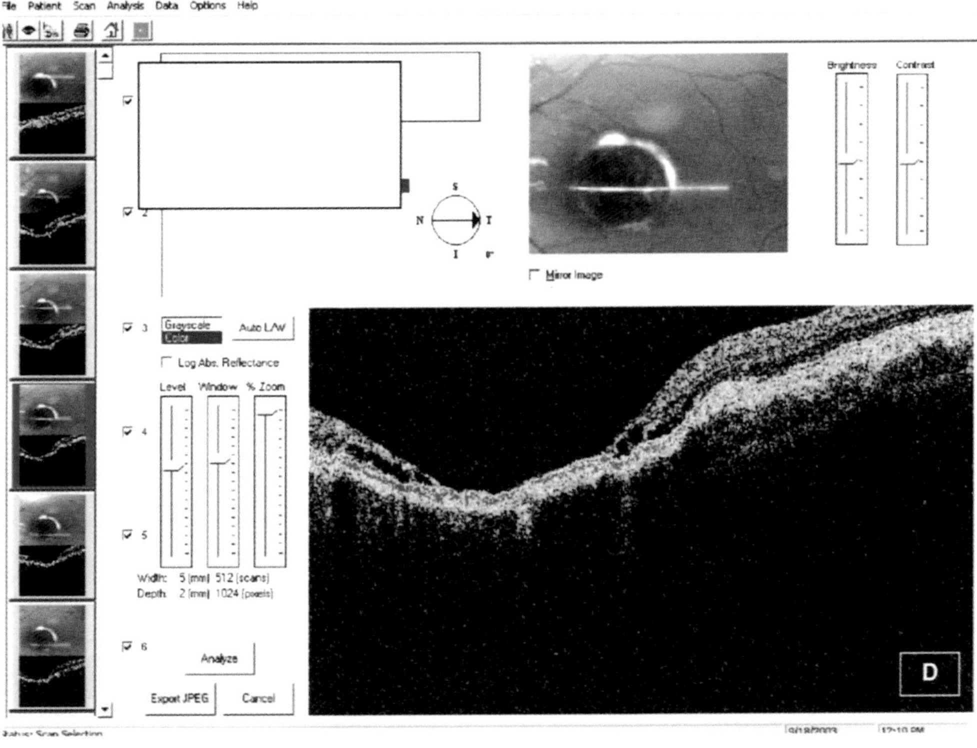

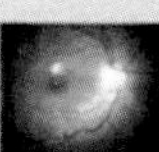

Case 18.2: Acquired Toxoplasmic Retinochoroiditis

Case Summary

A 26-year-old woman was seen with a patch of focal retinochoroiditis with overlying vitreous reaction (A). Fluorescein angiography showed initial hypofluorescence and late hyperfluorescence of the lesion indicating active inflammation (B, C). The visual acuity was reduced to 20/100.

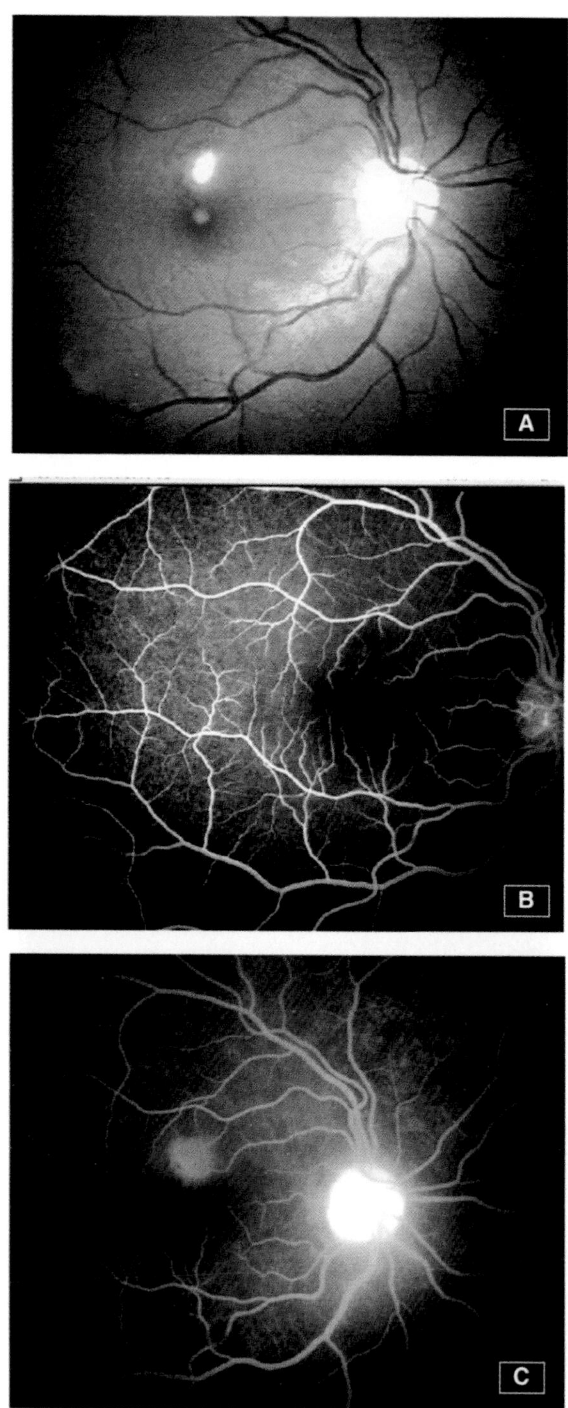

Optical Coherence Tomography

Horizontal OCT line scan through the lesion (D) showed a well-defined, raised area of hyper-reflectivity in the inner retinal layers. The hyper reflectivity from the lesion shadowed the signals from the underlying retina. The location of the lesion was consistent with the toxoplasmic retinitis that involves the inner retina primarily.

The patient was treated with oral bactrim and prednisolone.

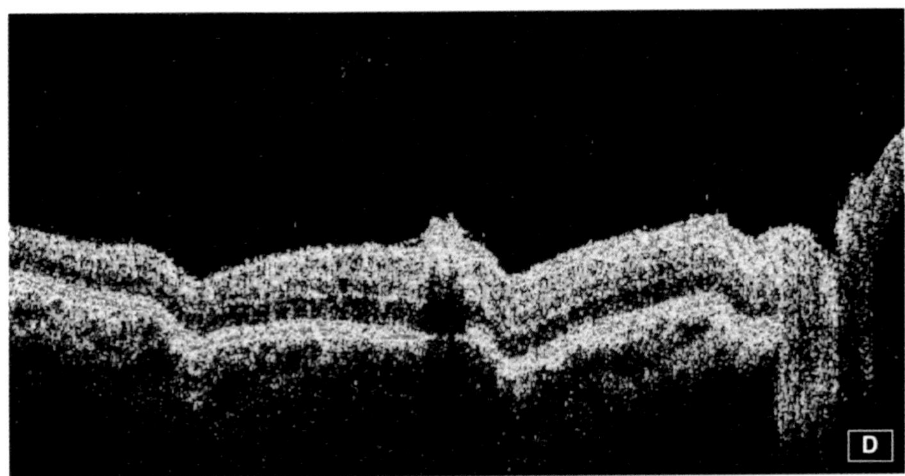

Ten days later, the visual acuity was improved to 20/80 and the lesion had become more organized (E). Repeat OCT showed that the area of hyper-reflectivity in the inner retina was smaller, and more localized than before (F).

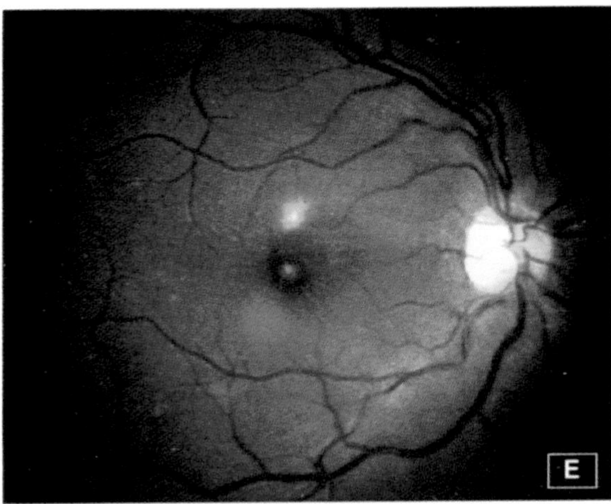

Three weeks later, her visual acuity had improved to 20/30 (G). Repeat OCT scan (H) showed flattening of inner retinal layer with reduced backscattering from the outer retinal layers. Focal areas of fragmentation were seen in the RPE, probably suggesting the RPE attempt to proliferate.

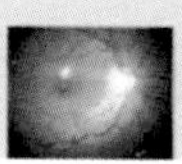

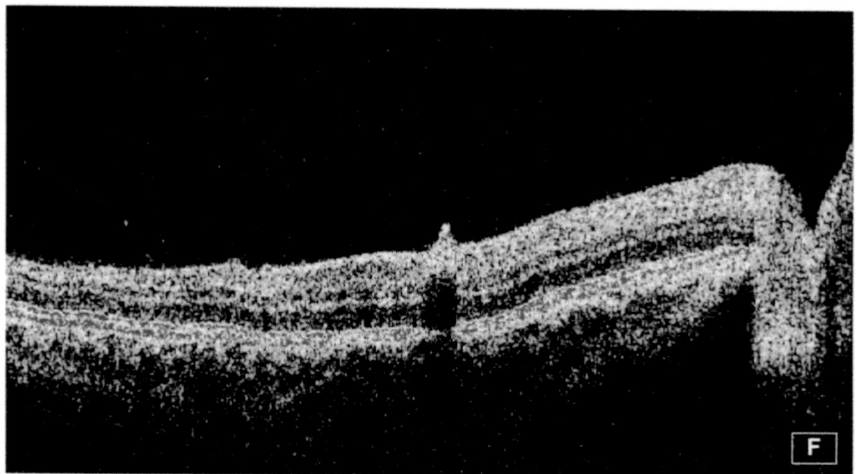
F

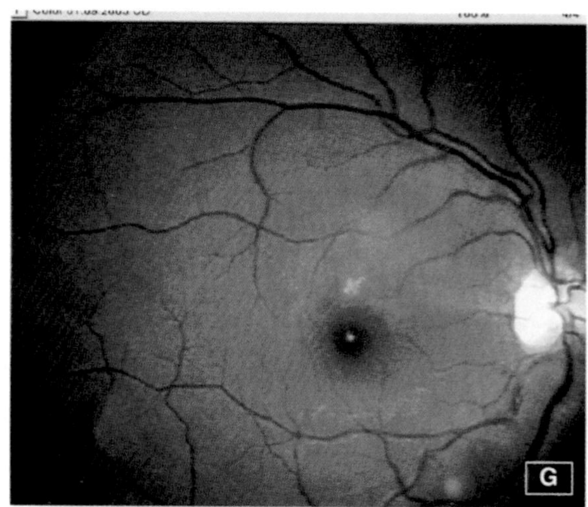
G

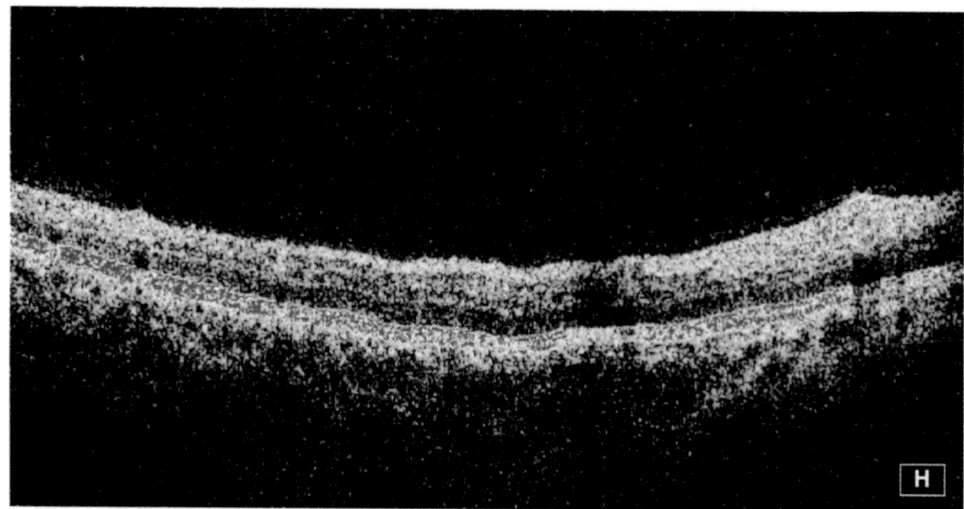
H

Case 18.3: Type II Choroidal Neovascular Membrane (CNVM) in Toxoplasmosis

Case Summary

A 25-year-old woman was seen with decreased vision in her right eye of 8 months duration. Her best corrected visual acuity was 20/200 in the right eye. She was diagnosed as toxoplasmosic retino-choroiditis elsewhere and was receiving treatment for the same. Fundoscopy and fluorescein angiography revealed the presence of CNVM adjacent to the scar (A).

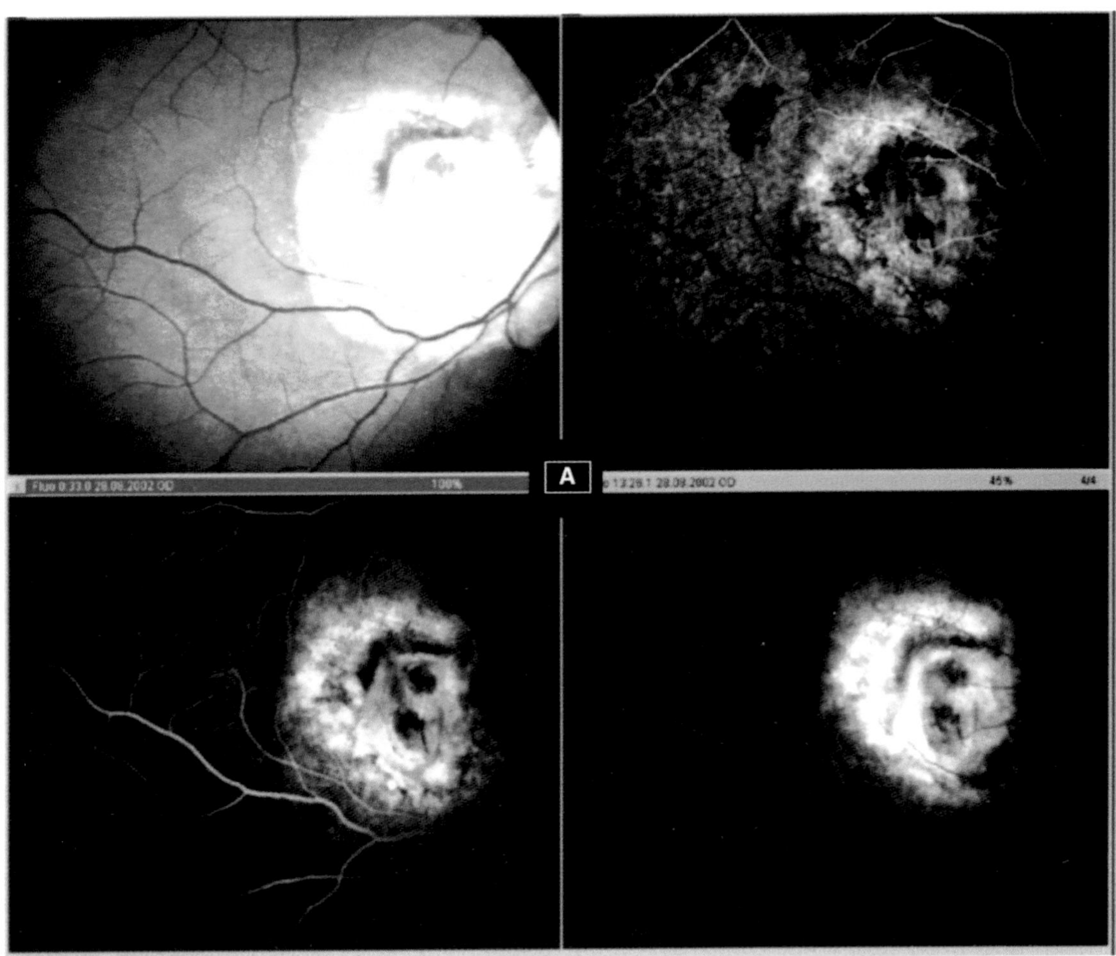

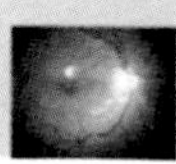

Optical Coherence Tomography

OCT scan through various levels of the CNVM (B,C) showed an area of moderately intense hyper-reflectivity in the outer retinal layers both nasal and temporal to the fovea (arrows) with hyporeflective area under the fovea suggestive of subretinal fluid.

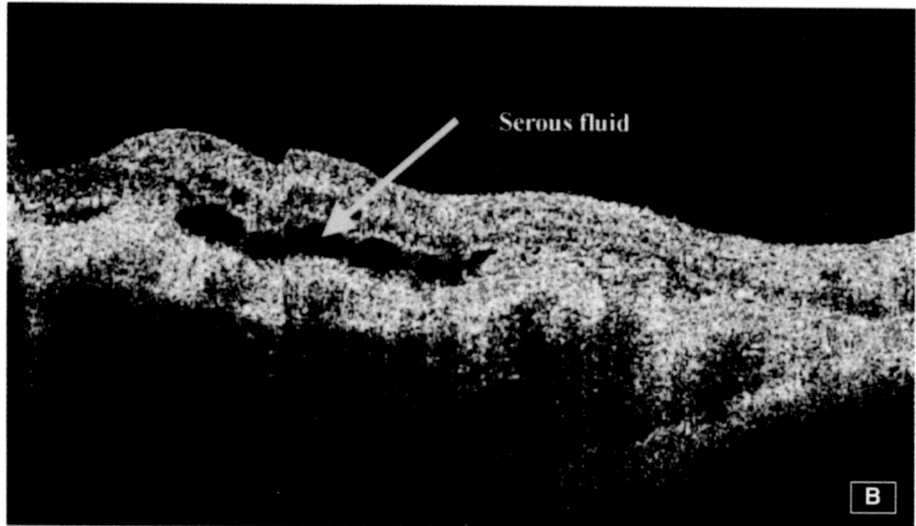

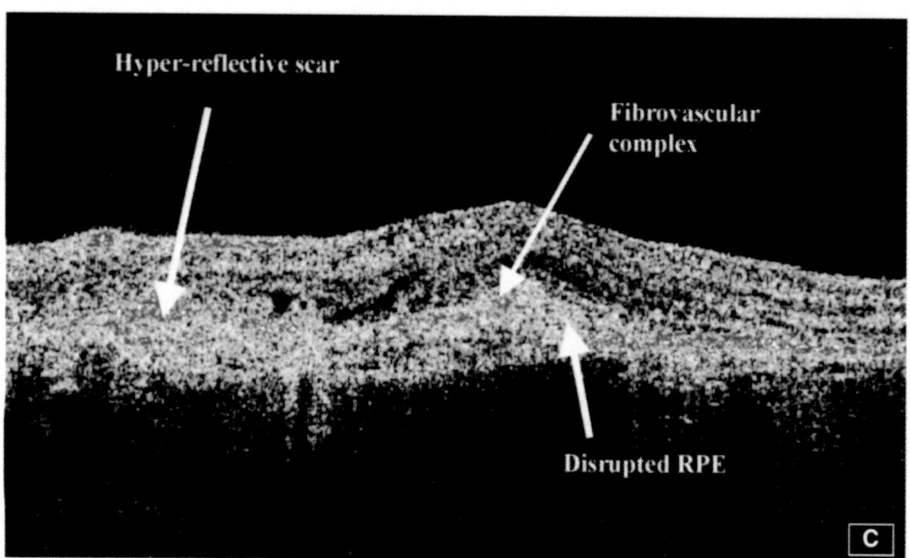

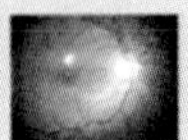

Case 18.4 Congenital Toxoplamsmosis Scar with Central Serous Chorioretinopathy (CSC)

Case Summary

A 20-year-old boy was seen with active toxoplasmic retinochoroiditis adjacent to a congenital toxoplasmosis scar which responded to oral clindamycin and prednisolone (not shown). Two years later he came back with complaints of blurred vision in his right eye of 10 days duration.

His best corrected visual acuity in this eye was 20/70. Fundus showed the presence of healed pigmented scar with surrounding serous retinal detachment. Since the patient was allergic to fluorescein dye, the angiography could not be performed. The indocyanine green angiography showed choroidal hyper-permeability with diffuse staining and silhouetting of retinal vessels suggestive of CSC. No neovascular membrane was seen on ICG (A).

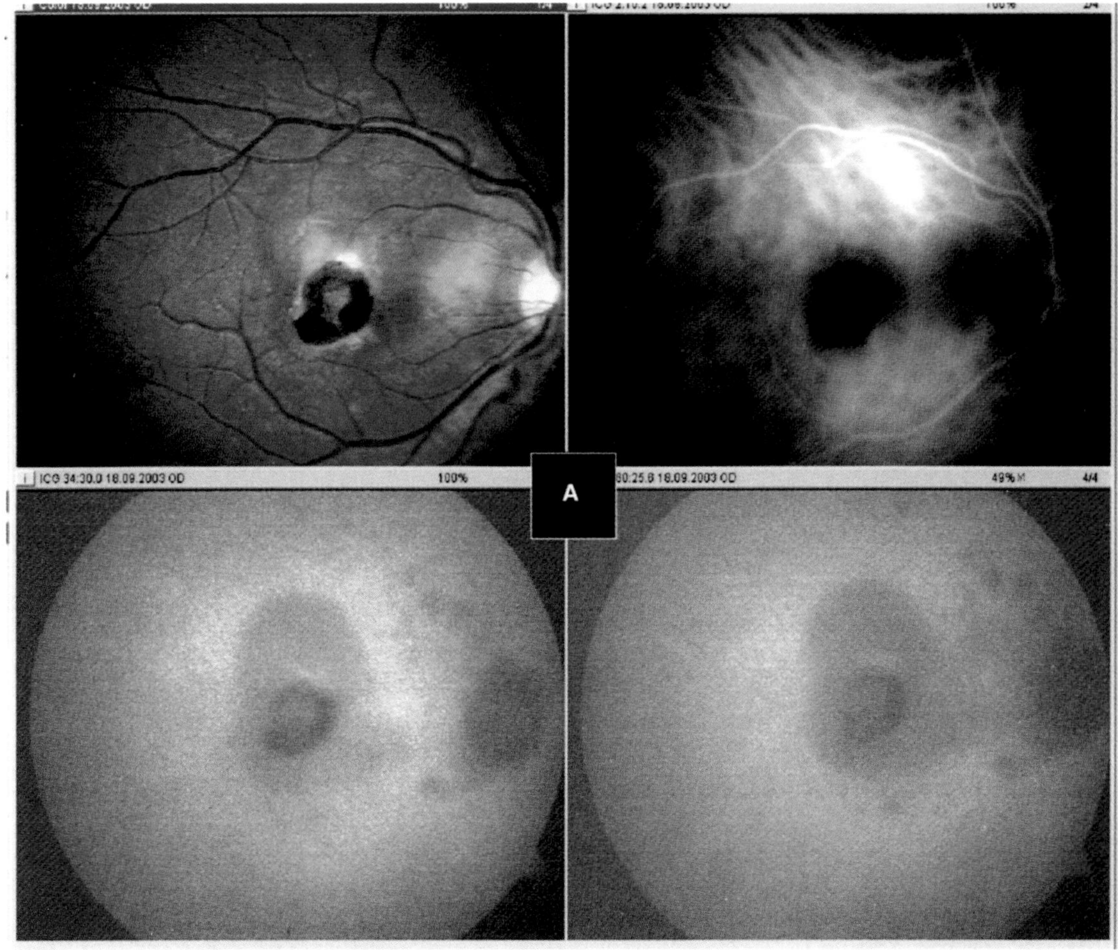

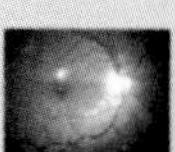

Optical Coherence Tomography

OCT line scan superior to the scar (B) showed an area of hyporeflectivity separating neurosensory retina from RPE suggesting the presence of serous retinal detachment. Note the absence of an underlying choroidal neovascular membrane.

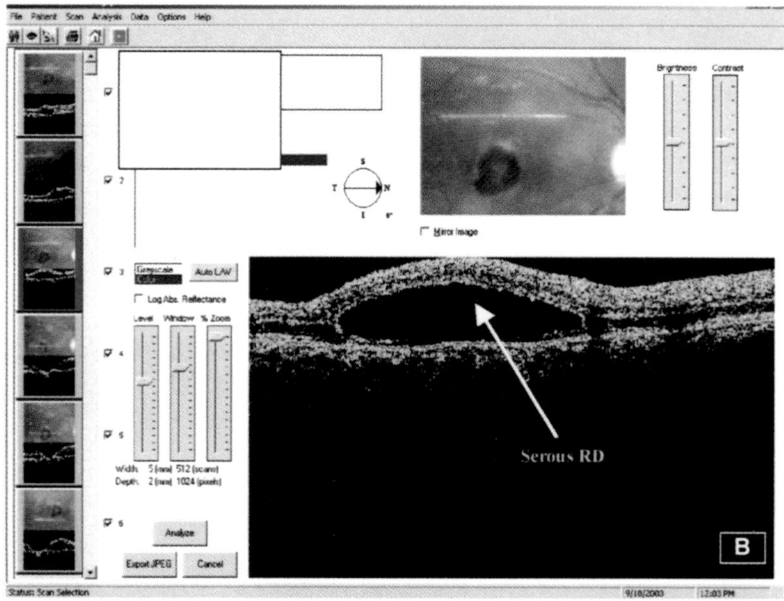

The OCT line scan through the scar (C) showed the presence of serous fluid nasally, absence of neurosensory retina overlying the central scar and a pocket of fluid temporal to the scar as well, indicating that serous fluid was straddling the previous scar. OCT helped in establishing the diagnosis of central serous chorioretinopathy in this patient.

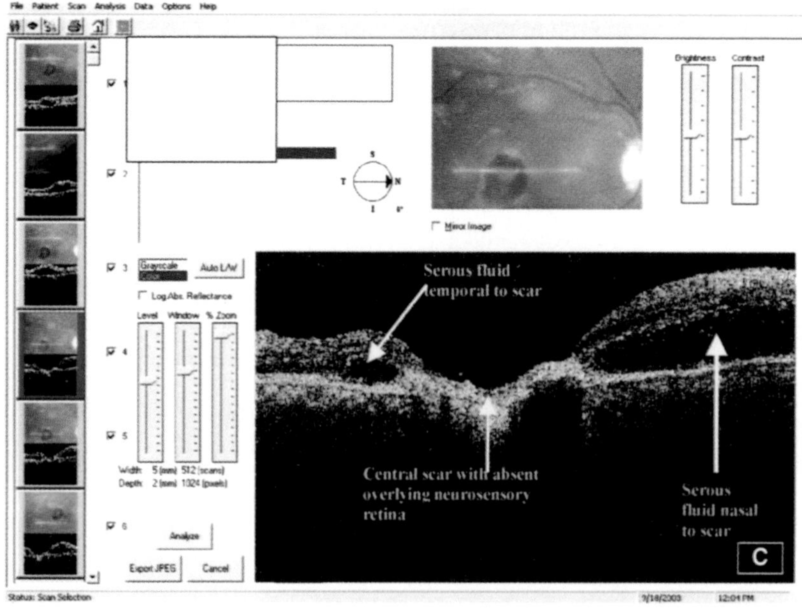

CONCLUSIONS

1. On OCT, the congenital toxoplsmic scar was seen as an area of atrophy with absence of overlying neurosensory retina.
2. The acute patch of retinochoroiditis was distinctly seen as hyper-reflective layers in the inner retina suggesting that the active inflammation was primarily in the inner retinal layers. OCT can be very useful tool in monitoring the response to therapy.
3. OCT can be useful in diagnosing the presence of choroidal neovascular membranes, if any.

SUGGESTED READING

1. Chorioretinal inflammatory Diseases Chapter 9. In Optical Coherence Tomography of Ocular Diseases Puliafito. CA, Hee MR, Schuman JS, Fujimoto JG (Eds). Slack Inc. 1996;249-68.

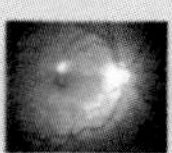

INTERMEDIATE UVEITIS

Case 18.5: Pars Planitis with Cystoid Macular Edema

Case Summary

A 40-year-old man was seen with a visual acuity of 20/40 in the right eye. He was diagnosed as a case of pars planitis with cystoid macular edema grade IV on fluorescein angiography (A). The patient had 1 + vitreous cells with snow balls inferiorly.

Optical Coherence Tomography

OCT line scan through the fovea showed the presence of cystoid macular edema (B).

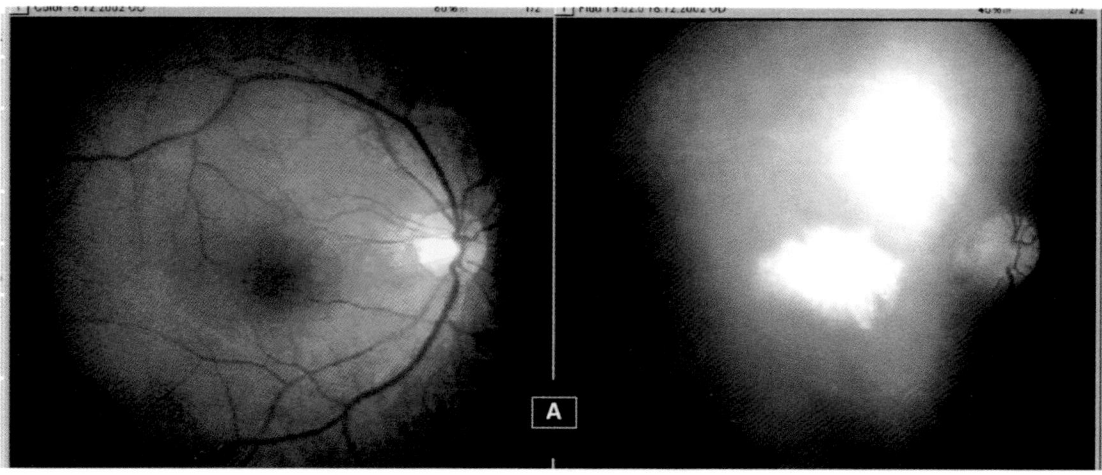

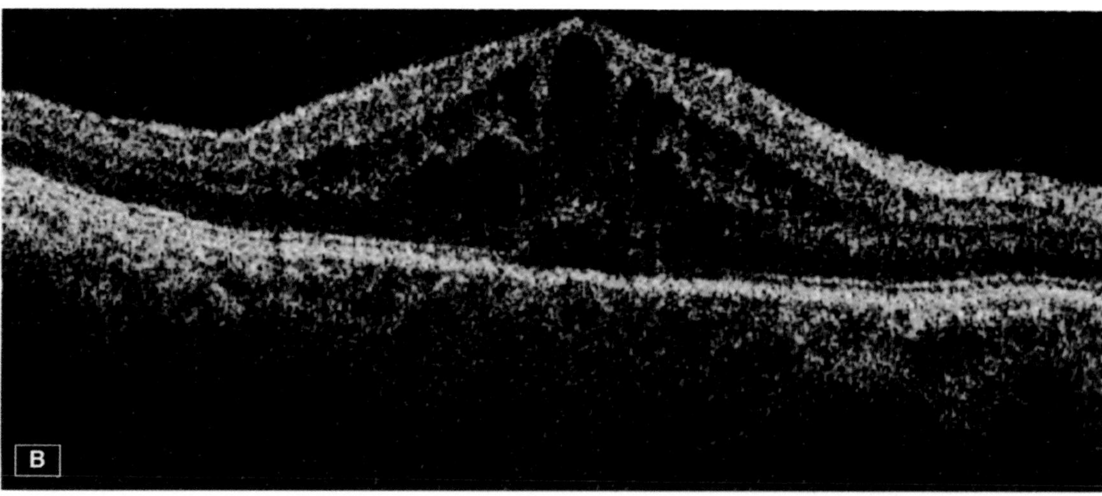

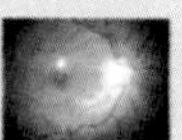

Central retinal thickness was measured on Retinal Map Analysis that showed the central retinal thickness measuring 496 μ (C). The patient was given posterior subtenon injection of triamcinolone acetonide 20 mg.

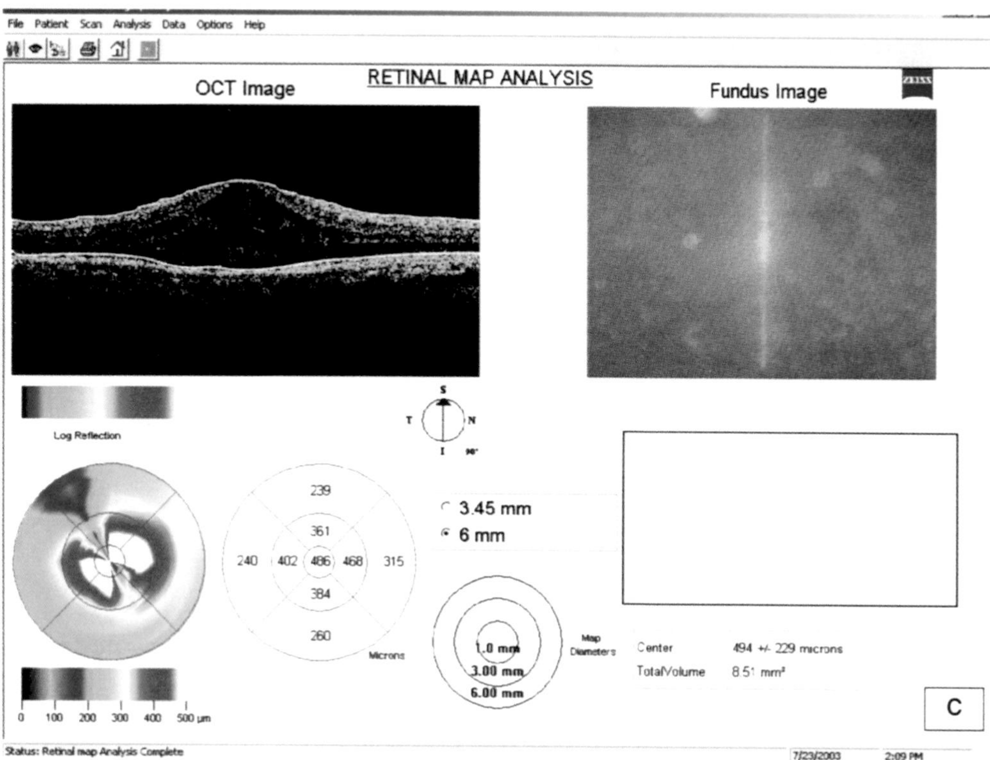

Four weeks later, repeat OCT scan (D) showed resolution of cystoid spaces with normal foveal contour. Repeat retinal map analysis showed central retinal thickness reduced to 256 μ (E).

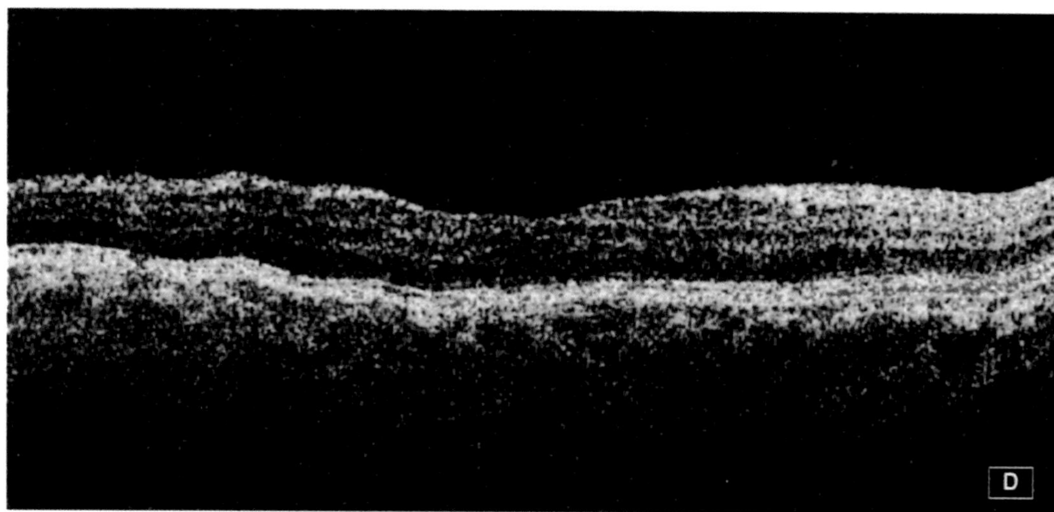

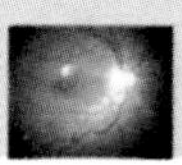

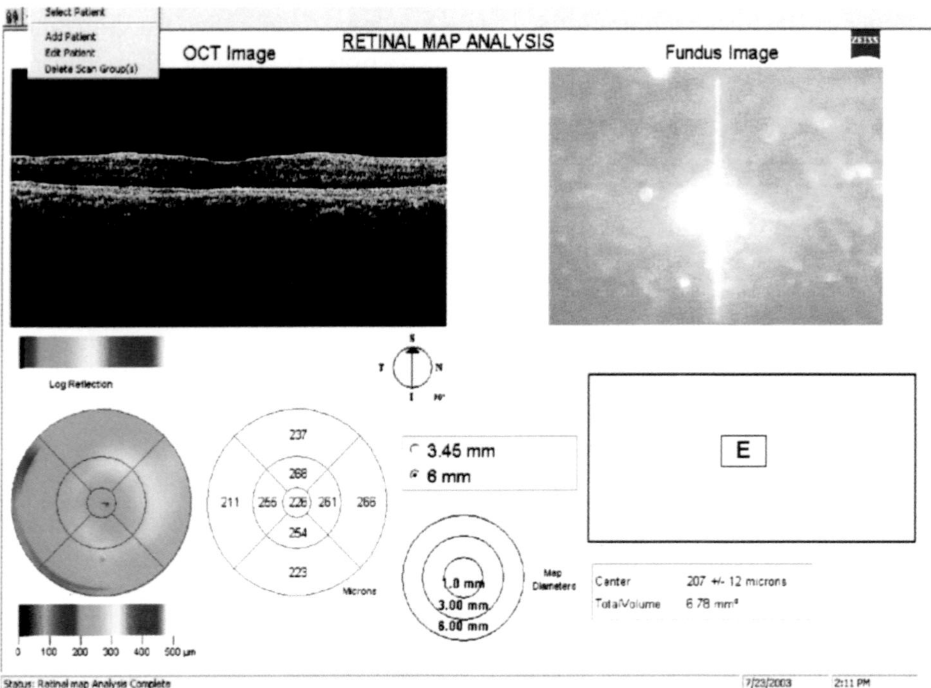

CONCLUSIONS

Cystoid macular edema (CME) is the most common cause of visual loss in intermediate uveitis. Its management includes corticosteroids (periocular, implant or oral), immunosupressives and pars plana vitrectomy. Quantification of CME by OCT helps in monitoring response to the therapy.

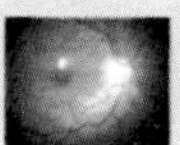

BEHÇET'S DISEASE

Case 18.6: Complete Beçhet's Disease with CME

Case Summary

A diagnosed case of complete Behçet's disease was seen with right eye anterior uveitis, vitritis, vasculitis and cystoid macular edema (CME) (A). The visual acuity in this eye was 20/80.

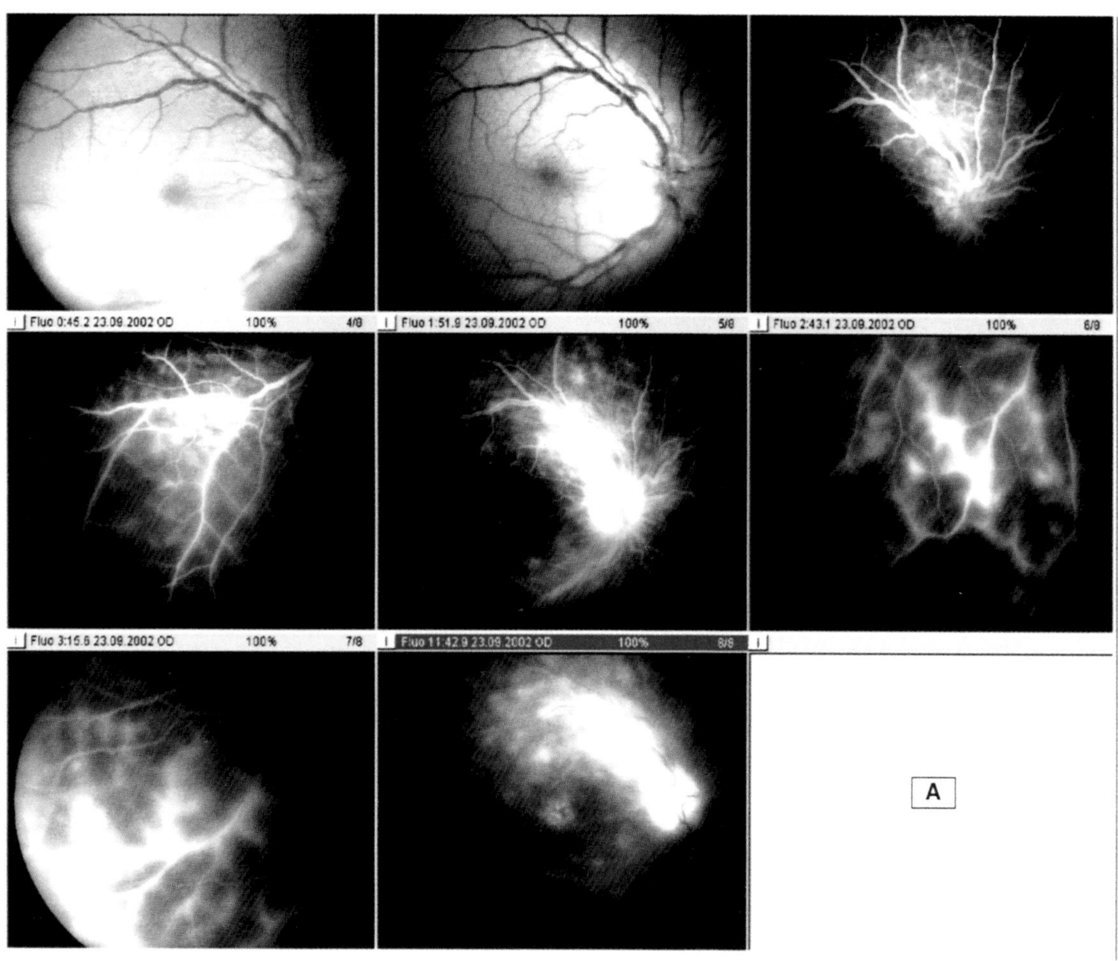

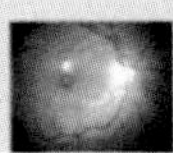

The left eye of the same patient showed vasculitis with cystoid macular edema grade IV (B). The visual acuity was reduced to 20/200. OCT confirmed the CME (C). The patient received intravitreal triamcinolone acetonide 4 mg in the left eye with immunosuppressive therapy.

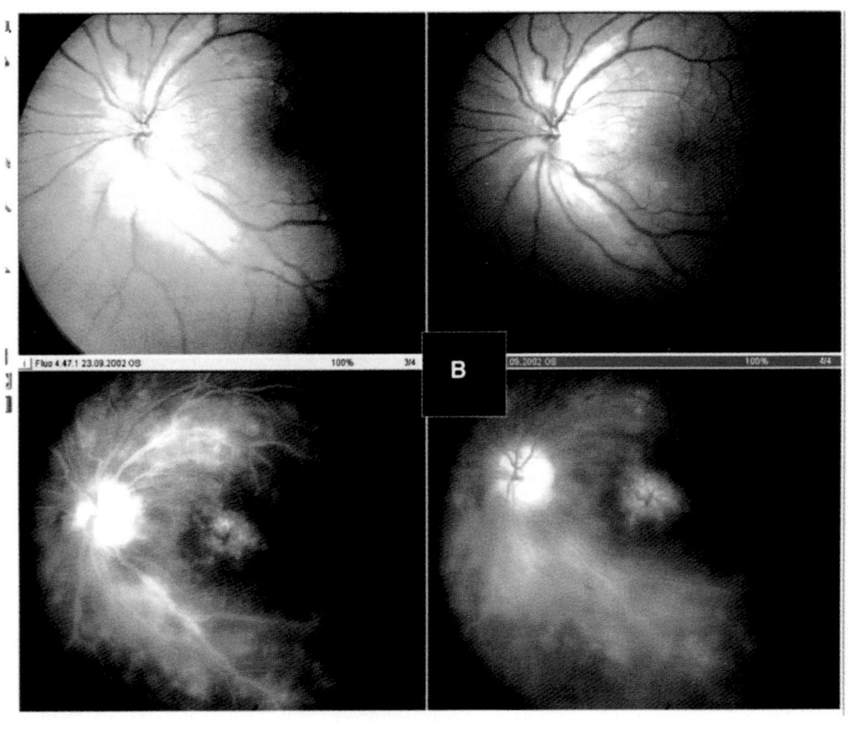

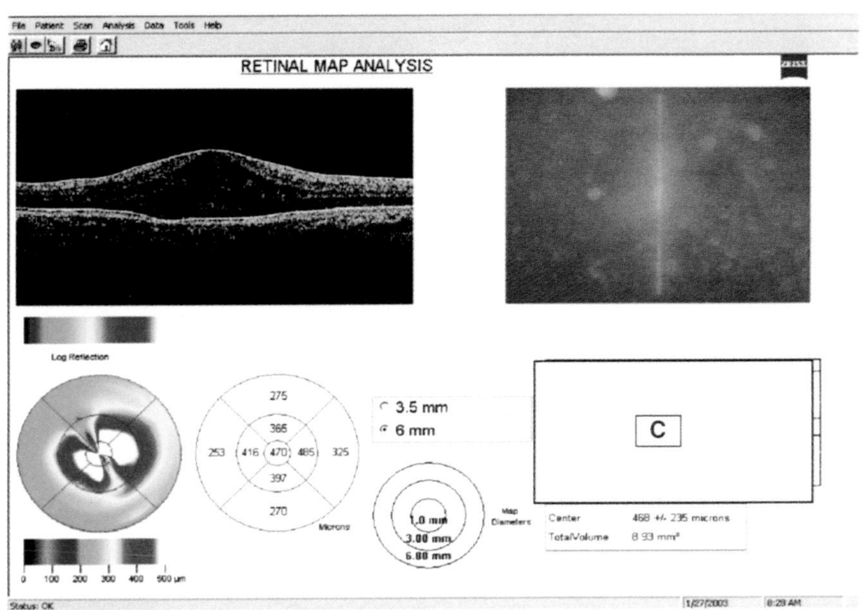

The left eye showed a severe fibrinous reaction following intravitreal triamcinolone and his visual acuity dropped to counting fingers within 24 hours of injection (D). The patient was treated as sterile endophthalmitis and received oral and topical corticosteroids.

Three days later, his visual acuity had improved to 20/50 and media clarity had improved to grade I. Repeat fluorescein angiography showed minimal CME (E).

Repeat OCT scan done at this stage confirmed resolution of CME (F).

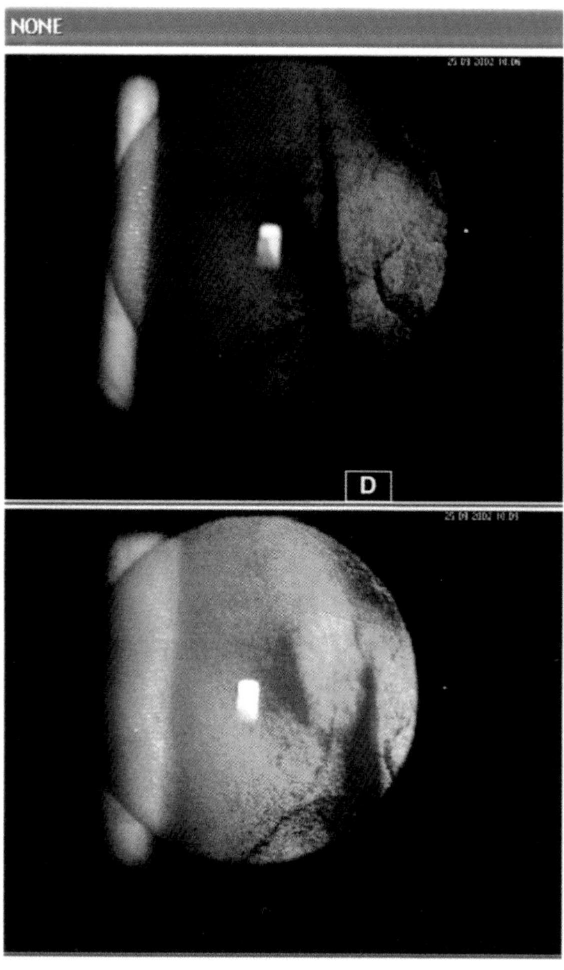

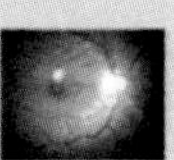

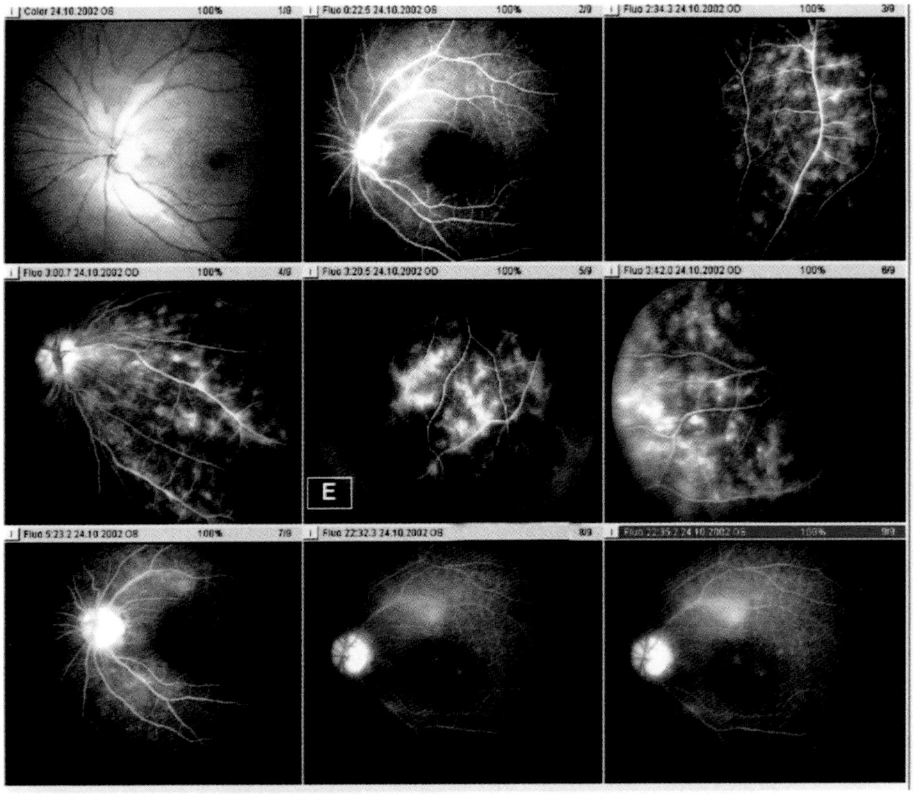

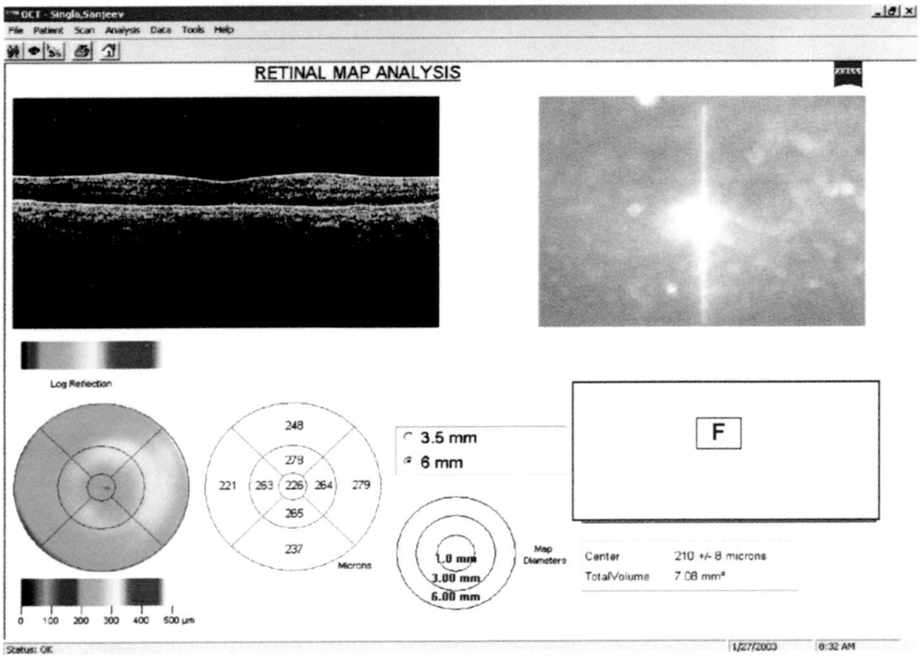

CONCLUSIONS

OCT helps in monitoring cystoid macular edema in patients with Beçhet's disease. It can also help in monitoring epiretinal membrane formation,development of macular hole and neurosensory atrophy in these patients.

VOGT-KOYANAGI-HARADA SYNDROME (VKH SYNDROME)

VKH syndrome is characterized by anterior uveitis, exudative retinal detachment with yellowish white lesions. Systemic findings may include headache, hair and skin changes including poliosis and vitiligo, and sensorineural deafness. The condition responds well to corticosteroids. Choroidal neovascularization and subretinal fibrosis may occur in few patients.

Case 18.7: VKH Syndrome

Case Summary

A 25-year-old woman was seen with multiple serous detachments of neurosensory retina and pigment epithelium in the right eye (A). Fluorescein angiography (B) showed multiple hyperfluorescent areas initially with dye pooling in the late phase conforming to multiple detachments. Visual acuity in this eye was 20/200.

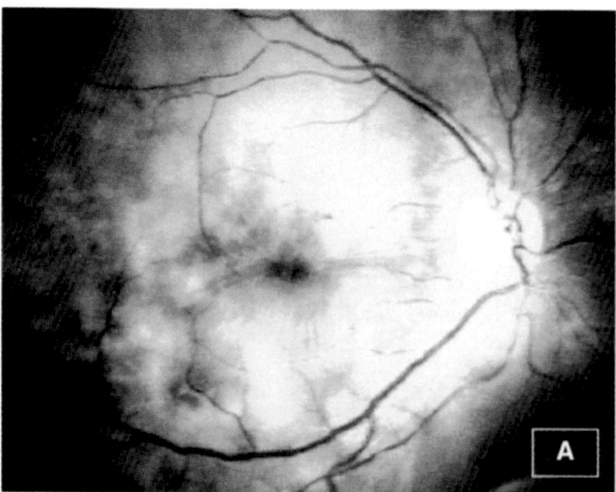

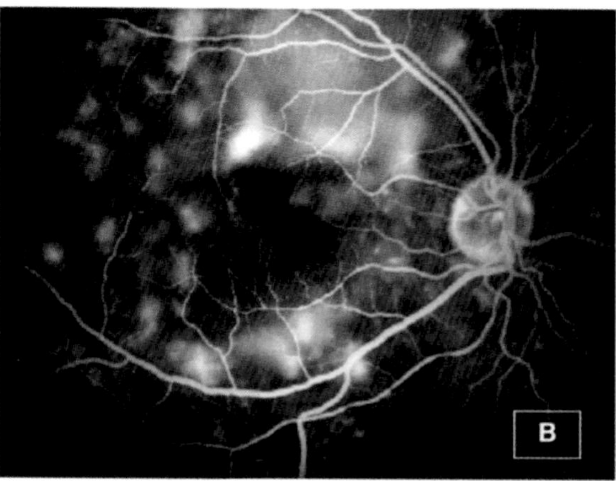

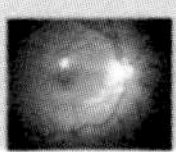

OCT scan through different levels (C) showed multiple areas of serous detachment with intraretinal pockets of fluid. The pigment epithelial detachment was not picked up, though RPE was found to be irregular on OCT.

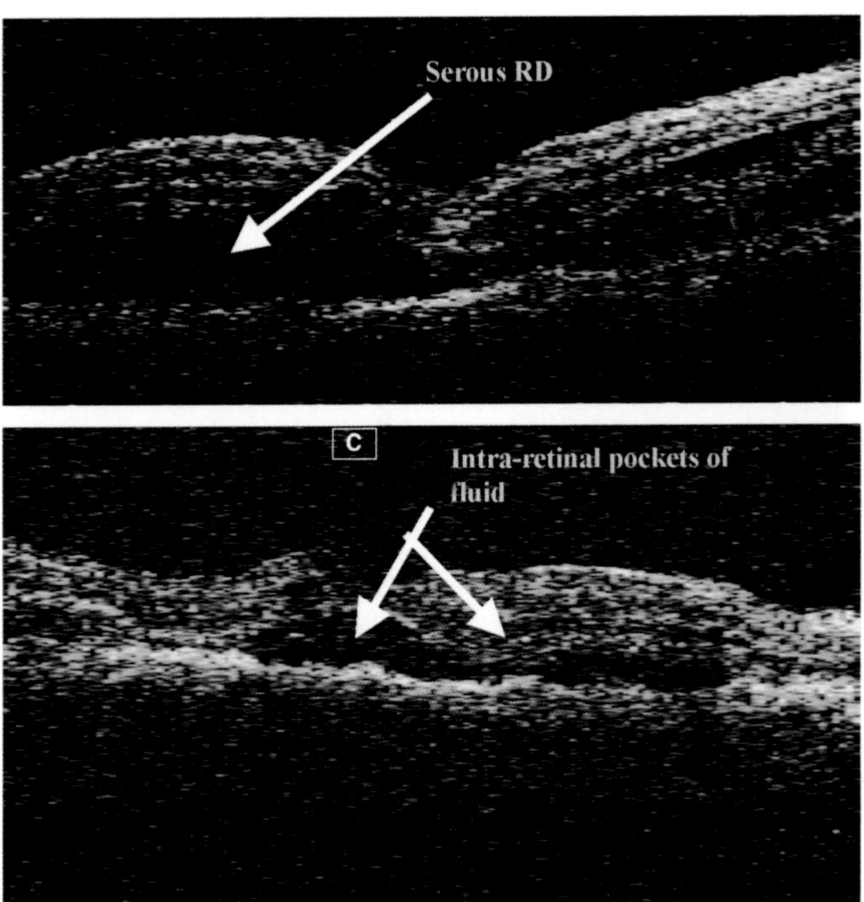

The left eye of the patient also showed similar features of VKH disease with multiple detachments seen clinically as well as angiographically (D, E). The visual acuity was reduced to 20/200.

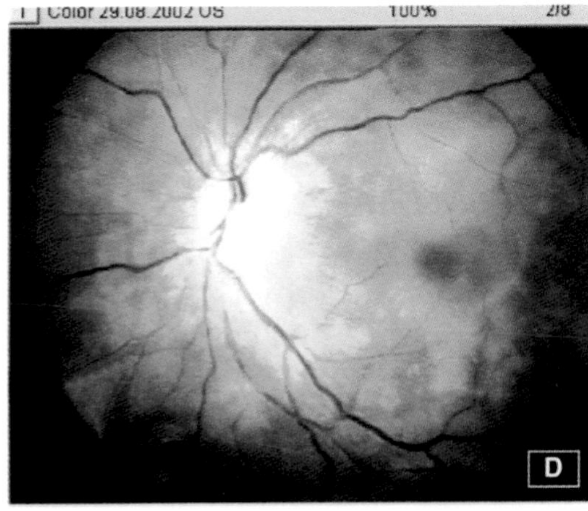

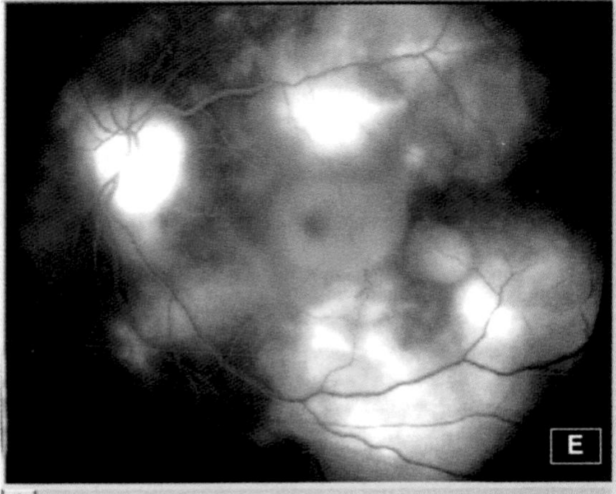

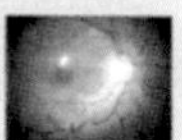

OCT line scan of the left eye (F, G) showed subretinal serous detachment with moderate backscattering suggesting the presence of turbid fluid. The fluid was seen as multiple pockets and the retinal pigment epithelium was irregular under the detachment.

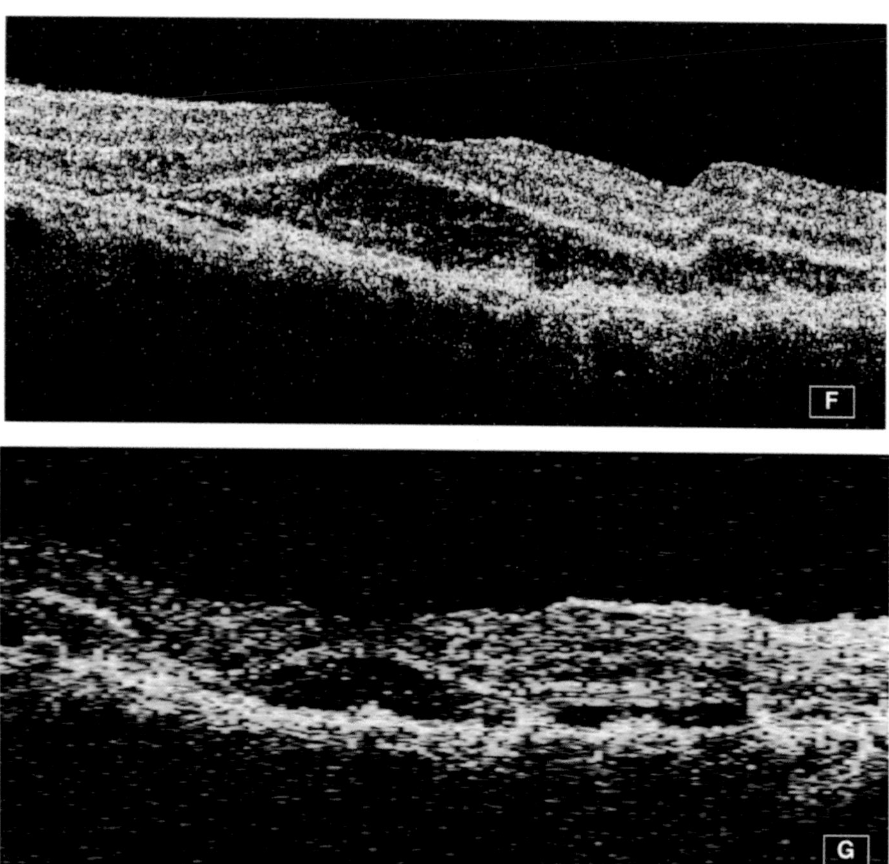

Following treatment with corticosteroids, the visual acuity improved to 20/20 in the right (H) and 20/30 in the left eye (I). Repeat OCT scans of both eyes did not show any residual changes in the right eye (J) while the left eye showed increased hyper-reflectivity temporal to the fovea (K).

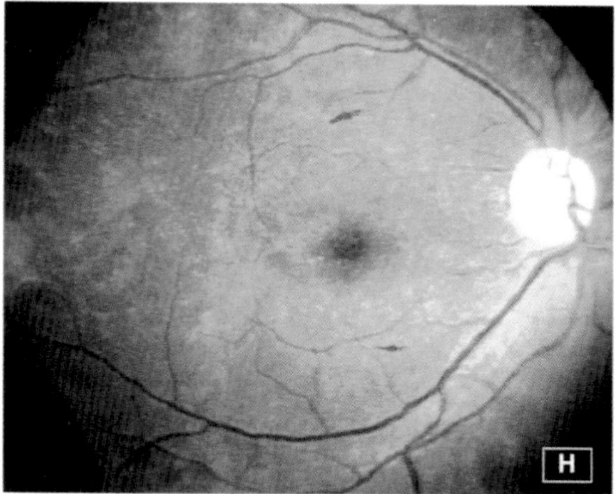

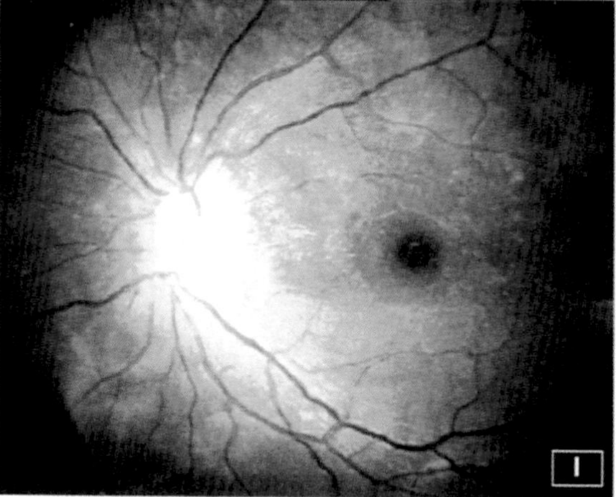

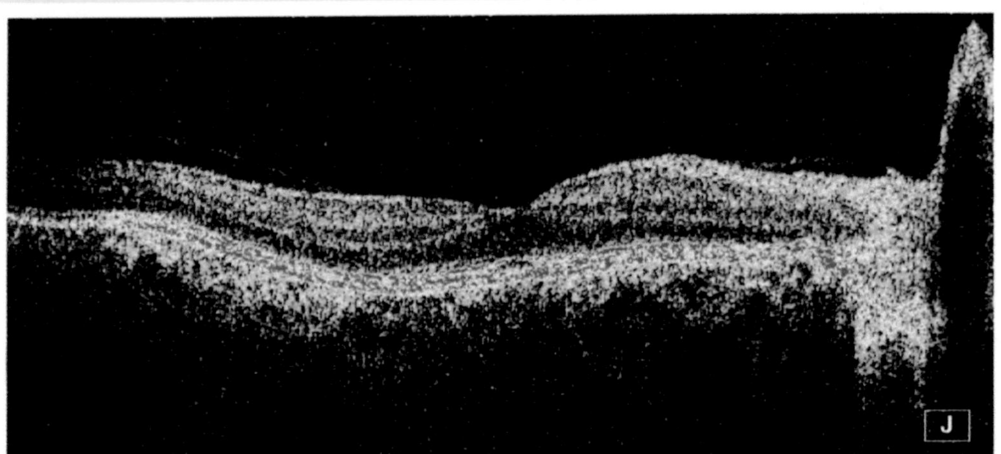
J

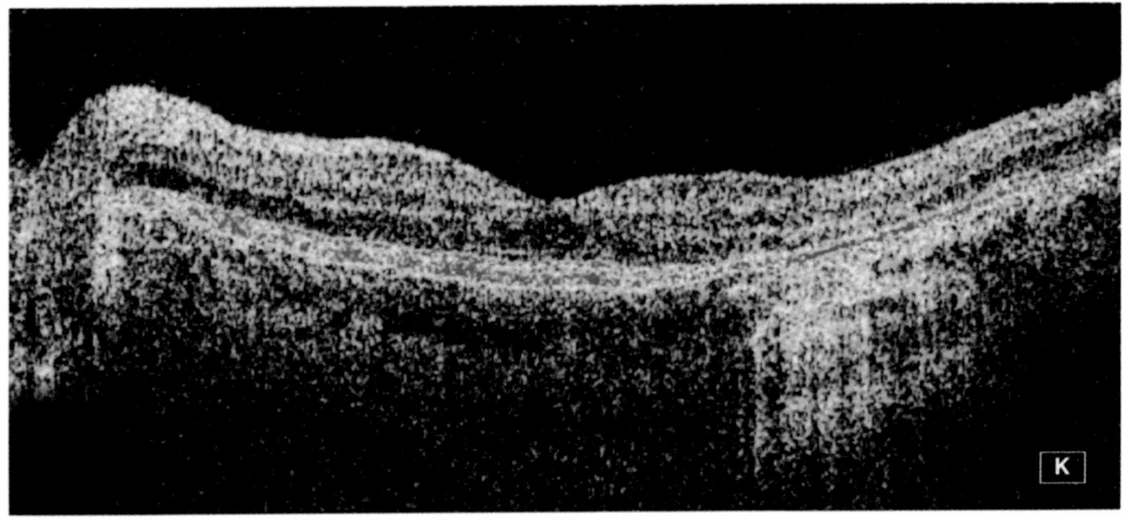
K

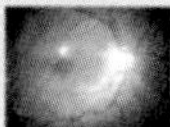

Case 18.8: Localized Ocular Harada's Disease

Case Summary

A 26-year-old boy was seen with decreased vision in both his eyes of 12 days duration. His best corrected visual acuity was 20/200 in the right eye. Right eye fundus (A) showed whitish spots in the posterior pole. The fluorescein angiography showed multiple hypofluorescent spots that showed hyperfluorescence in the late phase with two areas of dye pooling suggesting small neurosensory detachments (B-D).

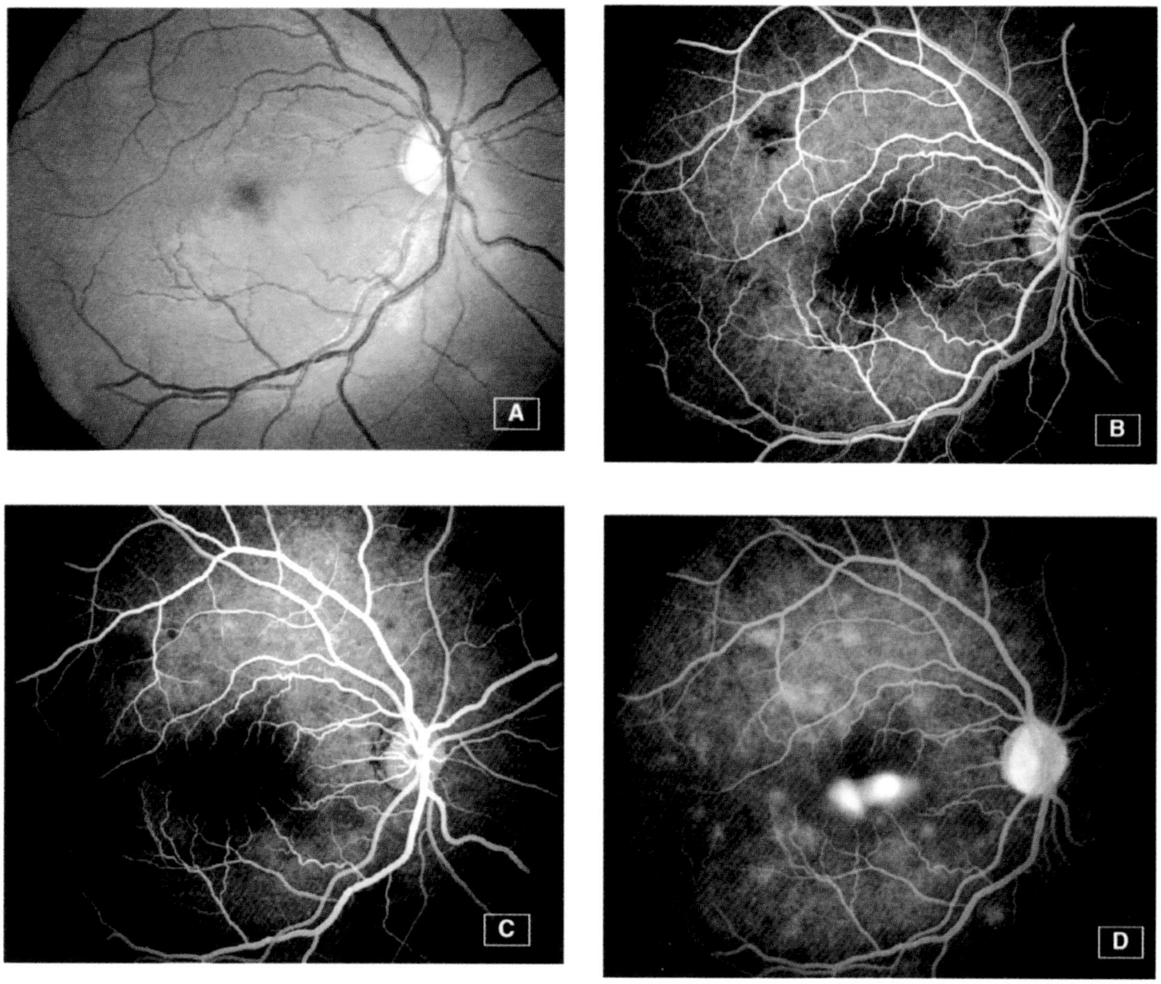

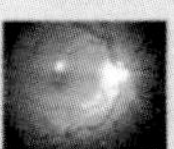

Digital indocyanine green (ICG) angiography showed a plethora of hypofluorescent spots (E) with masking of underlying choroidal vasculature in the late phase by neurosensory detachment (F). Note the area of neurosensory detachment seen on ICG is larger than seen on fluorescein angiography suggestive of Vogt-Koyanagi-Harada disease.

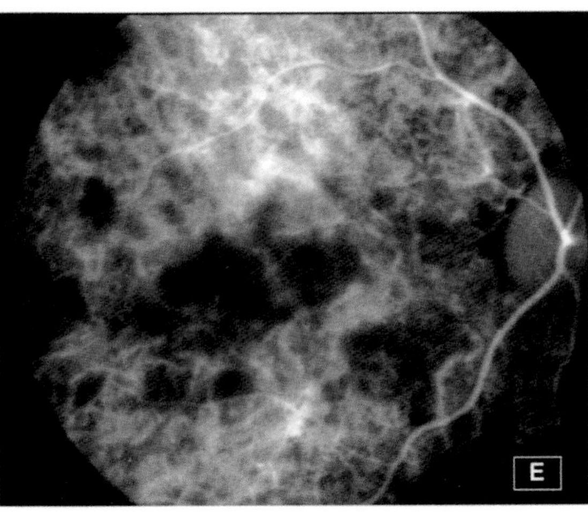

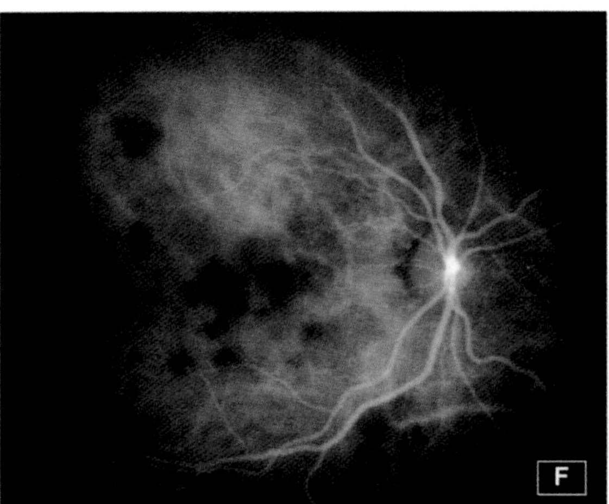

Optical Coherence Tomography

OCT line scan of the right eye (G) showed an intraretinal pocket of fluid accumulation (arrow). Though the underlying choroid showed moderately increased hyper-reflectivity from the choroid, the increased choroidal thickness could not be appreciated. Ultrasound B scan showed diffuse thickening of choroid in the posterior pole (not shown).

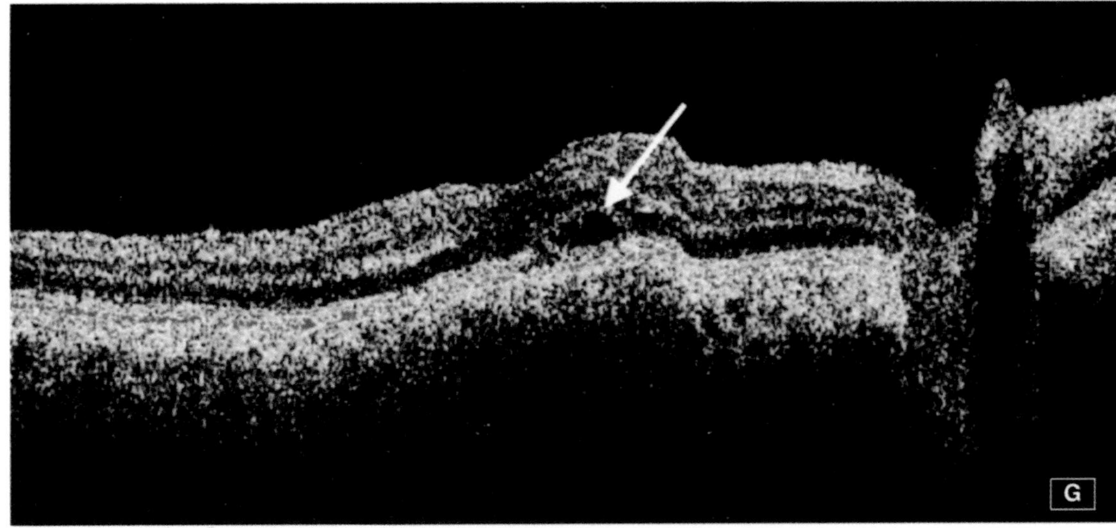

The left eye of the patient also showed similar whitish lesions that were hypofluorescent initially and hyperfluorescent in the late phase of fluorescein angiography (H). The visual acuity was reduced to 20/90. More hypofluorescent spots were noticed on indocyanine green angiography than on fluorescein angiography (I).

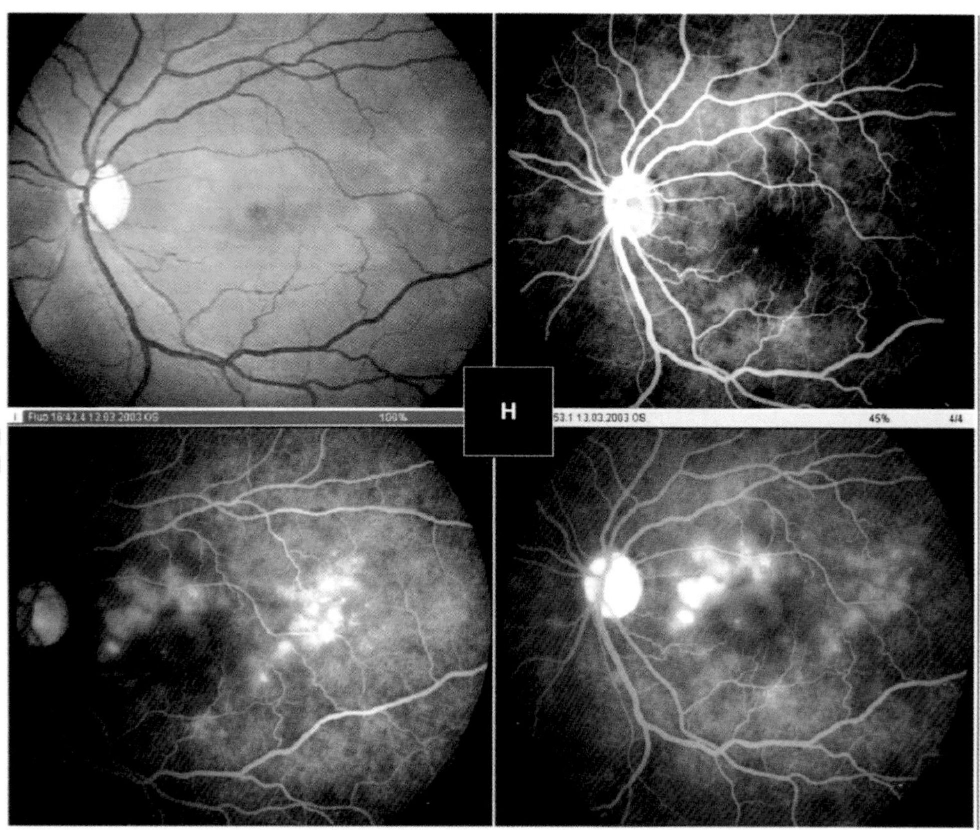

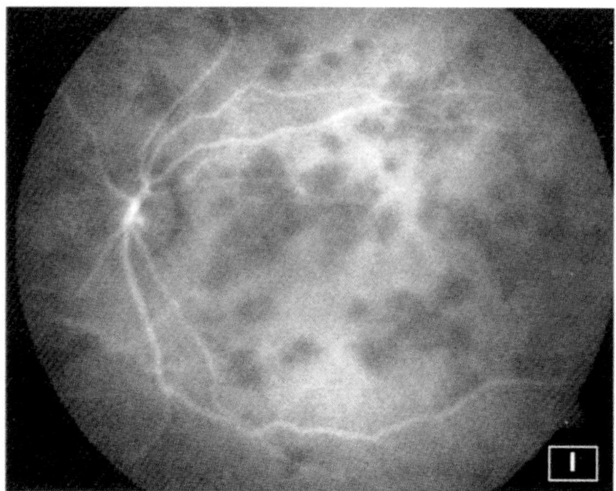

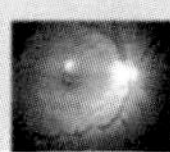

Optical Coherence Tomography

OCT line scans (J, K) showed a hyporeflective area nasal to the fovea corresponding to serous retinal detachment. Though retinal pigment epithelium was irregular at some places, no choroidal thickening was appreciable.

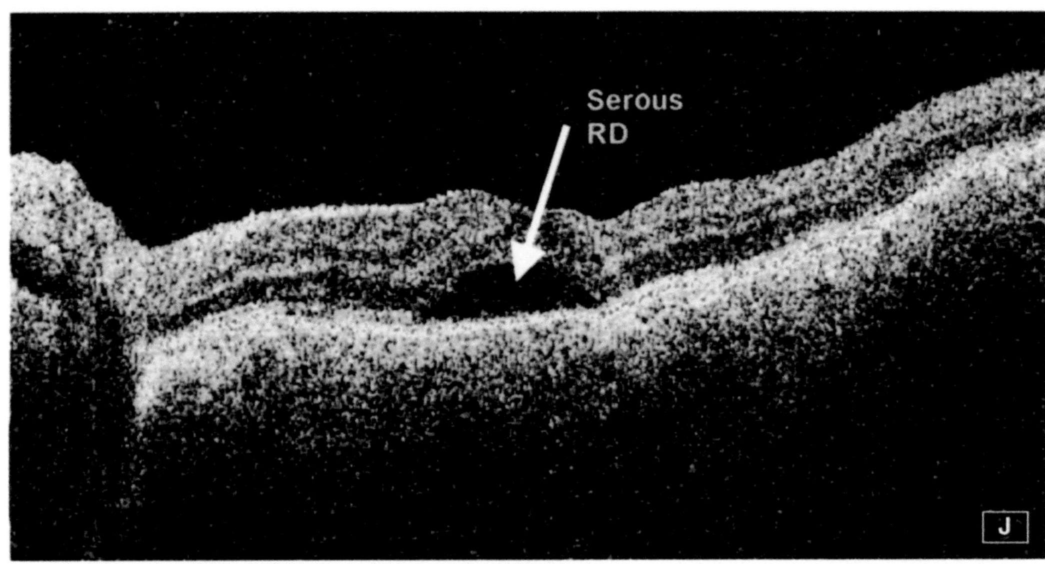

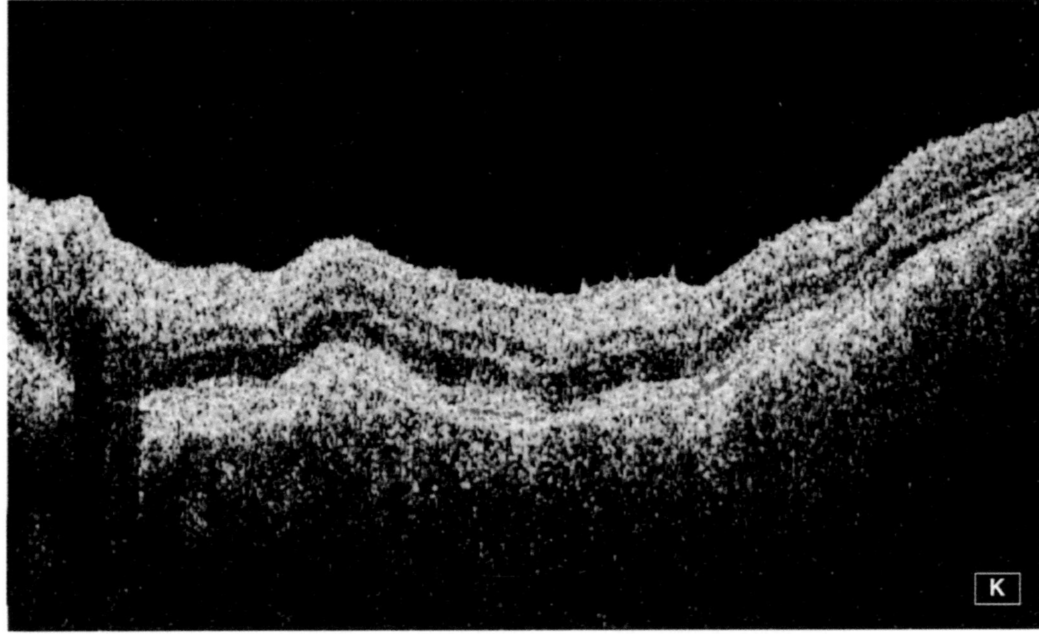

Follow-up

After 4 weeks of oral corticosteroid therapy, there was a significant clinical improvement with visual acuity improving to 20/30 in the right and 20/20 in the left eye. The repeat fluorescein angiography was unremarkable in both eyes (L).

Repeat OCT line scan of both eyes was normal (M, N). No residual changes were seen.

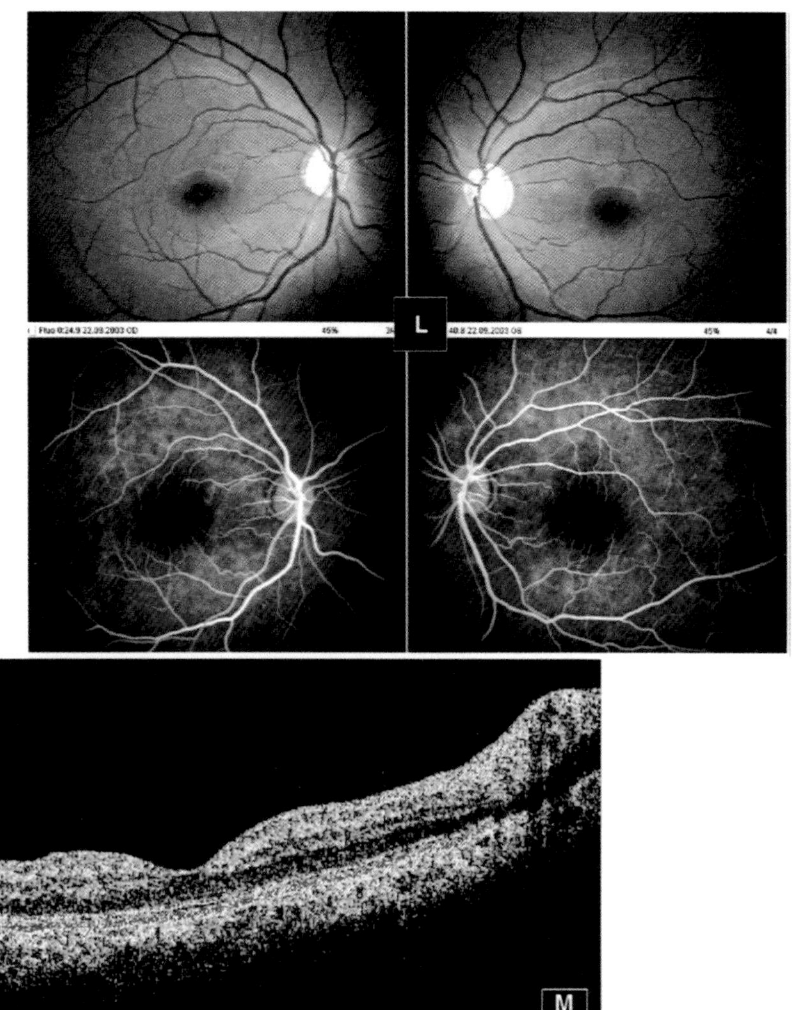

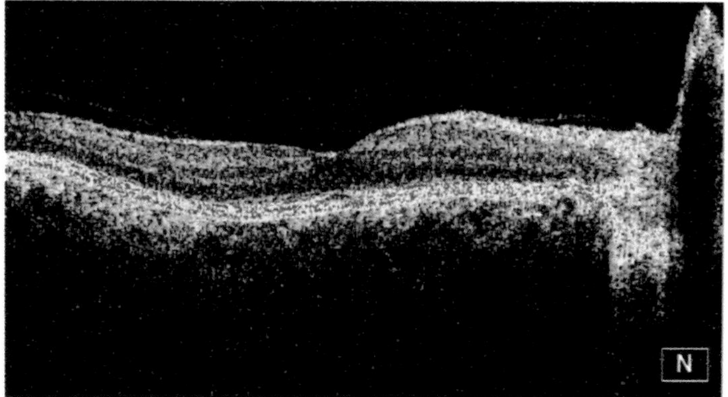

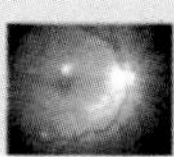

SYMPATHETIC OPHTHALMIA

The manifestations of this disease resemble those of Harada's with multiple neurosensory and pigment epithelial detachments

Case 18.9: Sympathetic Ophthalmia

Case Summary

A 62-year-old man was being treated elsewhere as a case of sympathetic ophthalmia in the right eye 6 months following glaucoma filtration surgery in the left eye (A). His best corrected visual acuity was hand motions in the left and 20/200 in the right eye. Right eye showed sunset glow indicating chronicity of the disease (B). The patient was on the maintence dose of corticosteroids and wanted to know whether he could stop them.

Fundus right eye showed widespread atrophic lesions throughout the fundus. No residual serous detachment was seen on fluorescein angiography (C).

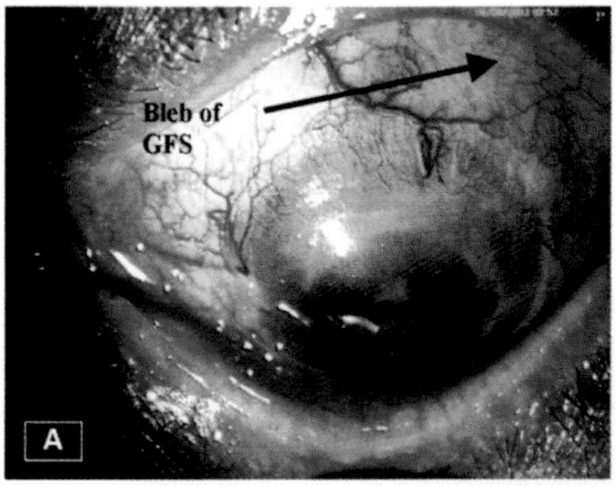

Bleb of GFS

A

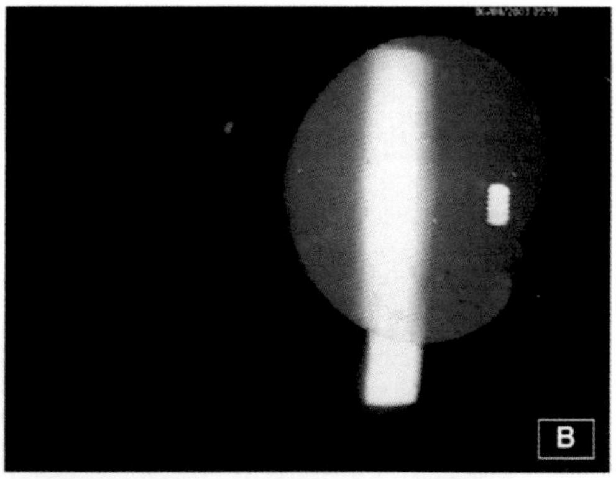

B

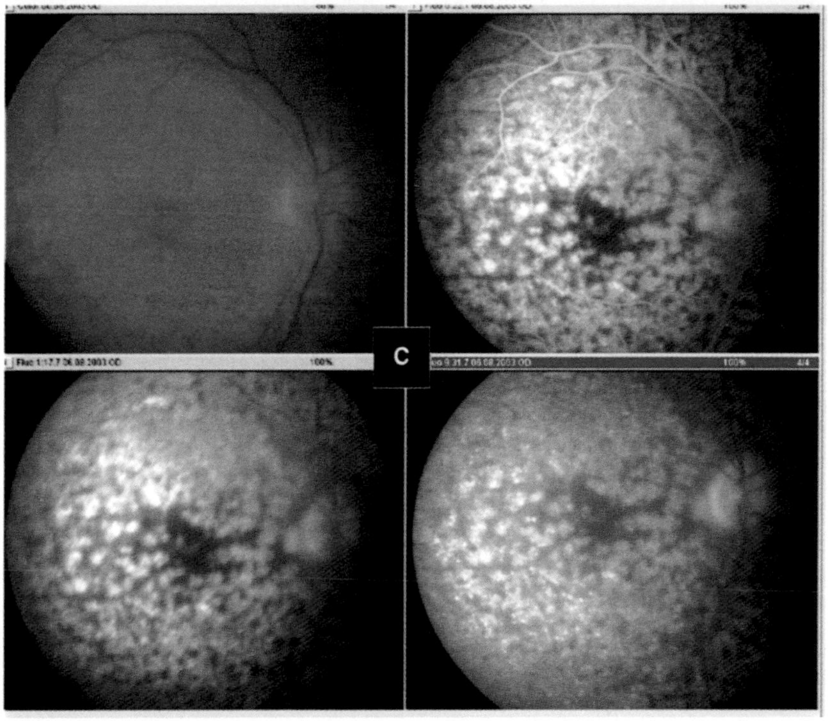

C

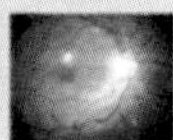

Optical Coherence Tomography

OCT line scans (D, E) showed the presence of small hyporeflective streak (arrows) between retinal pigment epithelium and neurosensory retina suggesting the presence of residual retinal detachment. In view of persistent detachment, the patient was advised to continue oral corticosteroids. **OCT was helpful in diagnosing residual subretinal fluid that was not seen on fundoscopy and fluorescein angiography.**

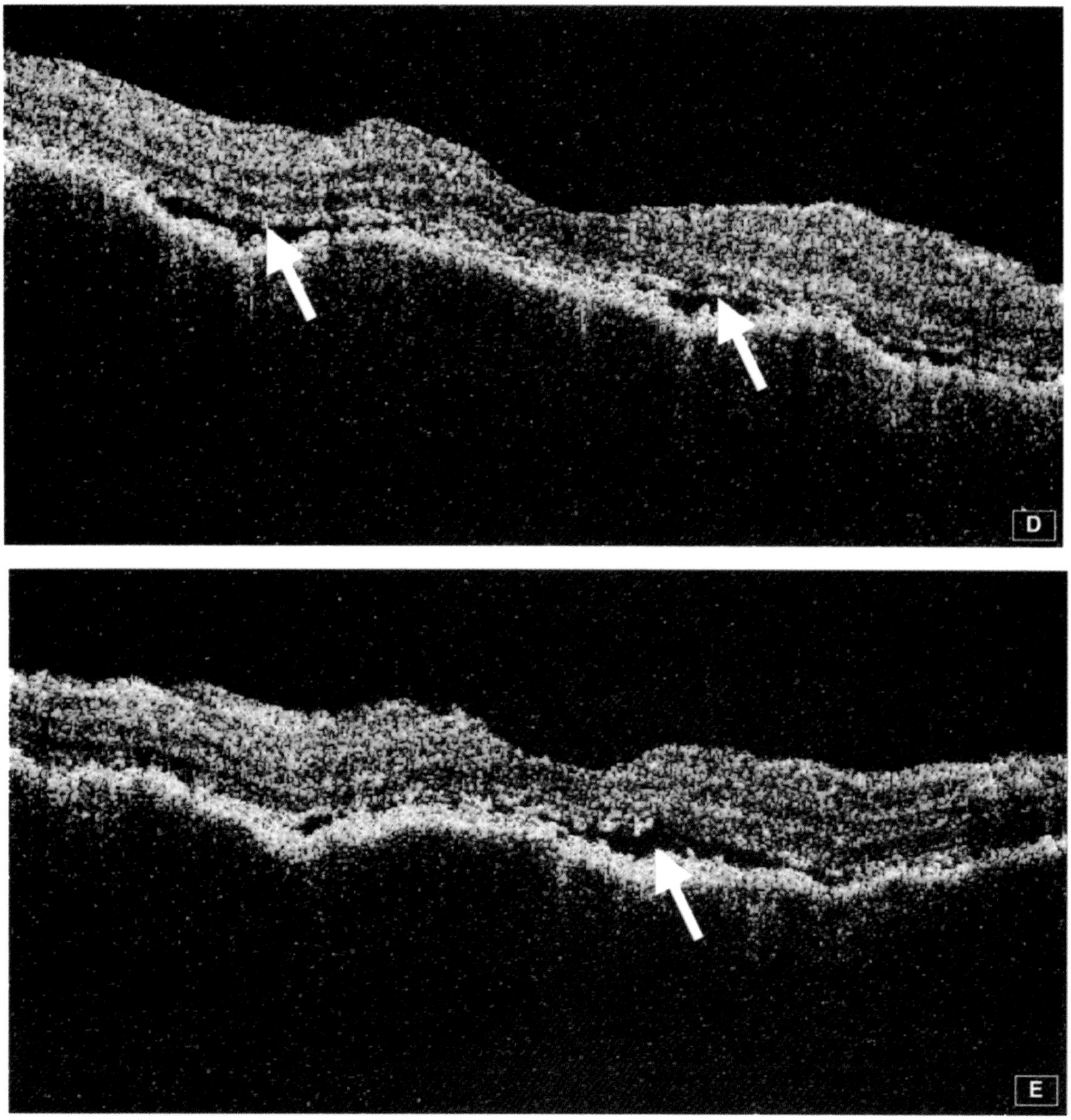

D

E

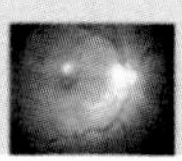

CONCLUSIONS

Both sympathetic ophthalmia and Vogt-Koyanagi –Harada's disease are characterized by the presence of multiple retinal detachments that tend to involve macula and posterior pole. Both need to be treated with oral corticosteroids/immunosuppressive agents and premature termination of oral corticosteroids could result in recurrent episodes. OCT could be a useful tool in monitoring serous retinal detachment in these patients. Over a long-term follow-up, it might be useful in defining the end point for stopping oral corticosteroids/immunosuppressive agents. However, in our experience, we did not find OCT helpful in monitoring choroidal thickness in these patients.

SUGGESTED READINGS

1. Vogt- Koyanagi-Harada syndrome. Chapter 60. In The Retina Atlas by Yannuzi LA, Guyer DR, Green WR (Eds). Mosby-Year Book, Inc. 1995;673-79.
2. Rao NA, Marak GE. Sympathetic ophthalmia simulating Vogt- Koyanagi-Harada's disease: A clinicopathologic study of four cases. Jpn J Ophthalmol 1983 ;27:506-511.
3. Sympathetic Ophthalmia. Chapter 59. In The Retina Atlas by Yannuzi LA, Guyer DR, Green WR (Eds). Mosby-Year Book, Inc. 1995;667-671.
4. Goto H and Rao NA. Sympathetic ophthalmia and Vogt-Koyanagi-Harada syndrome. Int Ophthalmol Clin 1990 ; 30:279-285.

ACUTE POSTERIOR MULTIFOCAL PLACOID PIGMENT EPITHELIOPATHY (APMPPE)

Acute posterior multifocal placoid pigment epitheliopathy (APMPPE) is characterized by the presence of multiple cream-colored, plaque like lesions seen at the level of Retinal pigment epithelium. The disease affects primarily young patients and is preceded by a viral illness. The disease is self limiting and vision returns to normal within weeks to months with no recurrences.

In our population, we found a variant of APMPPE where lesions show progression and recurrences, eventually resembling serpiginous choroiditis.

Case 18.10: APMPPE

Case Summary

A 38-year-old woman was seen with complaints of decreased vision in her right eye of 15 days duration. Her best-corrected visual acuity was 20/30 in the right eye. Fundoscopy showed healed lesions with two active lesions that were hypofluorescent initially with late hyperfluorescence (arrows) (A). These lesions resemble serpiginous choroiditis because of the simultaneous presence of active and healed lesions and hyperfluorescence of one of the lesions at the edge with central healing. They also resembled APMPPE morphologically.

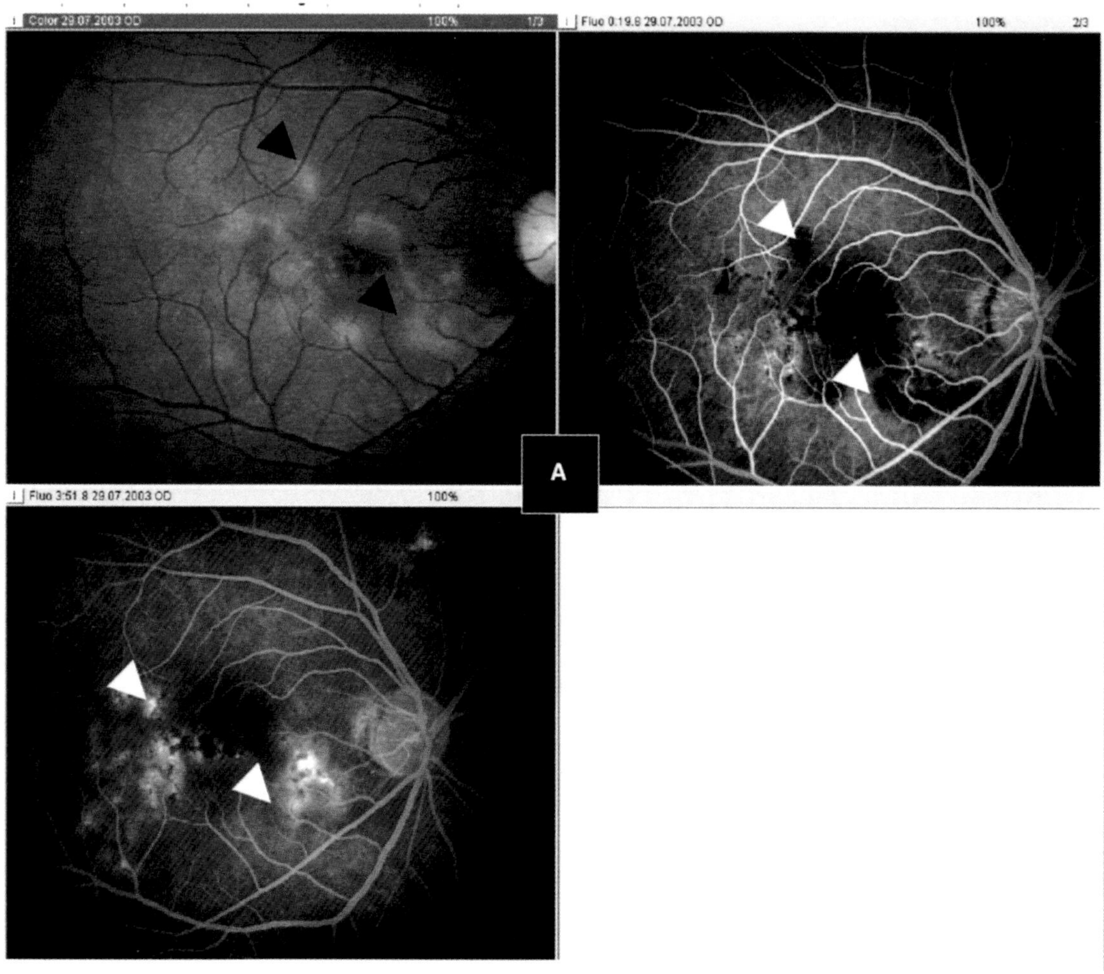

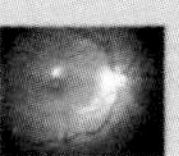

Optical Coherence Tomography

Horizontal OCT line scans passing through the fovea (B, C) showed an area of moderate backscatter nasal to the fovea in the outer retinal layers (arrows), corresponding to the plaque seen clinically. The scars did not show any abnormality on OCT.

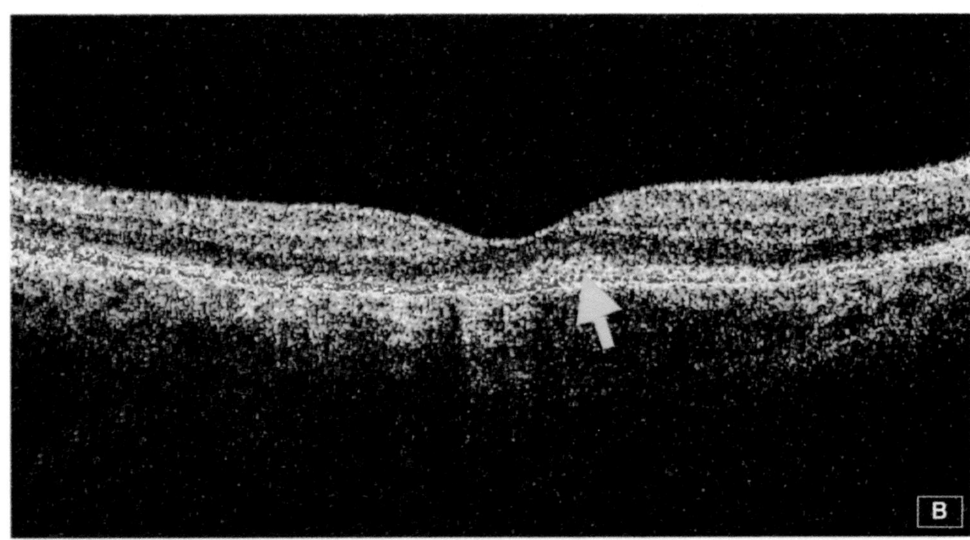

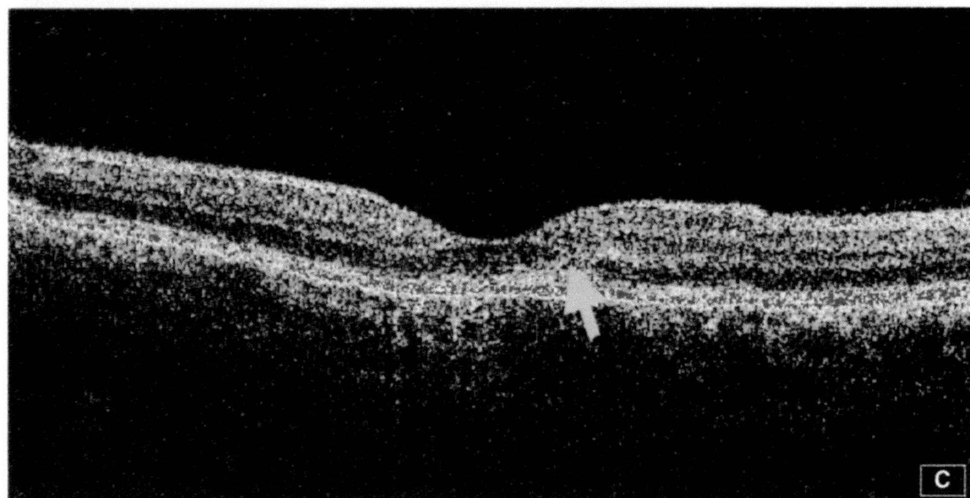

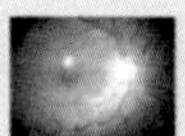

The patient received oral corticosteroids.Two weeks later, her visual acuity had improved to 20/20. The lesions were still active on fluorescein angiography (D). OCT showed reduced height of the area of moderate backscatter in the outer retina (E) (arrow).

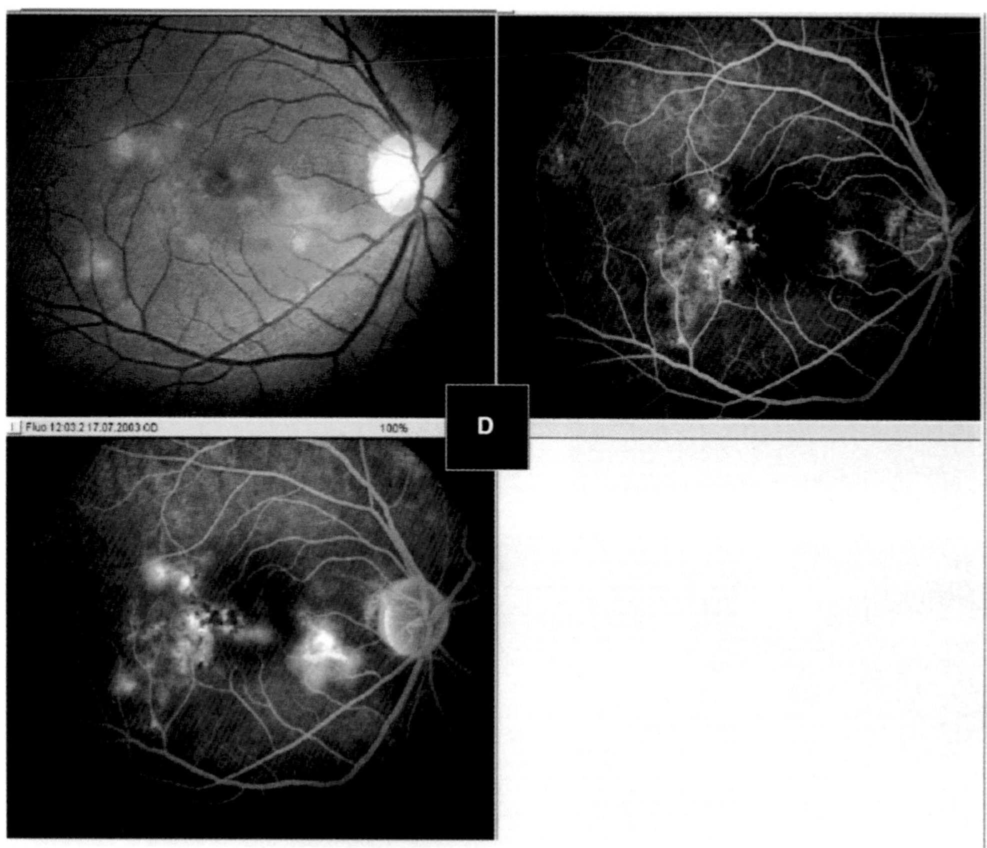

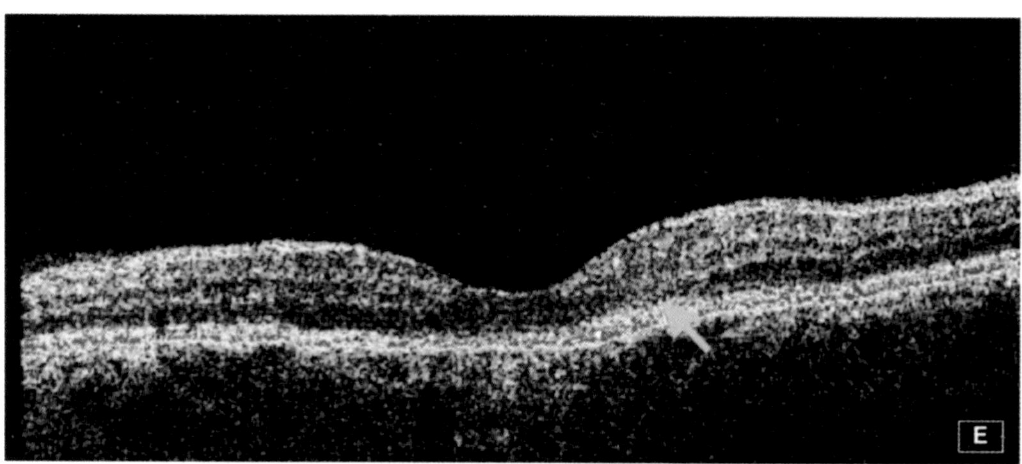

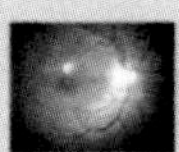

Three months later, her best-corrected visual acuity was 20/20. Note the depigmented scar has shown progression and become confluent resembling the scar of serpiginous choroiditis (F). The visual fields were normal. The repeat OCT (G) showed a normal scan with no residual changes.

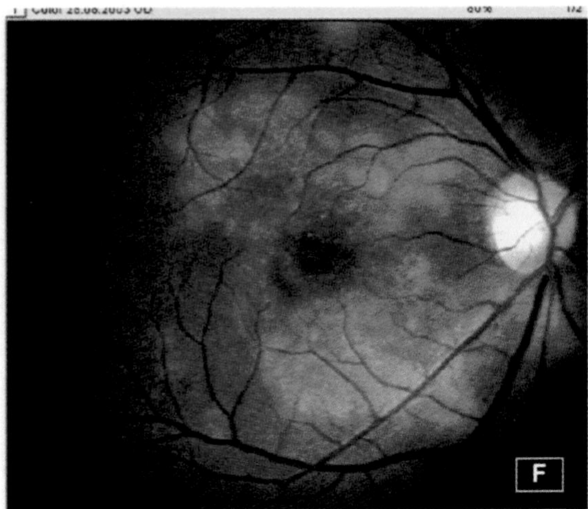

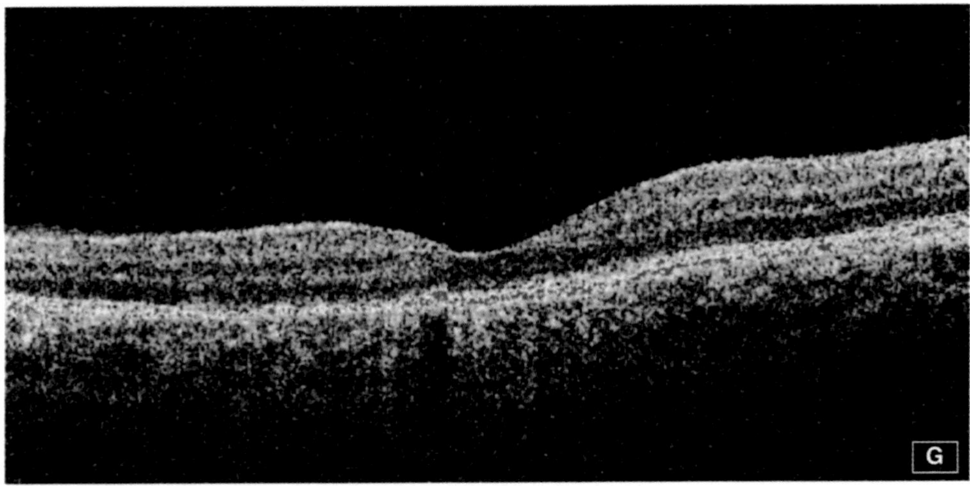

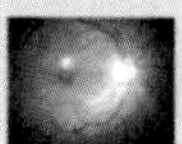

The patient had a visual acuity of 20/16 in the left eye that showed healed lesions resembling APMPPE (H). The OCT scan (I) showed few areas of irregular retinal pigment epithelial hypertrophy (arrow).

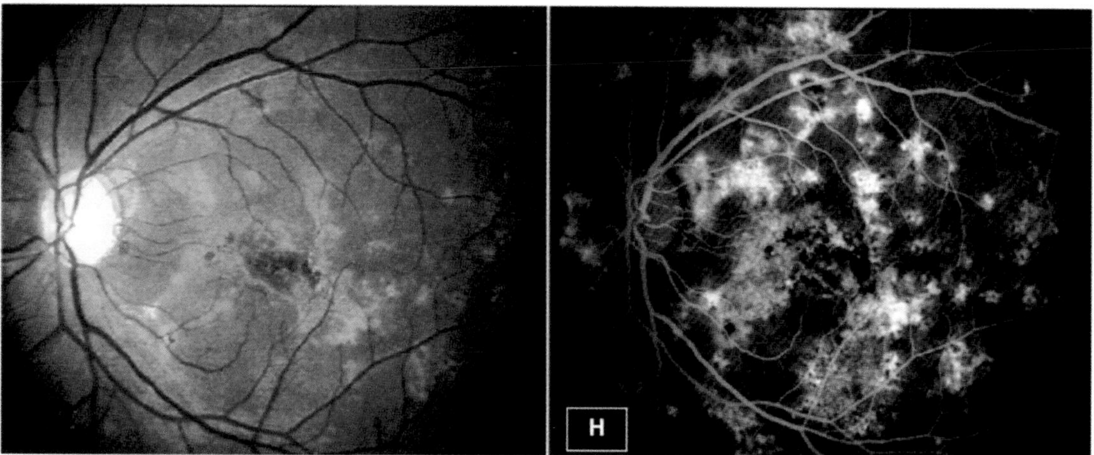

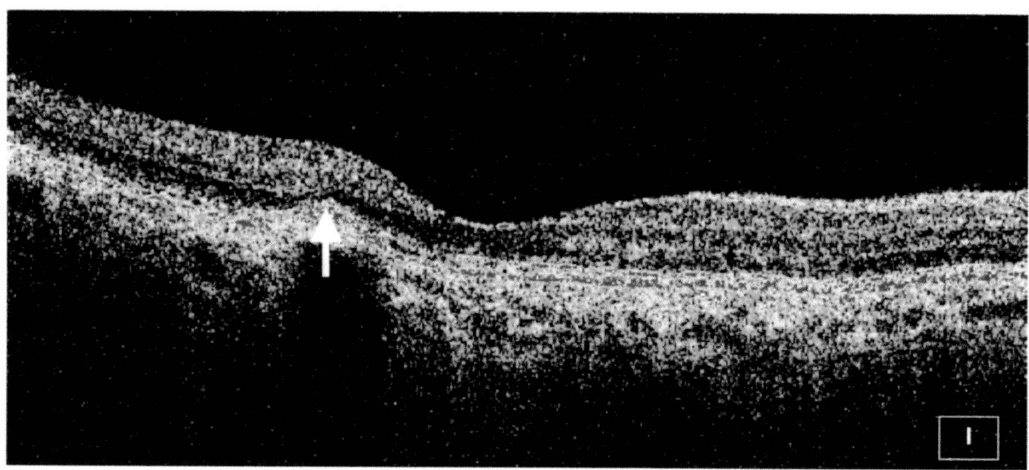

CONCLUSIONS

Acute posterior multifocal placoid pigment epitheliopathy (APMPPE) probably has a different presentation and course in our population. The disease tends to have a recurrent course with multifocal patches becoming confluent over a period of time and resembling sepiginous choroiditis. In our experience, the OCT scans were not much contributory in the diagnosis and management of APMPPE and may often be normal. However, it could be useful in diagnosing complications like choroidal neovascular membranes and subretinal fibrosis.

SUGGESTED READINGS

1. Gass JDM. Acute posterior multifocal placoid pigment epitheliopathy. Arch Ophthalmol 1968;80:177-185.
2. Gupta V, Agarwal A, Gupta A, Bambery P, Narang S. Clinical characteristics of serpiginous choroidopathy in North India. 2002; Am J Ophthalmol,134:47-56.

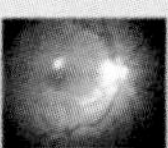

RECURRENT MULTIFOCAL CHOROIDITIS/ MULTIFOCAL CHOROIDITIS AND PANUVEITIS

Recurrent multifocal choroiditis is seen in 2nd-4th decade of life and is characterized by the presence of multiple, discrete lesions at the level of choriocapillaries and retinal pigment epithelium (RPE). The main cause of visual loss is the development of choroidal neovascular membrane or subretinal fibrosis. These CNVMs often respond to oral corticosteroids.

Case 18.11: Multifocal Choroiditis with Choroidal Neovascular Membrane

Case Summary

A 40-year-old man was seen with multifocal choroiditis and panuveitis with CNVM in the left eye. Fluorescein angiography confirmed the same (A).

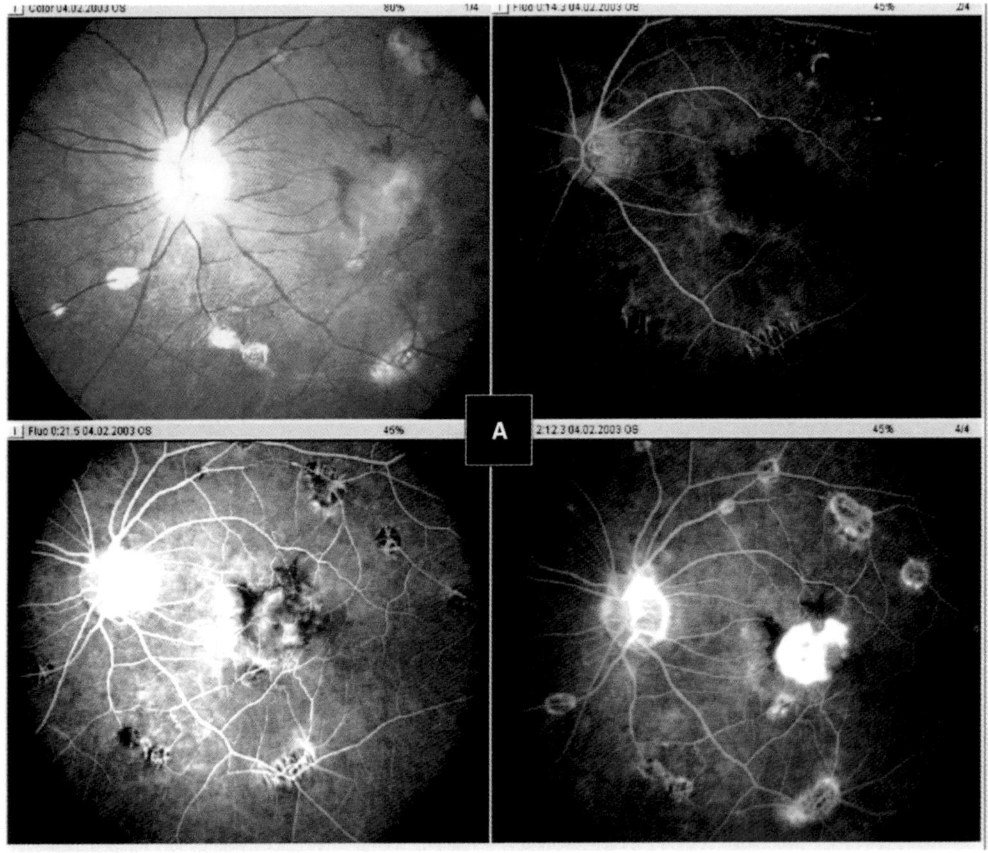

A

OCT line scan through the fovea (B) showed an area of disrupted retinal pigment epithelium with increased hyper-reflectivity from the outer retinal layers with adjacent hyporeflective area suggesting the presence of intraretinal fluid. These findings were consistent with the presence of a classic choroidal neovascular membrane (CNVM). The retinal surface showed a moderately hyper-reflective epiretinal membrane.

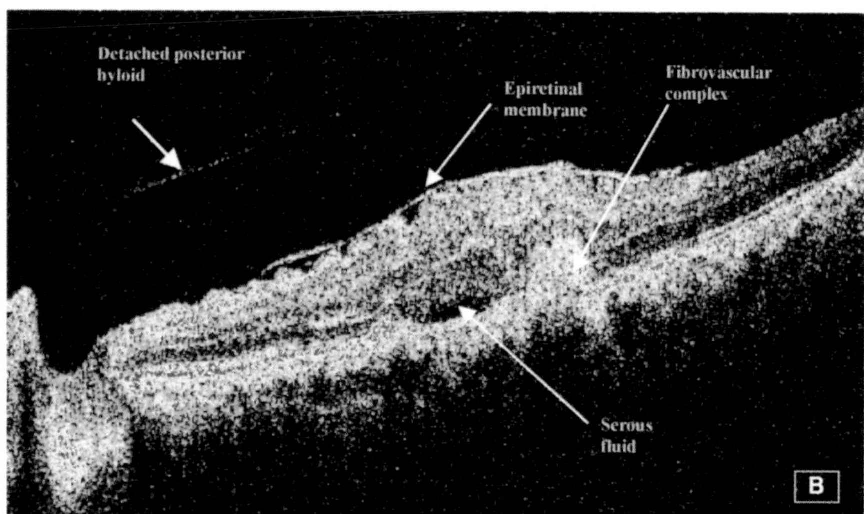

The Choroidal neovascular membrane continued to progress despite corticosteroid and immunosuppressive treatment (C).

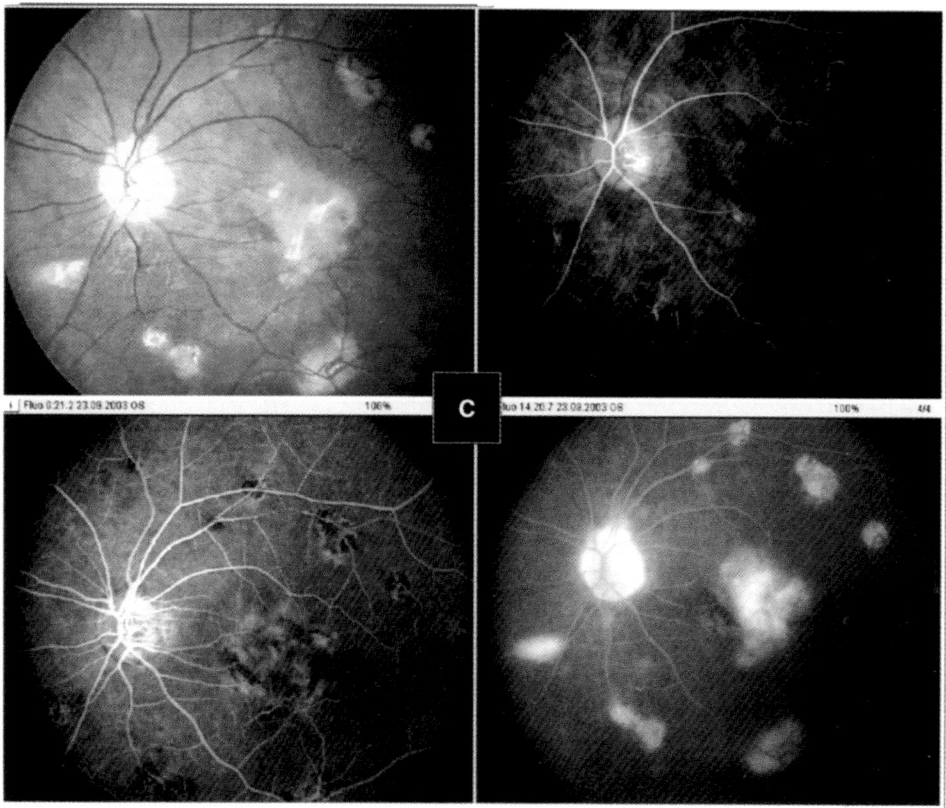

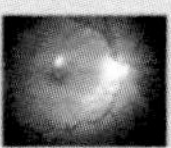

Repeat OCT line scan (D) showed increase in the area of fibrovascular complex as well as in the overlying intraretinal hyporeflective areas indicating the presence of fluid. The posterior hyloid was attached to the optic disc. The epiretinal membrane was seen with traction on underlying retinal tissues.

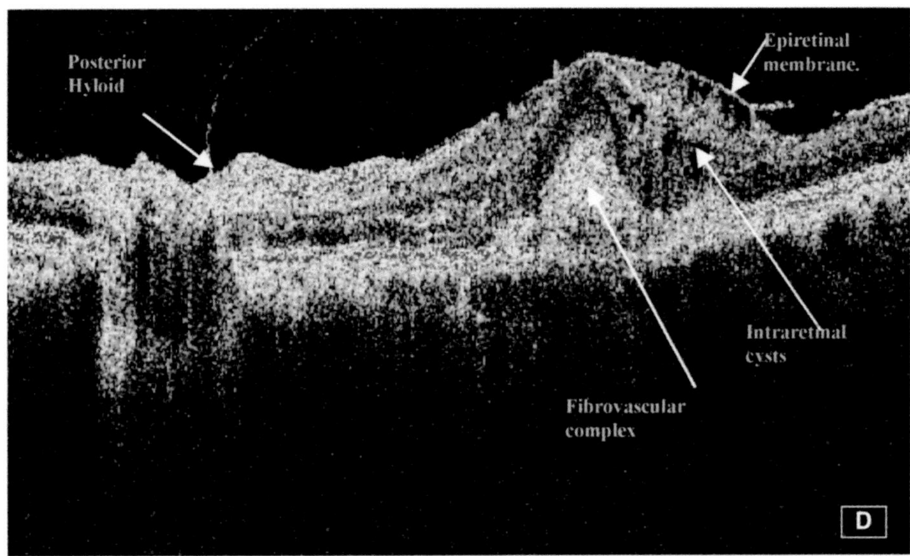

CONCLUSIONS

The multifocal lesions are small, punched-out lesions seen mostly in the mid-peripheral and peripheral fundus. These lesions are best seen on fluorescein angiography. OCT is helpful in monitoring other associated lesions including choroidal neovascular membranes and subretinal fibrosis.

SUGGESTED READING

1. Rao NA, Forster DJ, Spalton DJ. WhiteDot Syndromes. Chap 7 In Podos SM and Yanoff M (Eds) The Uvea Uveitis and Intraocular Neoplasms. Mosby-Wolfe 1995; 7.17-7.20.

MULTIPLE EVANESCENTWHITE DOT SYNDROME

Multiple evanescent White Dot Syndrome (MEWDS) is characterized by the presence of small white dots at the level of retinal pigment epithelium or deeper retina. These lesions show spontaneous resolution with minor residual changes.

Case 18.12: MEWDS

Case summary

A 34-year-old woman was seen with visual acuity of 20/30 in the right eye. Fundus showed the presence of small white dots in the posterior pole (A) that were hyperfluorescent on fluorescein angiography (B).

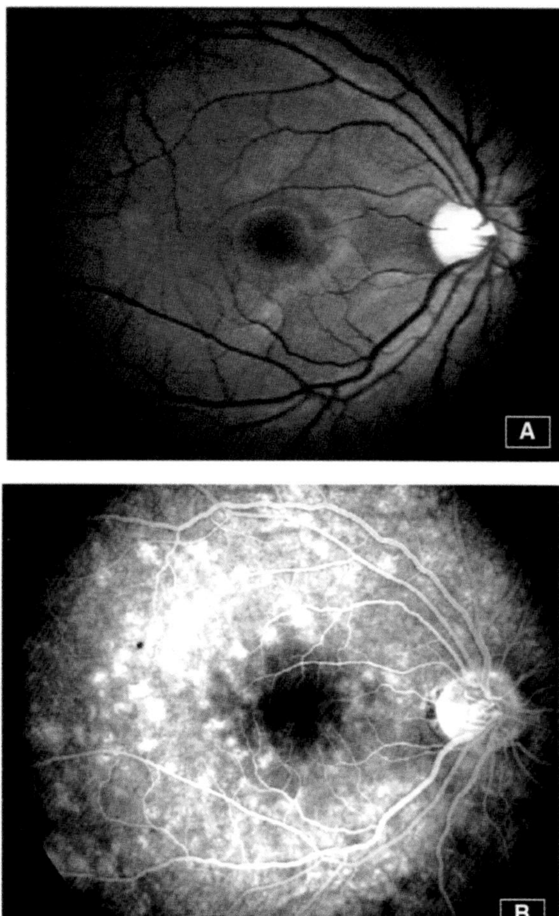

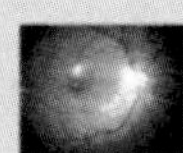

Optical Coherence Tomography

The horizontal OCT line scan (C) passing just above the fovea through the white dots did not show any abnormality.

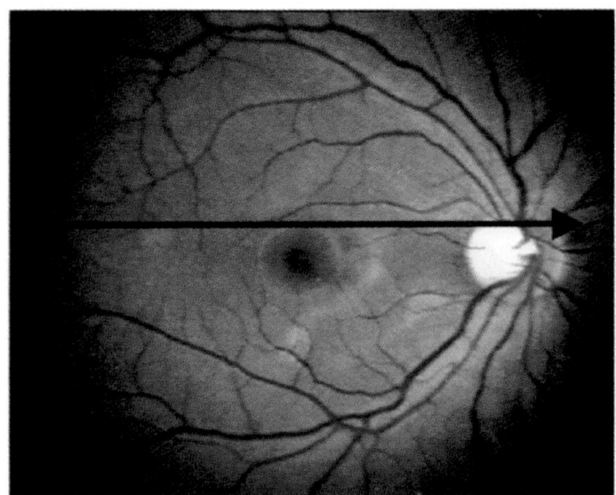

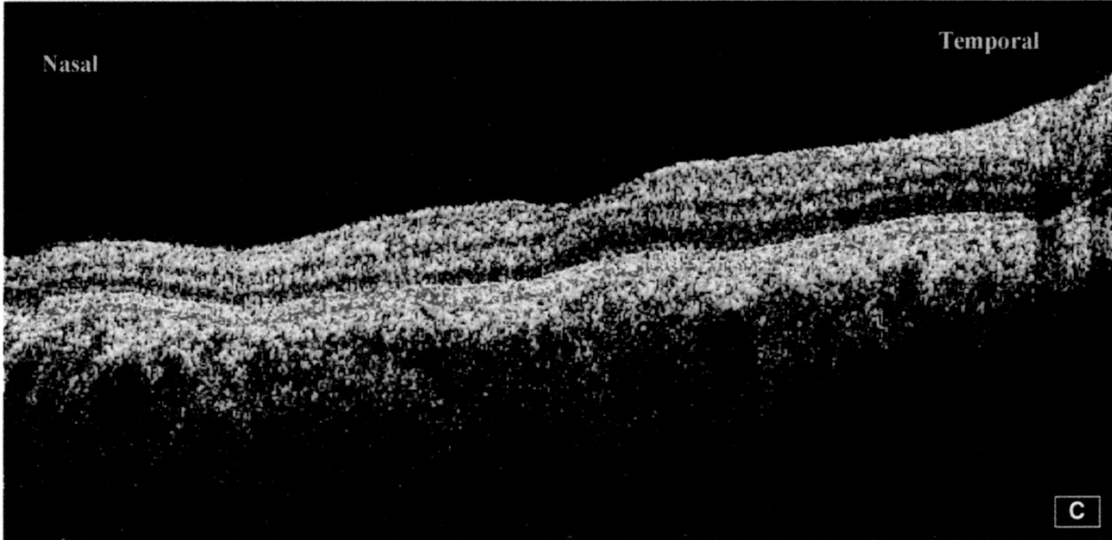

The left eye of the patient showed multiple white dots at the level of outer retina that were hyperfluorescent on fluorescein angiography (D). The OCT, however, was normal (E).

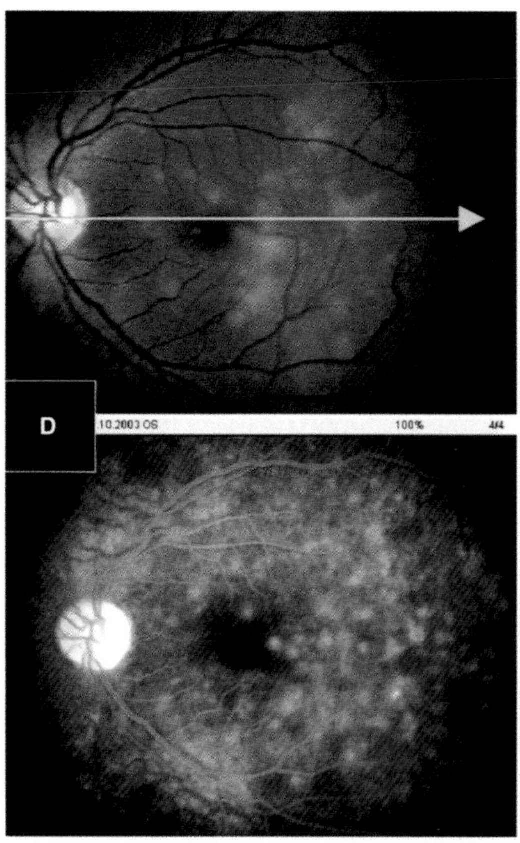

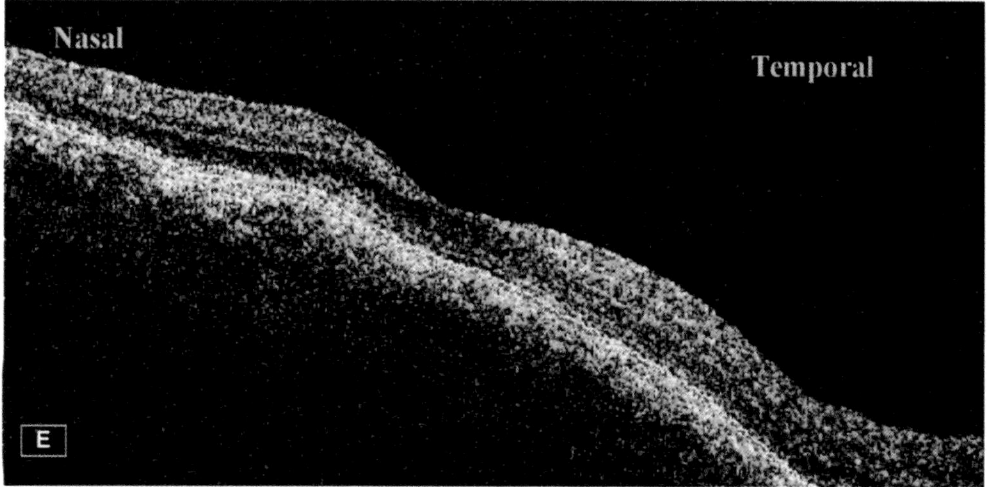

CONCLUSIONS

In our experience, OCT maybe normal in certain white dot syndromes.

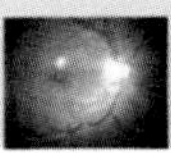

SERPIGINOUS CHOROIDOPATHY

This entity is also known as geographic or helicoid choroidopathy and is classically defined as bilateral disease with perpapillary grayish white lesions that grow centripetally towards the periphery. They spread with an active and heal with destruction of choroid and overlying retina and pigment epithelium edge. The disease tends to have a recurrent course and may be complicated with the development of choroidal neovascular membrane or subretinal fibrosis.

In our population from North India, we found that serpiginous choroidopathy had different course; the disease was seen in younger patients, had better outcome and few of these cases also had hypersensitivity to *Mycobacterium tuberculosis*.

Case 18.13: Serpiginous choroidopathy

Case Summary

A 39-year-old woman had serpiginous choroidopathy in the right eye. The fluffy, yellowish-white edge indicates active disease (A). The edge is hypofluorescent initially with late hyperfluorescence (B-C).

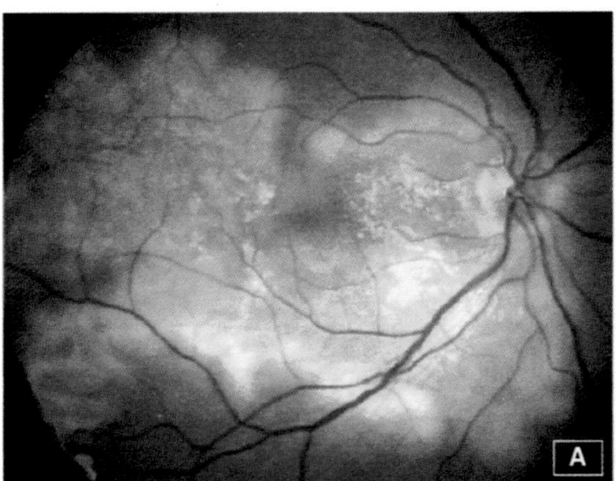

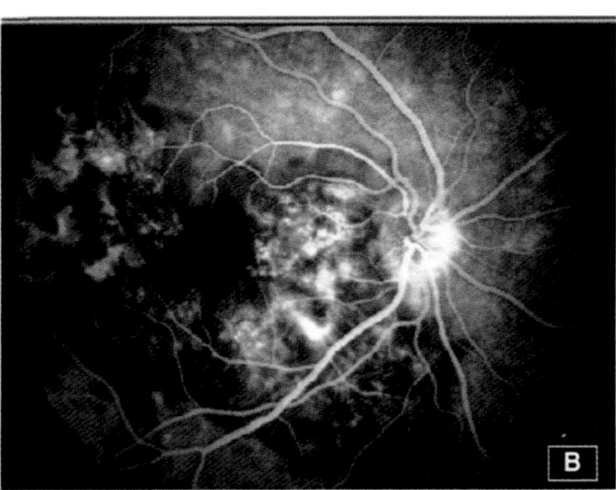

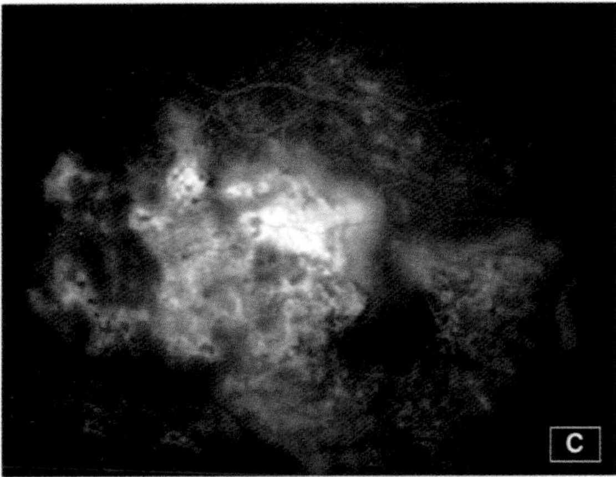

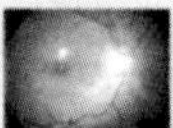

Optical Coherence Tomography

The OCT line scan (D) through the active inferior edge showed increased hyper-reflectivity from the underlying choroid with an area of hyporeflectivity in the outer retina that showed shadowing behind.

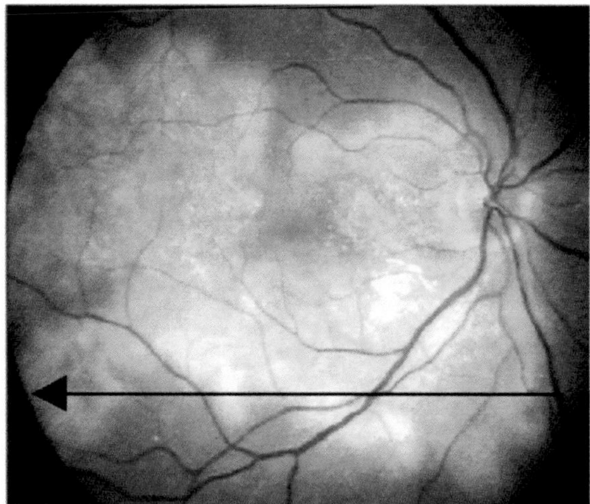

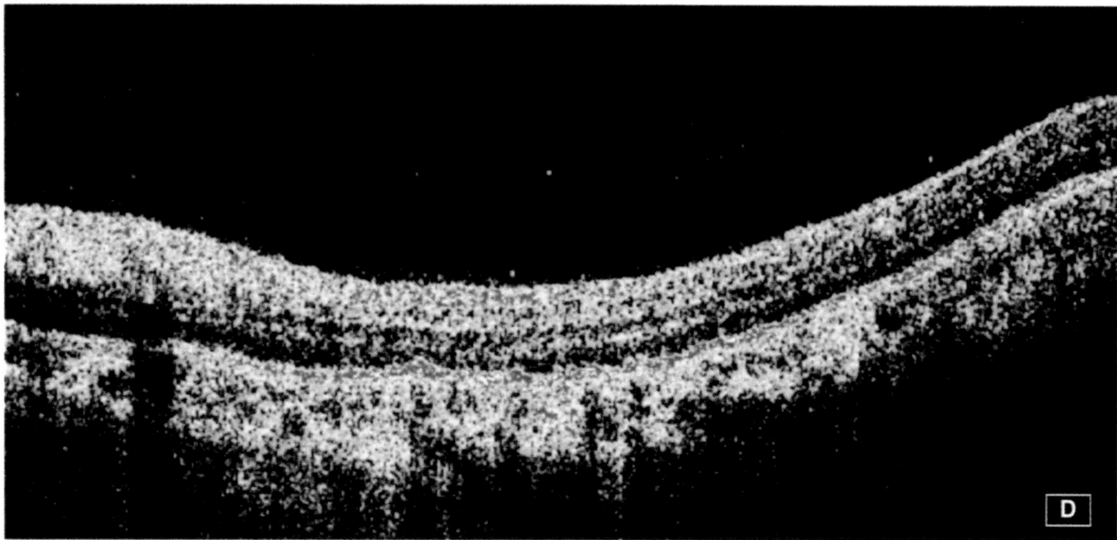

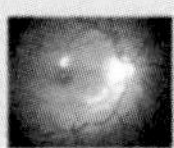

OCT line scan through the superior active edge (E) showed two hyporeflective areas in the outer retina in the peripapillary region with a trail of back shadow obscuring the details of underlying tissues.

The lesion healed with oral corticosteroids leaving an atrophic scar (F).

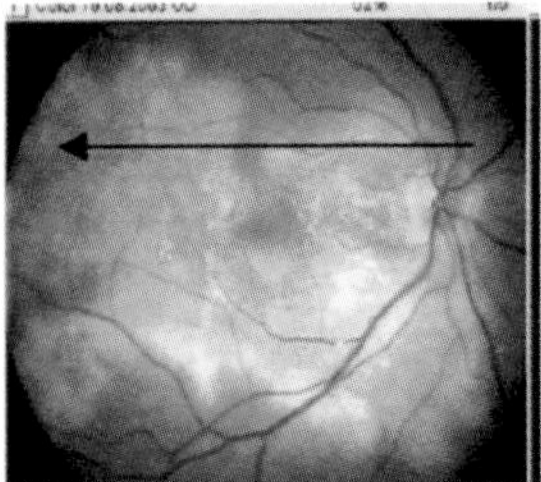

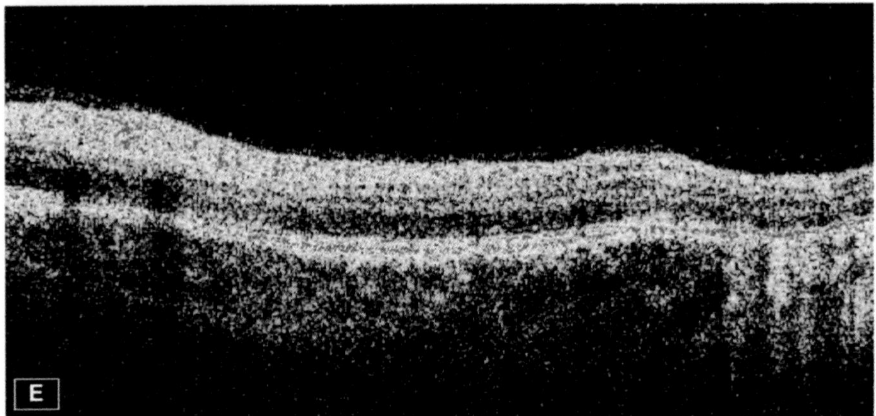

The repeat OCT scan through the fovea (G) showed increased hyper-reflectivity from the retinal pigment epithelium (RPE) under the fovea. The RPE was irregular nasal to the fovea whereas temporally, the RPE layer could not be differentiated from the underlying choroid, probably indicating areas of RPE atrophy.

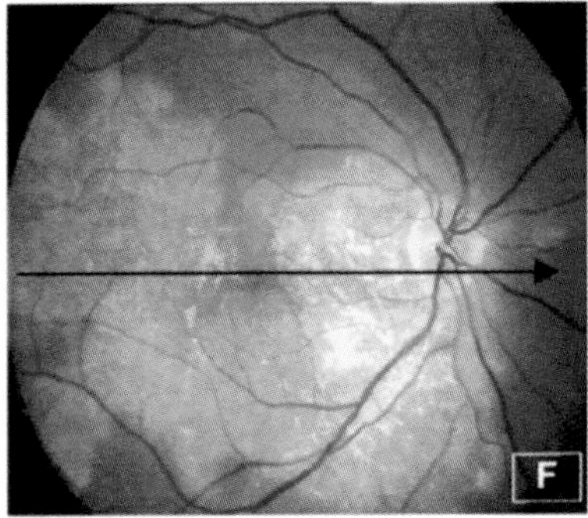

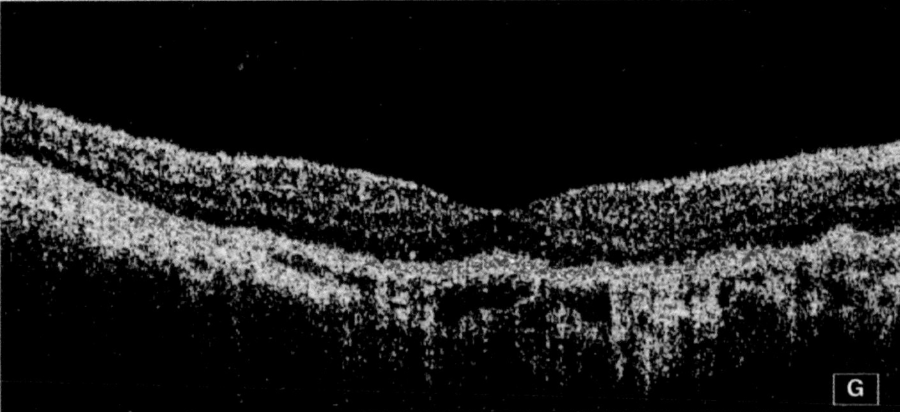

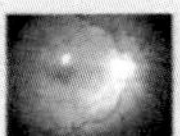

The repeat OCT scan done through the superior border showed resolution of areas of hypo-reflectivity with restoration of hyper-reflectivity from the underlying retinal pigment epithelium (RPE) (H). Note the absence of RPE or choroidal atrophy.

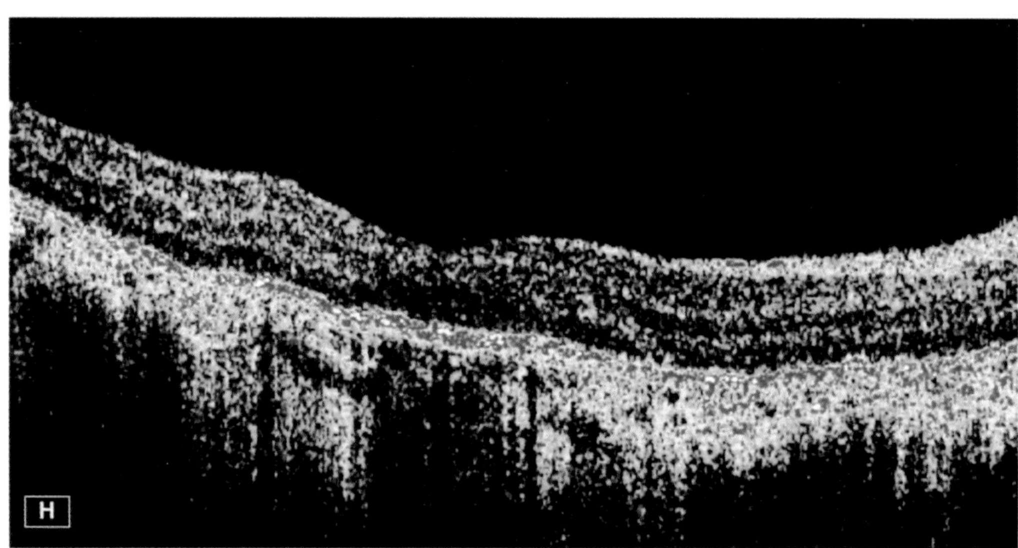

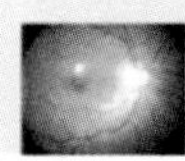

Case 18.14: Serpiginous choroidopathy with choroidal neovascular membrane (CNVM)

Case Summary

A 36-year-old woman was seen with healed lesions of serpiginous choroidopathy in her right eye (A). There were two small active lesions (arrows). The patient received posterior subtenon injection of triamcinolone acetonide 20 mg as she was intolerant to oral corticosteroids.

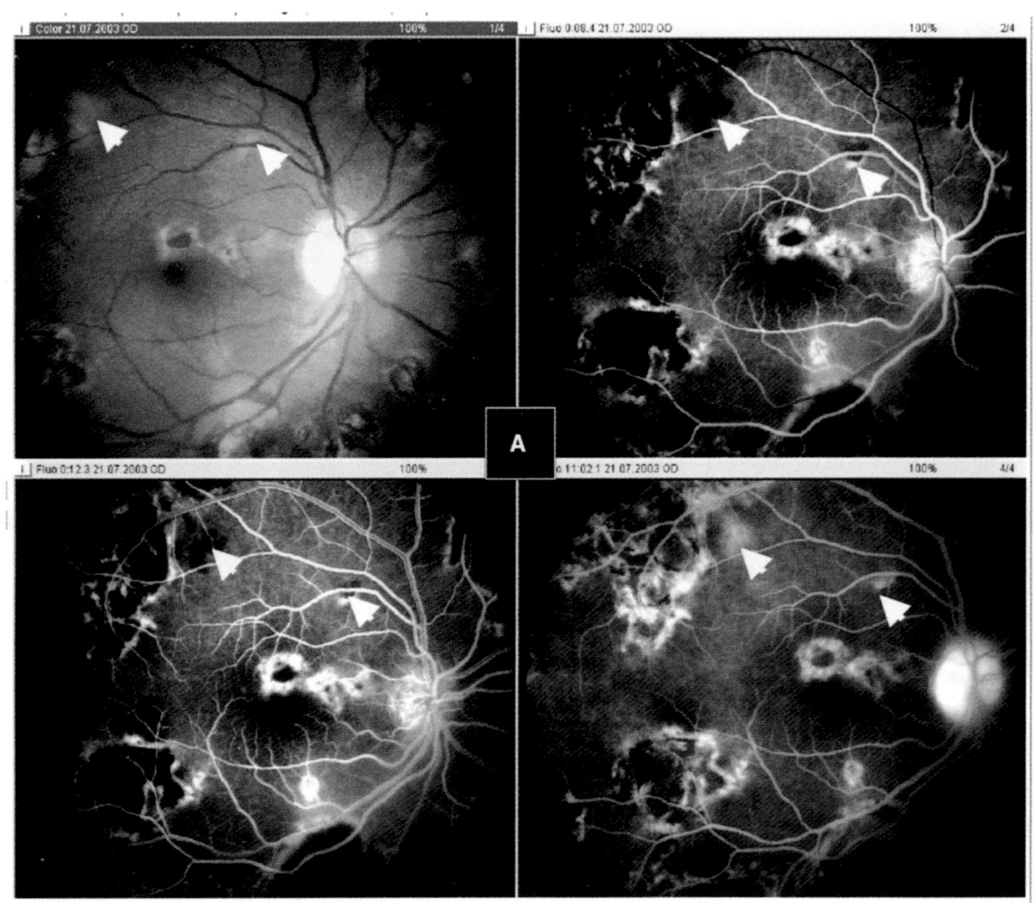

The vertical OCT scan (B) through fovea showed normal foveal contour with retinal pigment epithelial thickening in the area corresponding to the pigmented scar superior to the fovea.

The patient returned ten days later with complaints of blurred vision of 3 days duration. Her best corrected visual acuity was reduced to 20/40. The right eye now showed the appearance of new active lesions (arrows) that showed early hypo and late hyperfluorescence on fluorescein angiography and hypofluorescence on indocyanine green (ICG) angiography (C-F). The fovea also showed the presence of hemorrhage (black arrow) that was seen as a choroidal neovascular membrane on fluorescein angiography with hyperfluorescence in late phase of ICG (not shown).

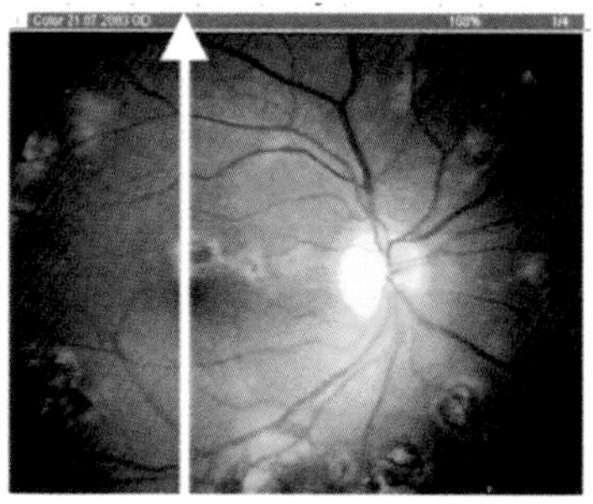

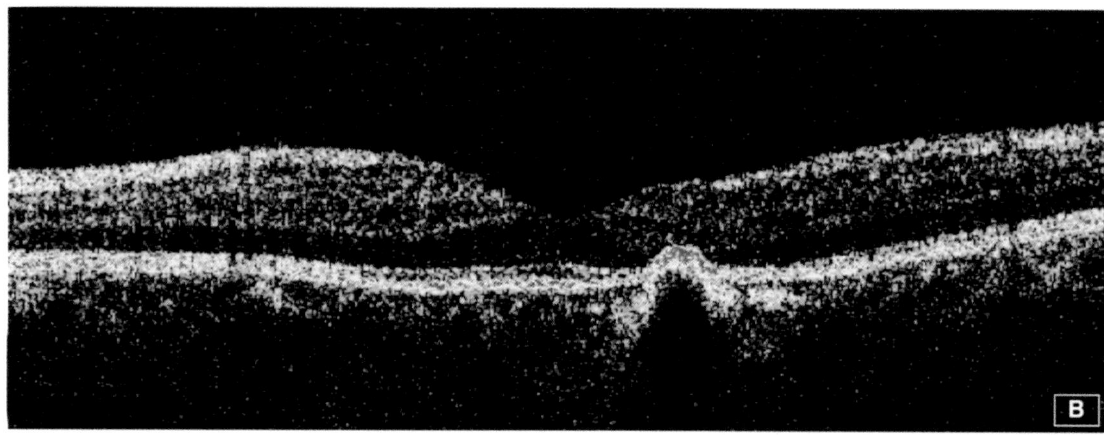

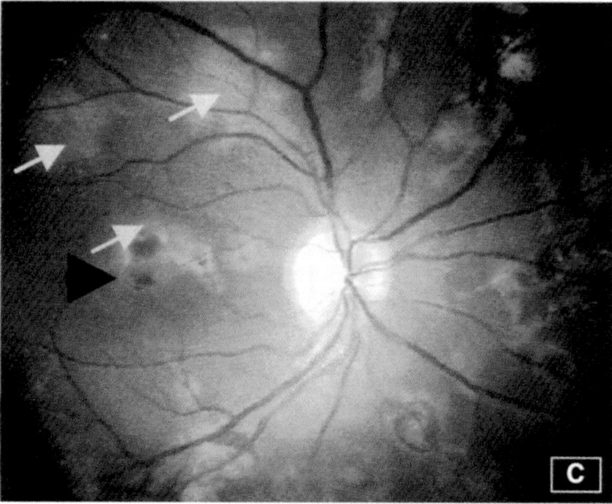

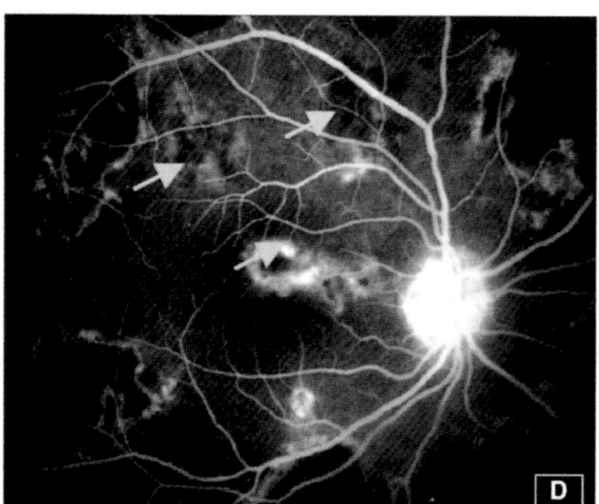

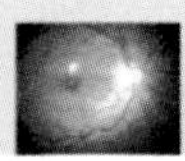

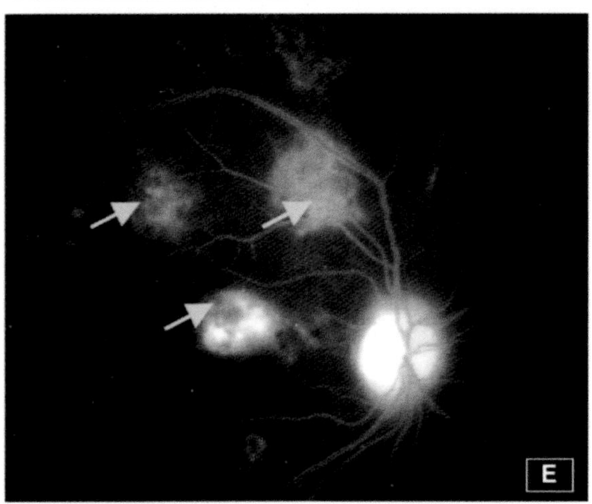

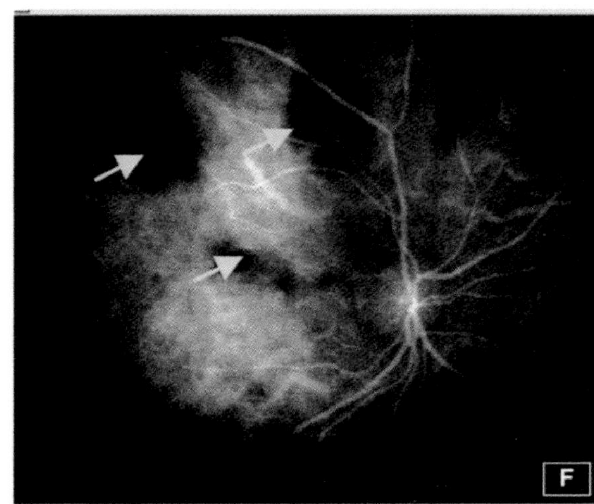

Optical Coherence Tomography

The vertical line scan through the fovea (G) showed a disruption in the retinal pigment epithelium (RPE) adjacent to the RPE hyperplasia with an area of moderate backscatter corresponding to the fibrovascular complex of choroidal neovascular membrane.

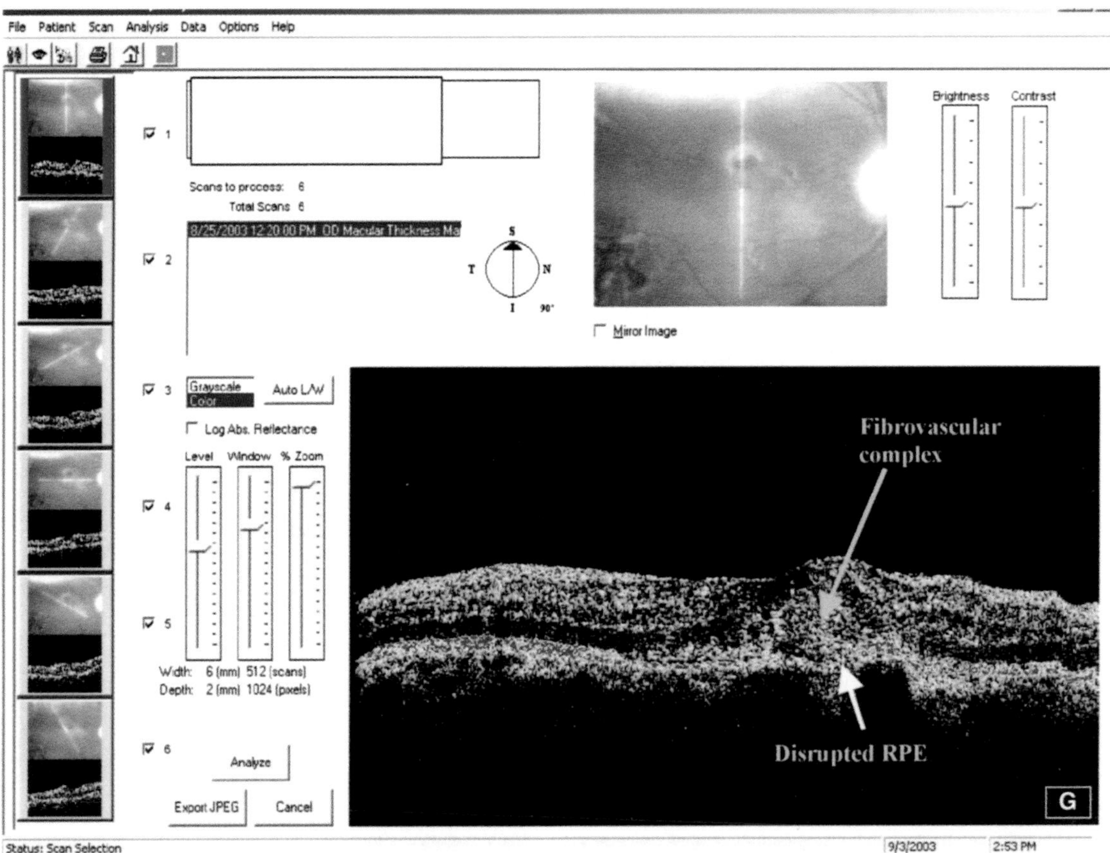

The oblique line scan passing through the same area (H) showed increased retinal thickness, disrupted retinal pigment epithelium and hyporeflective space suggestive of intraretinal fluid.

The patient underwent photodynamic therapy (PDT) with verteporfin.

Three weeks later, repeat OCT (I) showed stage III response showing choroidal neovascularization as hyper-reflective zone seen anterior to red outer band representing retinal pigment epithelium. The hyporeflective strip adjacent to it represents subretinal fluid. The hyporeflective spaces seen anterior to this represent intraretinal accumulation of fluid.

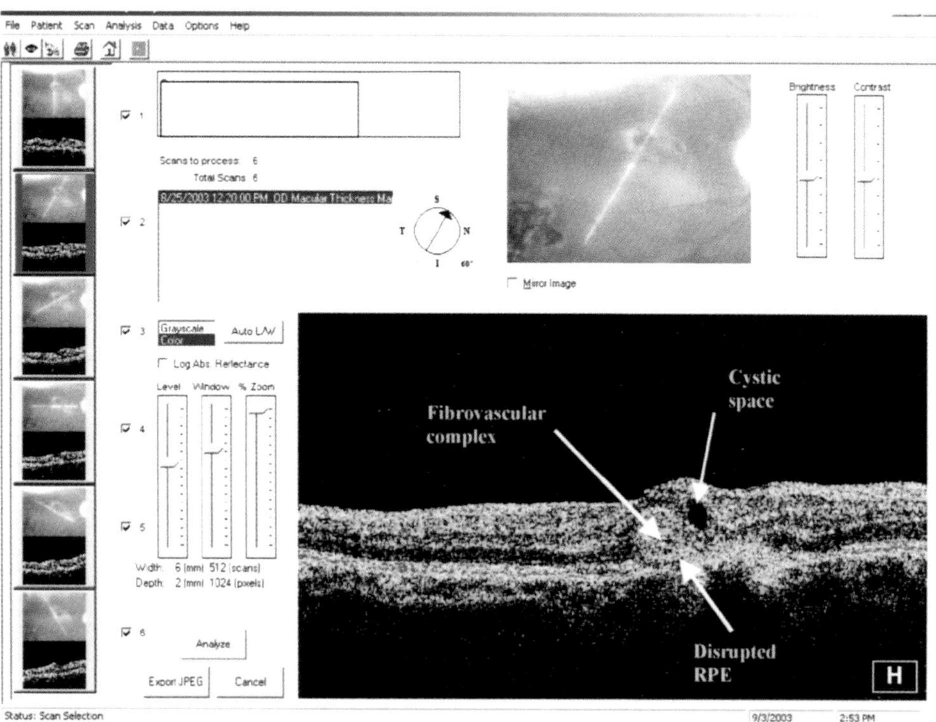

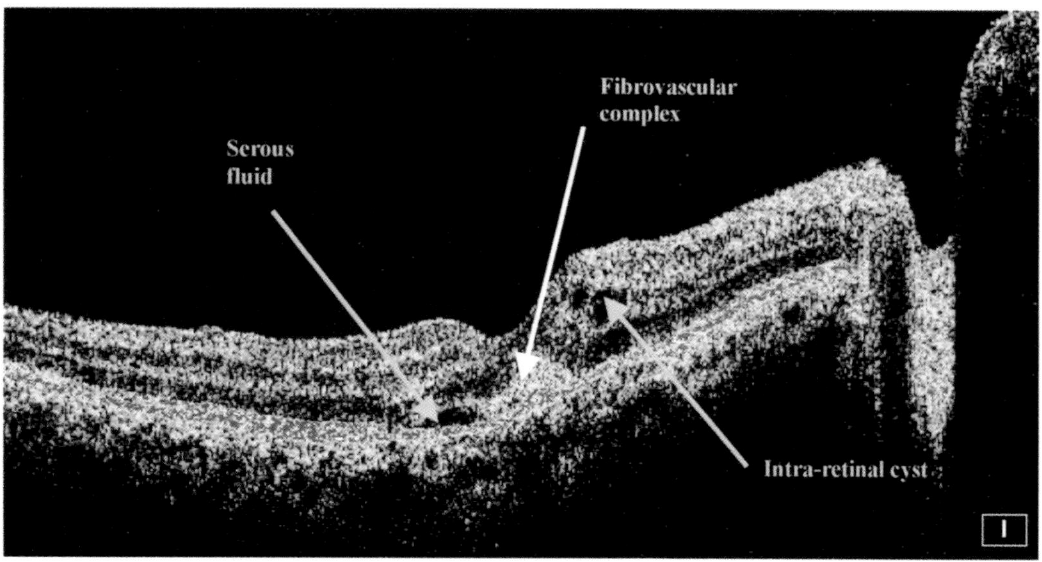

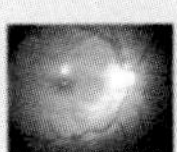

Case 18.15: Serpiginous choroidopathy with cystoid macular edema

Case Summary

A 24-year-old man was seen with healed atrophic scar of serpiginous choroidopathy (A) that showed pooling of dye in small cystic spaces in the late phase of fluorescein angiography (B-D).

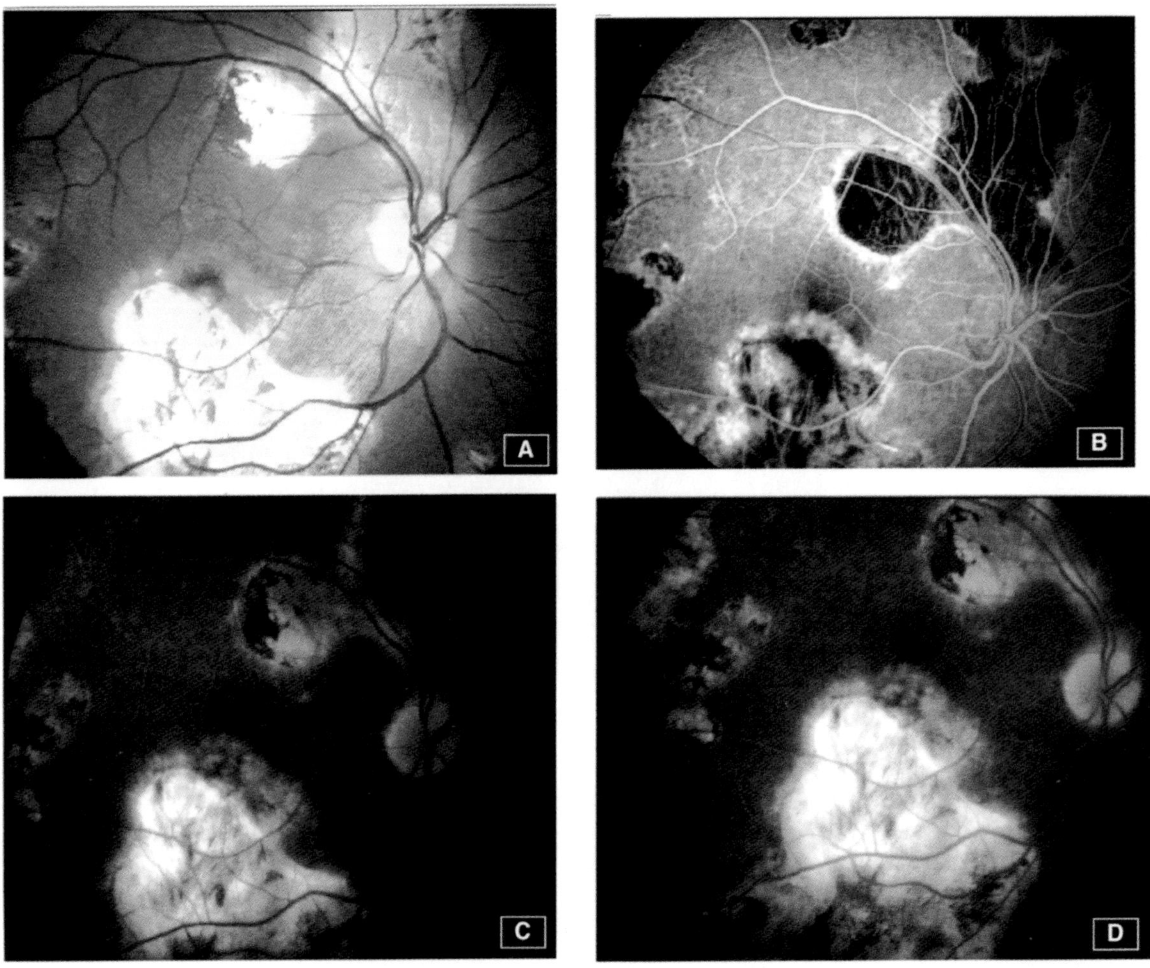

The OCT line scans (E, F) showed the presence of hyporeflective areas with intervening septae suggesting the presence of cystoid spaces at the edge of the healed serpiginous choroiditis scar.

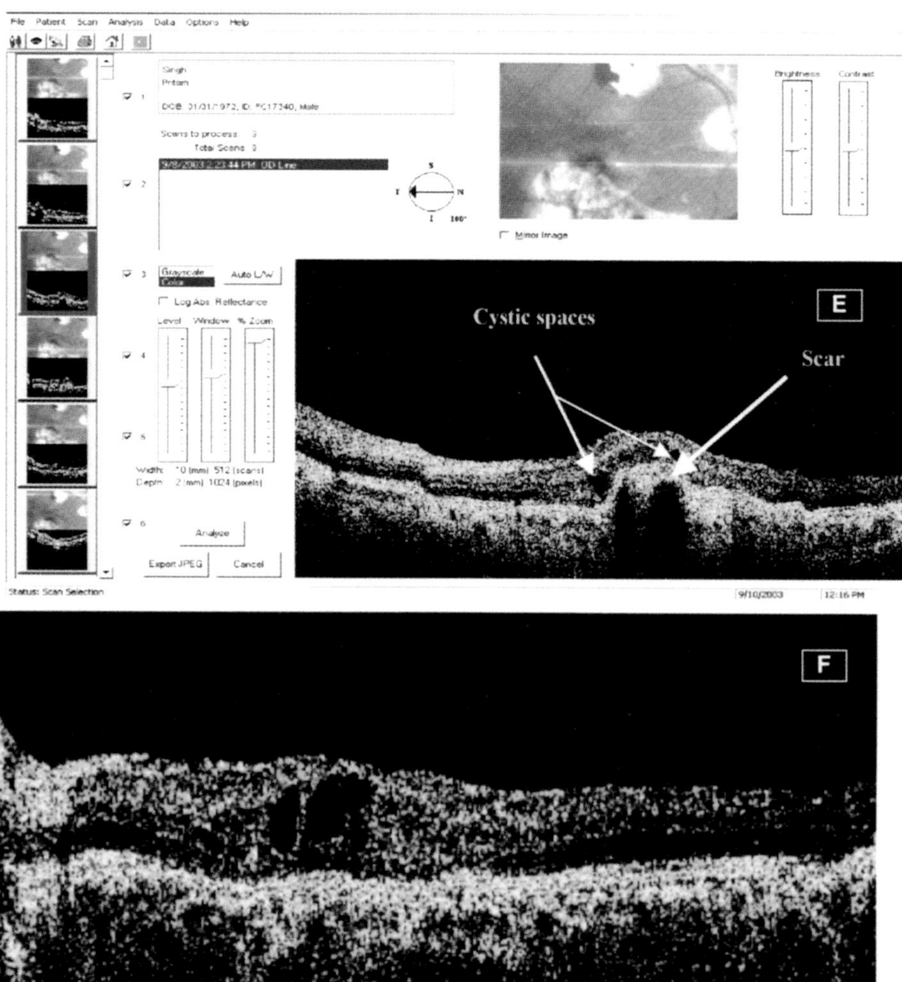

CONCLUSIONS

In our own experience, we did not find any consistent OCT findings in monitoring choroiditis. Though it shows changes in the overlying retinal pigment epithelium and neurosensory retina, we were not able to identify the patterns of changes in the choriocapillaries. Maybe with more experience, we shall be able to define choroiditis patterns with more certainty. However, it was found to be a very useful tool in diagnosing the associated changes occurring in the overlying neurosensory retina and the development of choroidal neovascular membrane.

SUGGESTED READINGS

1. Gass JDM. Inflammatory diseases of the retina and chroid. In : Steroscopic Atlas of Macular Disease : Diagnosis and treatment, 4th ed. St. Louis Mo: C.V. Mosby Co.; 1997 :158-65.
2. Gupta V, Agarwal A, Gupta A et al. Clinical characteristics of serpiginous choroidopathy in North India. Am J Ophthalmol 2002; 134: 47-56.
3. Gupta V, Gupta A, Arora S et al. Presumed Tubercular Serpiginouslike Choroiditis Clinical Presentations and Management. Ophthalmology 2003;110:1747-52.

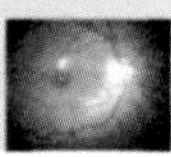

Case 18.16: Intraocular Cysticercosis

Case Summary

A 24-year-old boy was seen with subretinal cysticercus in the right eye. The fundus showed a subretinal cyst with central whitish area suggesting an invaginated scolex (A,B). The scar seen just above the cyst probably represented the site of entry. The fluorescein angiography showed well demarcated hyperfluorescent boundary with central areas of hyperfluorescence (C, D).

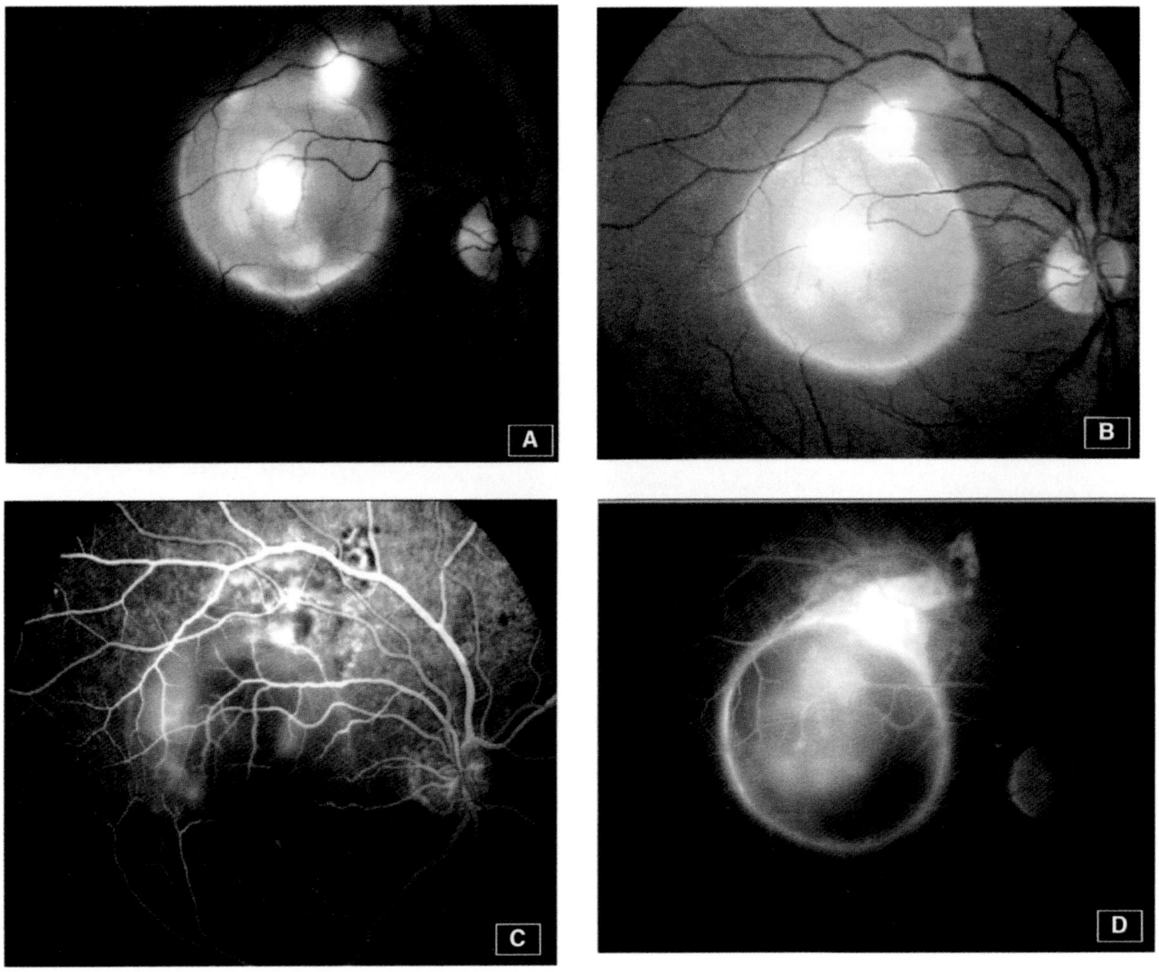

Optical Coherence Tomography

OCT scan through the cyst showed the subretinal location of the cyst (E).

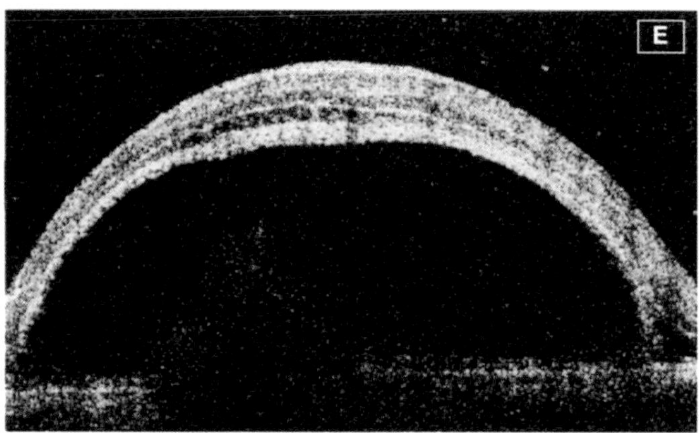

When seen 3 days later, the cyst had migrated from the subretinal location into the vitreous (F). The patient was subjected to pars plana vitrectomy. Behind the cyst was seen a large fibrotic scar (G) that was seen as hyper-reflective area on OCT associated with an overlying epiretinal membrane (H).

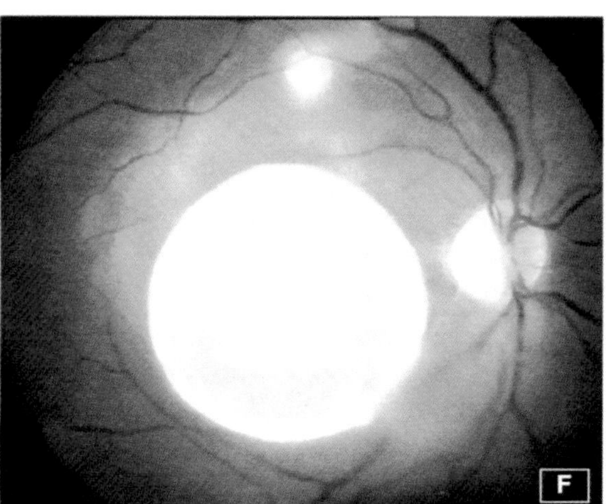

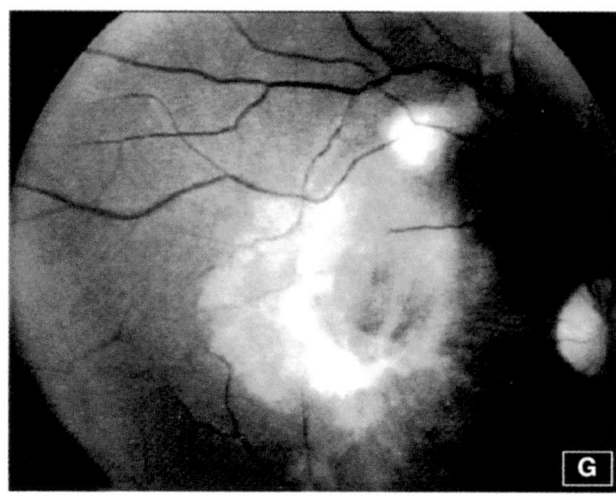

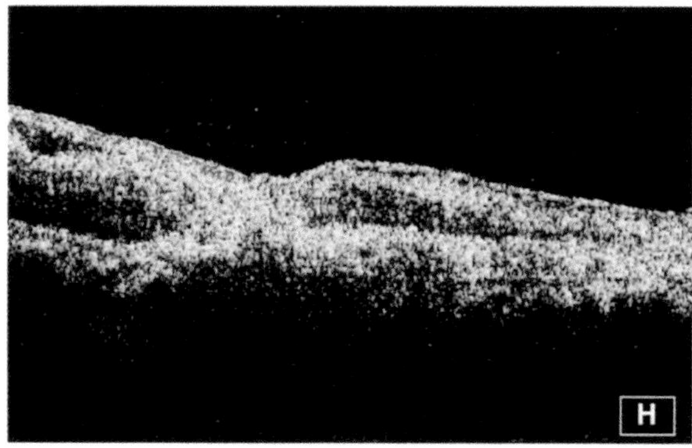

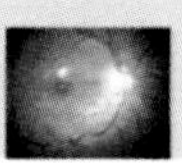

CONCLUSIONS

On OCT, intraocular cyst was seen as hyporeflective area due to the presence of fluid in the cyst cavity. The height of the cyst obscured the visualization of scolex on OCT.

SUGGESTED READING

1. Danis P. Intraocular cysticercus. Arch Ophthalmol 1974;91:238-39.

TUBERCULOMA

Case 18.17: Tuberculoma

Case Summary

A 24-year-old man with military tuberculosis was seen with tuberculoma in the left eye (A). The tuberculoma was hypofluorescent initially and became hyperfluorescent in the late phase. In addition, there were three more hypofluorescent areas that showed mild hyperfluorescence in the late phase (B-D).

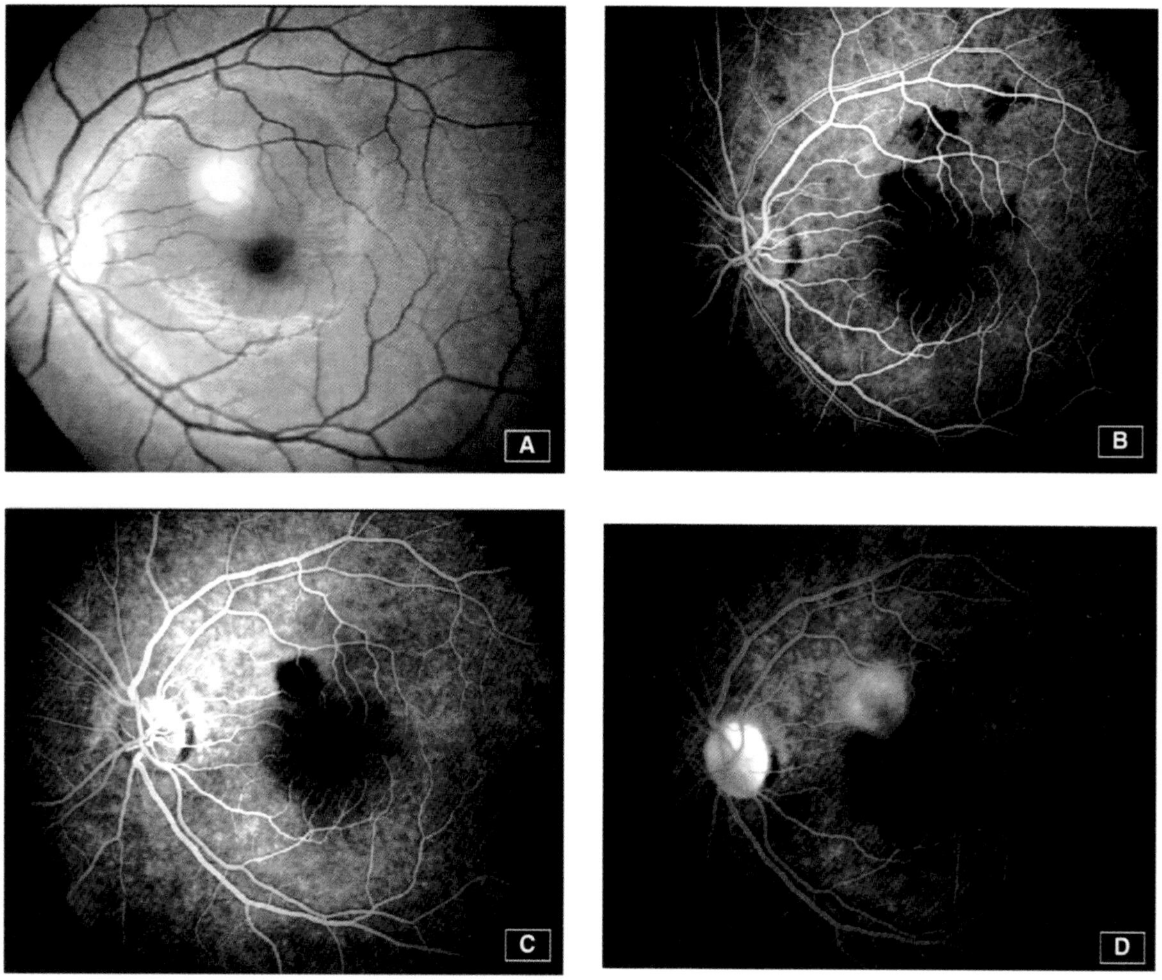

A

B

C

D

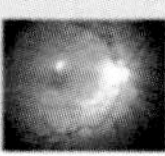

The horizontal OCT line scans (E, F) through the tuberculoma showed moderately increased hyper-reflectivity in the outer retinal layers with adjacent serous retinal detachment.

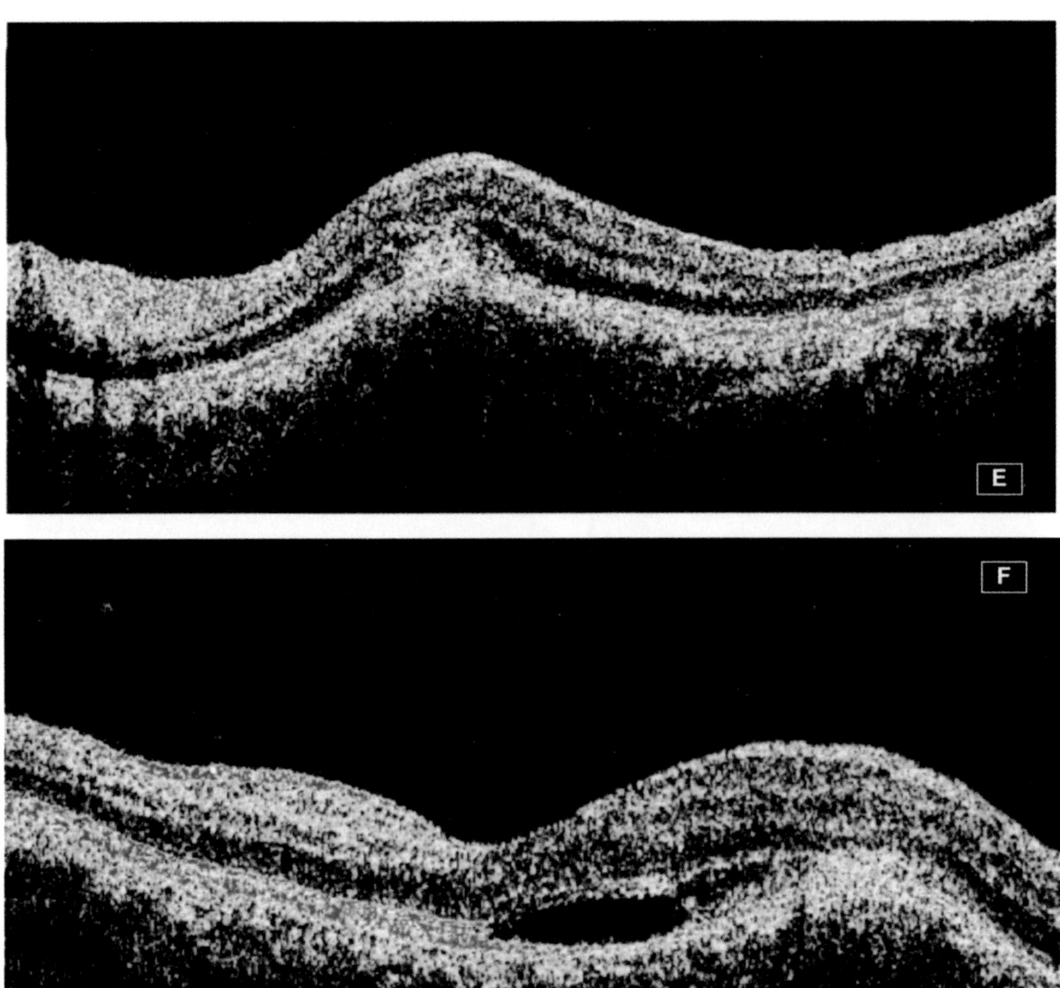

CONCLUSIONS

In patients with granulomas/tuberculomas, OCT helps in diagnosing associated pathologies like cystoid macular edema, serous retinal detachment, choroidal neovascularization and subretinal fibrosis. It can also help in determining the extent and location of granuloma and help in monitoring response to the therapy.

Chapter 19

Retinal Angiomatosis Proliferation

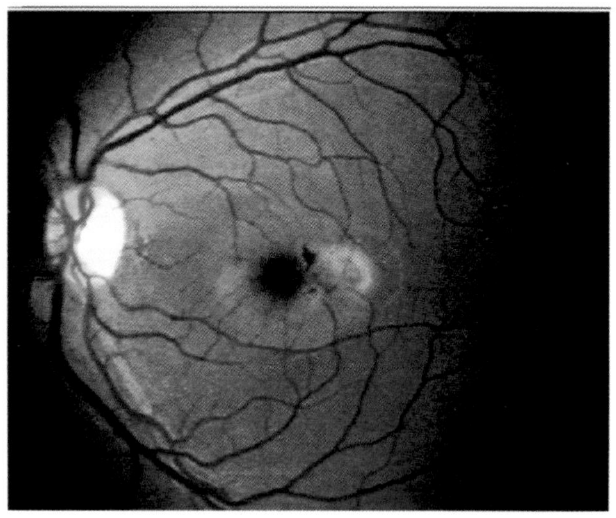

RETINAL ANGIOMATOUS PROLIFERATION

Retinal Angiomatous Proliferation (RAP) is a subgroup first defined in patients with age related macular degeneration (ARMD) where the neovascular process originates from the retina rather than choroid and then extends into the subretinal space. It has 3 distinct stages:

Stage 1: Intraretinal neovascularization (IRN): This begins as a small cluster of retinal capillaries in the neurosensory retina that develops into a mass of angiomatous tissue in the inner retina. These vessels may develop retinal-retinal anastomosis.

Stage 2: Subretinal neovascularization (SRN): In this stage, the intraretinal new vessels extend deep into the subretinal space creating a neurosensory detachment. As it advances and merges with the retinal pigment epithelium, a pigment epithelial detachment also develops.

Stage 3: Choroidal neovascularization (CNV): Here the subretinal neovascularization develops a connection with choroidal vessels termed as retinochoroidal anastomosis.

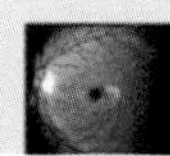

Case 19.1: Stage 2 RAP in Idiopathic Perifoveal Telangiectasia

Case Summary

A 34-year-old woman was seen with bilateral idiopathic perifoveal telangiectasia (A).

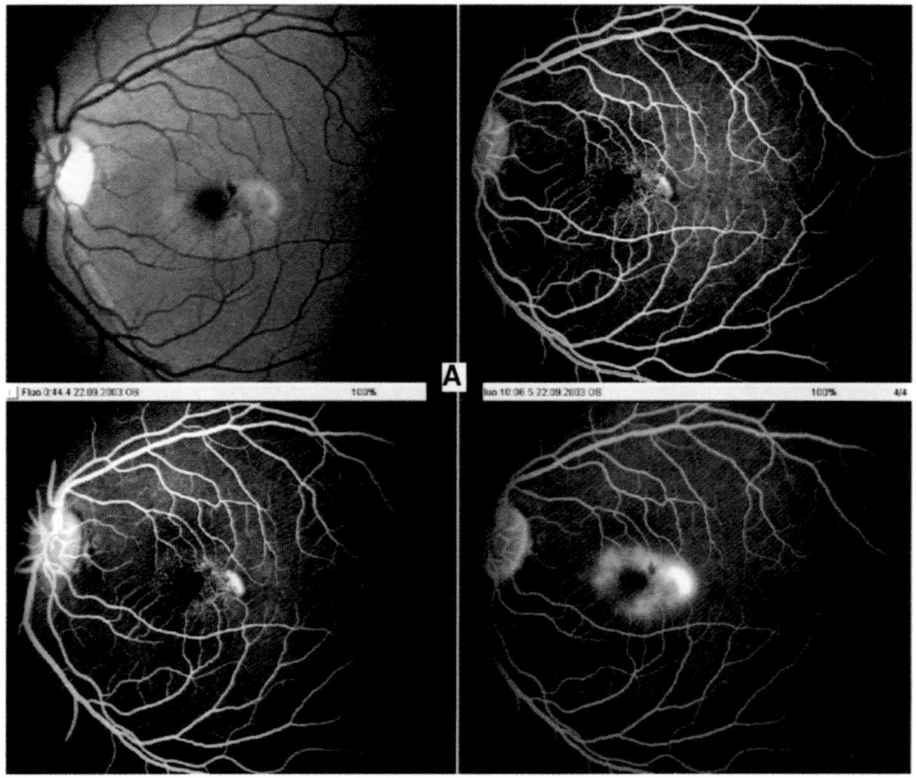

The fluorescein angiography (B) showed retinal-retinal anastomosis with arteriole and venule forming a hair-pin connection (arrows).

On OCT horizontal line scan (C), these new vessels were seen as hyper-reflective irregular intraretinal reflections.

Vertical line scan through the area of RAP (D) showed the growth of new vessels beneath the retinal pigment epithelium.

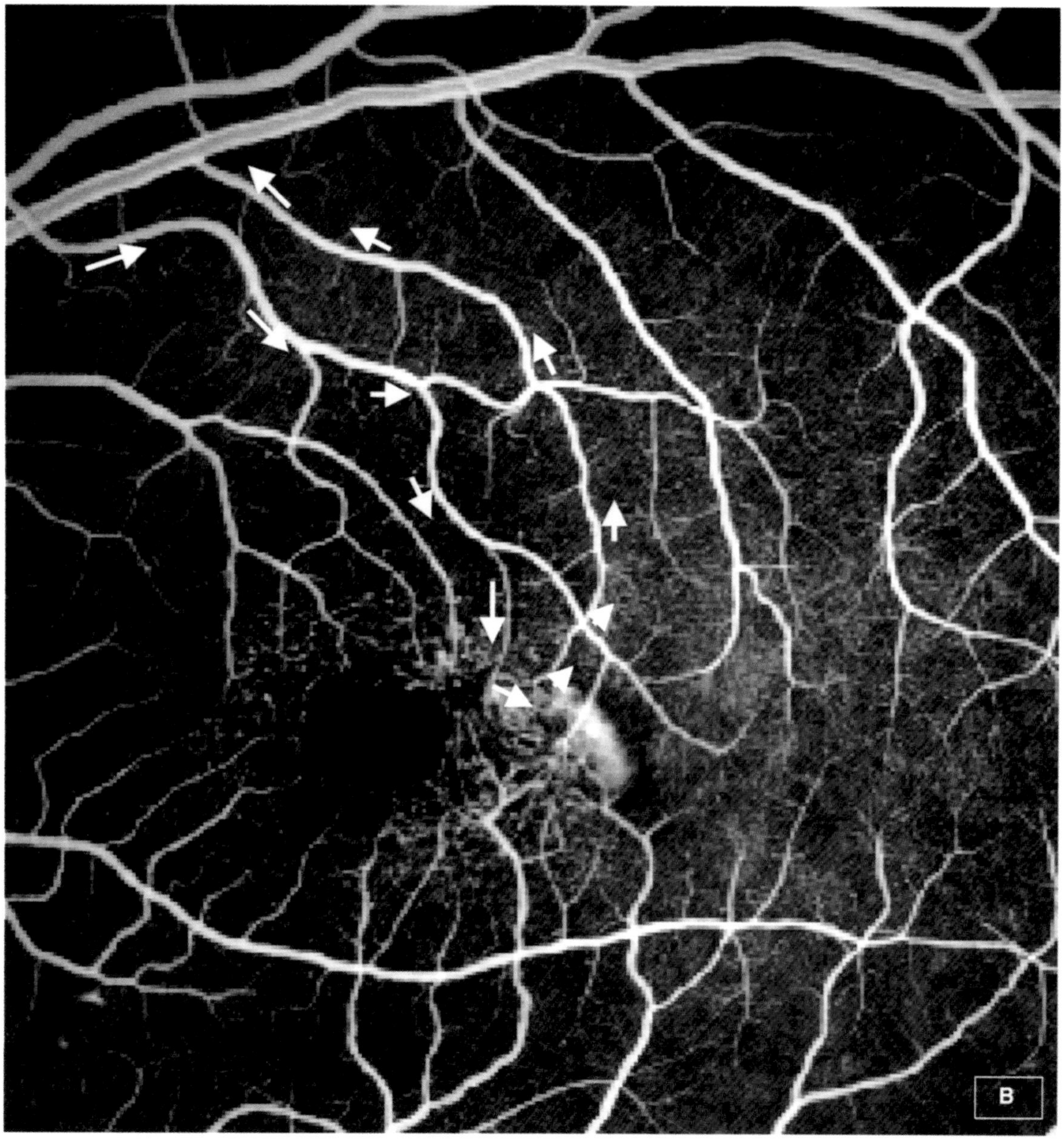

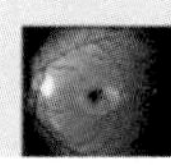

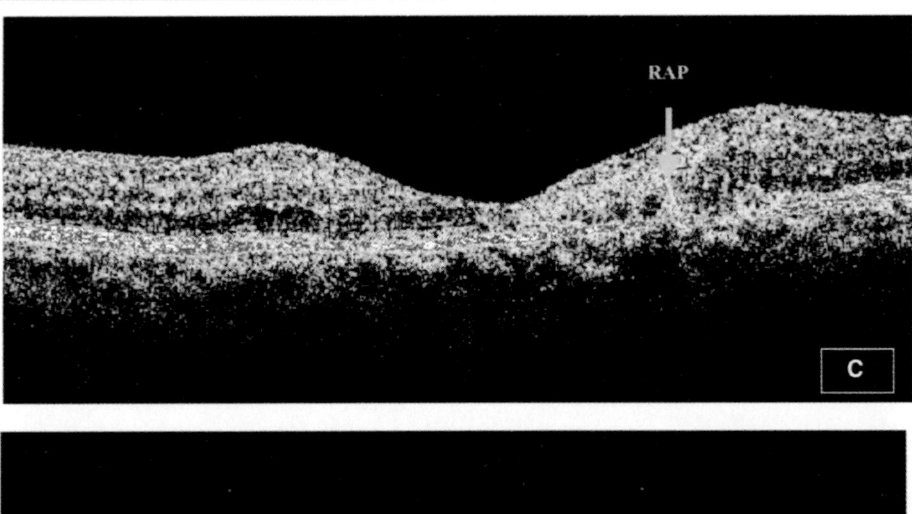

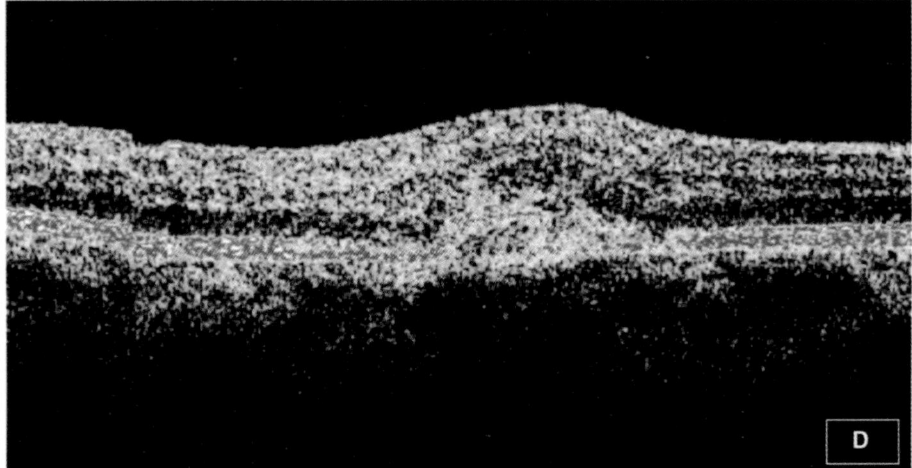

CONCLUSIONS

OCT provides the *in vivo* histopathology of retinal layers that helps in staging of the disease. It also helps in localizing other features including cystoid spaces, pigment epithelium and serous retinal detachments.

SUGGESTED READING

1. Yannuzi LA, Negrao S, IidaT et al. Retinal angiomatous proliferation in age-related macular degeneration. Retina 2001;21:416-434.

Chapter 20

Retinal Trauma

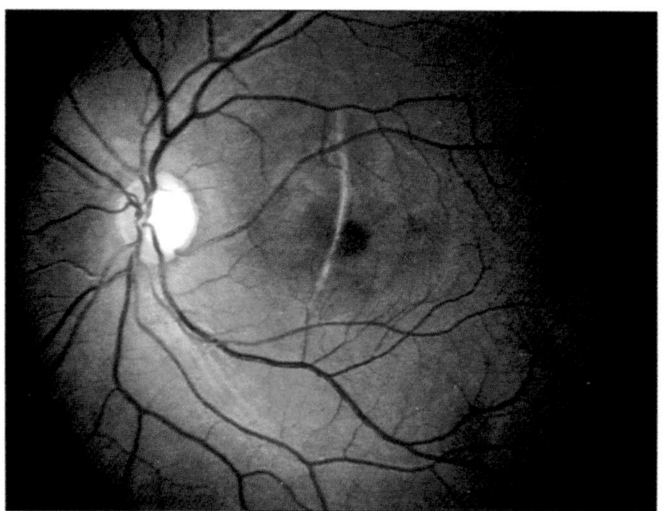

RETINALTRAUMA

Closed globe injuries can cause damage to the retina and underlying choroid and include commotio retinae, choroidal ruptures that may be associated with choroidal neovascular membrane, macular cyst, macular hole, retinal detachment, subretinal hemorrhage and so on. OCT is useful in the following ways:

1. It provides the ultrastructural information regarding the extent and degree of damage to the retina.
2. It can help in diagnosing changes that are not seen on fundoscopy and fluorescein angiography.
3. It can be used to monitor these patients for the development of new changes as well as monitoring response to the therapy.

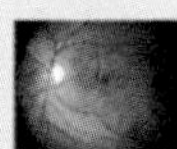

COMMOTIO RETINAE/ BERLIN'S EDEMA

Commotio retinae is characterized by the development of retinal whitening following blunt trauma. In the acute stage, there is disruption in the outer segments of photoreceptors. Subsequently the fluid accumulates in outer retina that might resolve or result in the formation of cystoid macular edema. The cysts then coalesce and might form a large cyst or a macular hole.

Case 20.1 : Commotio Retinae

Case Summary

A 24-year-old man suffered from blunt trauma in the left eye. His best-corrected visual acuity was 20/40 in this eye. Fundus showed mild disc edema with retinal edema in the posterior pole and internal limiting membrane folds (A), fluorescein angiography showed disc hyperfluorescence (B). Two days later, he developed peripapillary serous detachment (C,D).

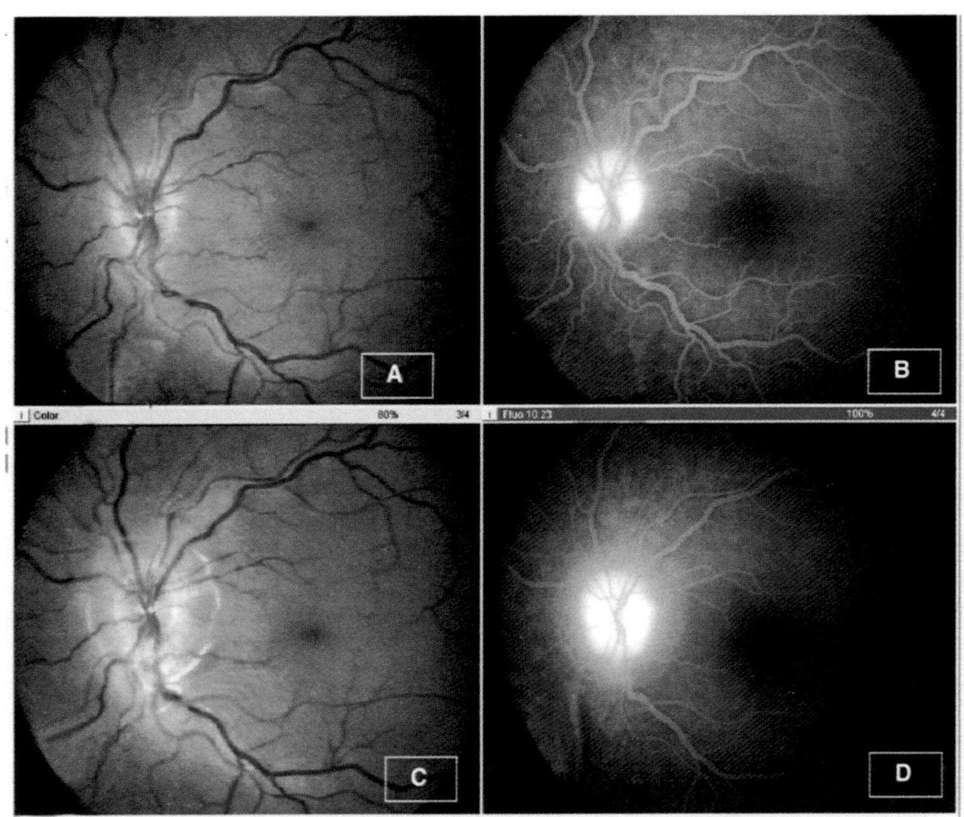

Optical Coherence Tomography of the left eye showed moderately increased hyper-reflectivity from the retinal layers just below the papillomacular bundle. No increase was noticed in the retinal thickness. Note mild disruption in the outer photoreceptor layer. These changes subsided over next two weeks and patient regained vision of 20/16 in this eye.

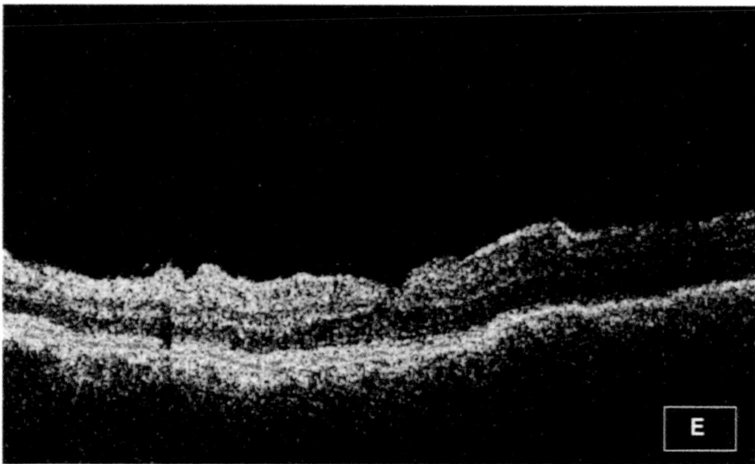

Case 20.2: Commotio Retinae with Intraretinal Cyst

Case Summary

A 20-year-old man was seen three weeks following trauma to the left eye with a stick. His best-corrected visual acuity was 20/100. Fundoscopy showed grayish-white opacification of retina adjacent to the fovea (A, B). The fluorescein angiography was normal (C, D).

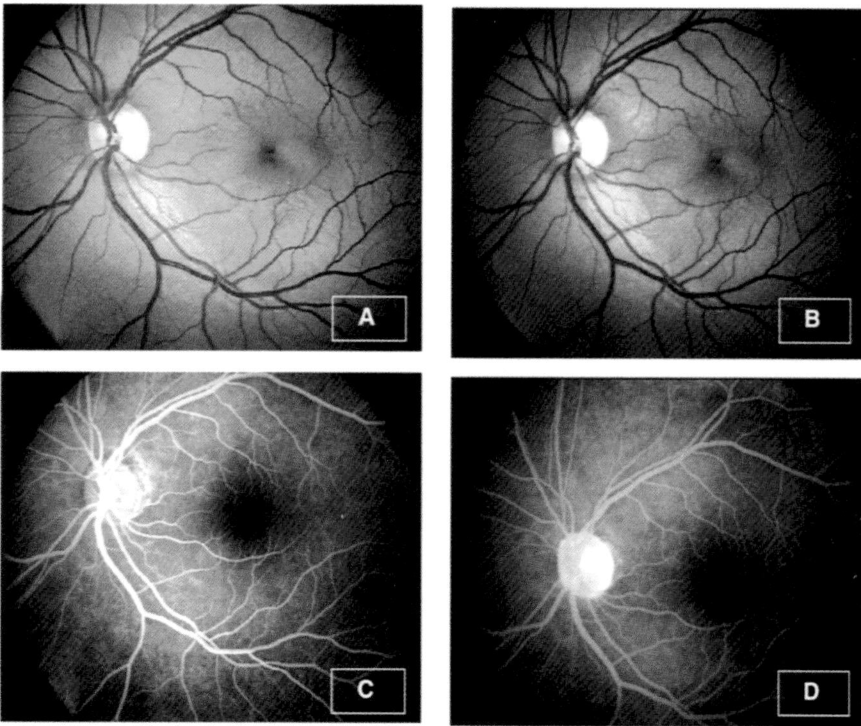

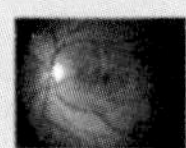

Optical Coherence Tomography

OCT line scan through the foveal center (E) showed the presence of a hyporeflective area within the retina suggesting the formation of an intraretinal cyst that precedes the development of a macular hole.

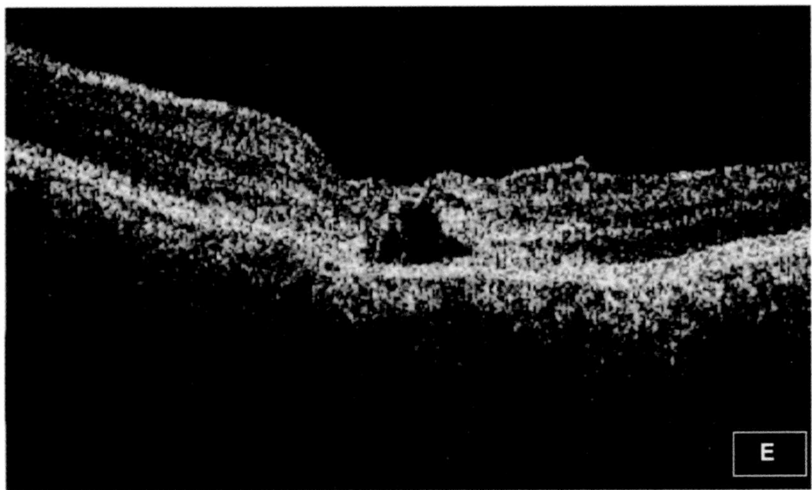

Case 20.3: Traumatic Macular Cyst

Case Summary

A 20-year-old woman was seen with decreased vision in her left eye following blunt trauma (A). The fluorescein angiography showed mild hyperfluorescence in the fovea (B).

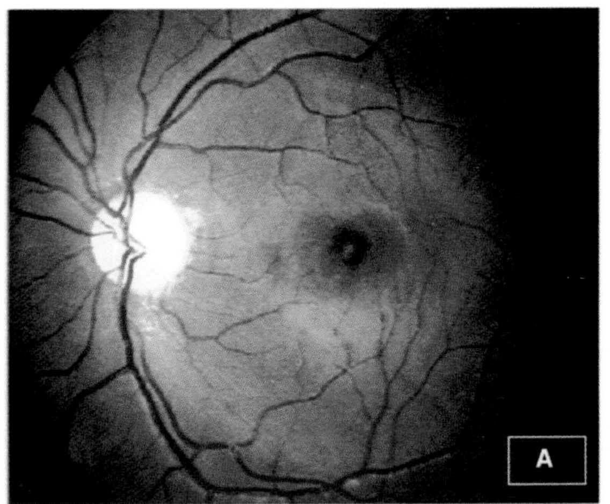

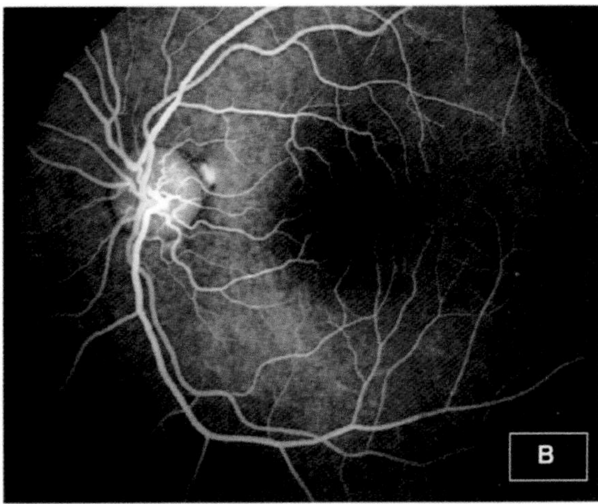

Optical Coherence Tomography

OCT line scan through the fovea showed the development of a macular cyst in the inner retinal layers (C).

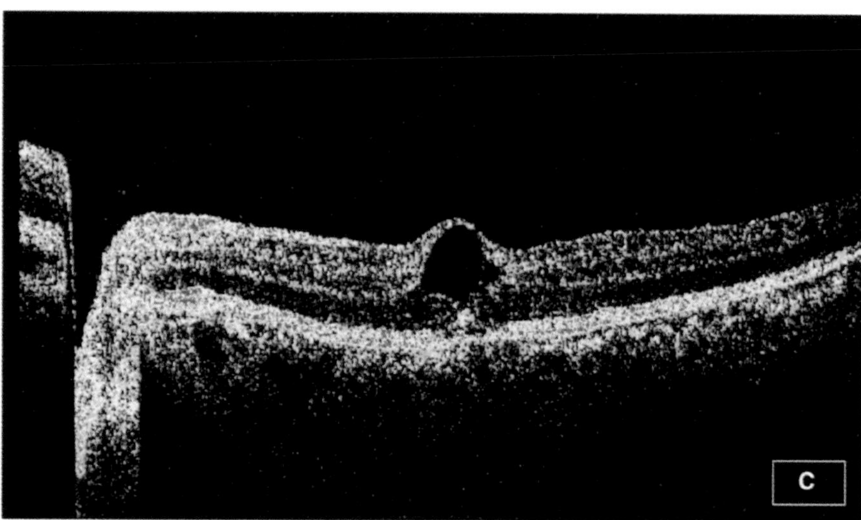

TRAUMATIC MACULAR HOLES

Case 20.4: Traumatic Macular Hole

Case Summary

A 32-year-old man was seen with traumatic macular hole in the left eye (A). Optical Coherence Tomography of the left eye showed full thickness macular hole (B).

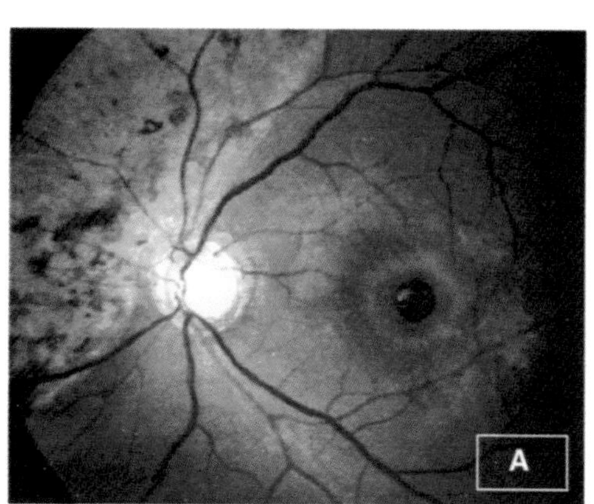

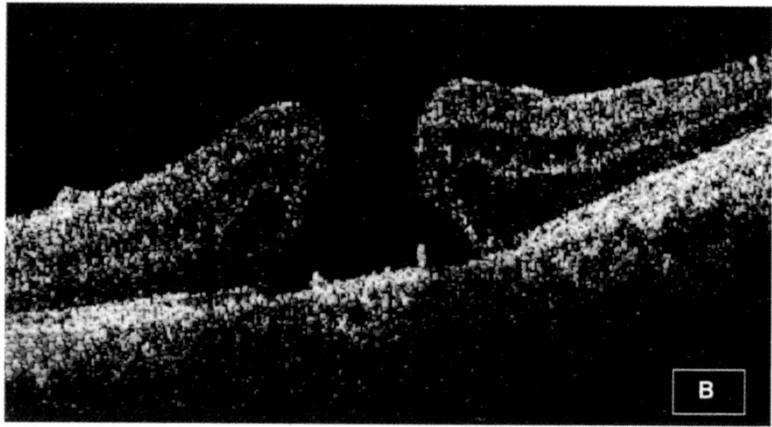

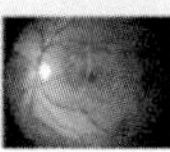

The patient underwent pars plana vitrectomy with $C_3 F_8$ gas temponade. Postoperatively, one edge of the hole got attached to underlying retina (C) but a month later, the edge reopened (D). The patient underwent repeat pars plana vitrectomy.

The macular hole closed after re-surgery as was seen on fundoscopy (E) and OCT (F).

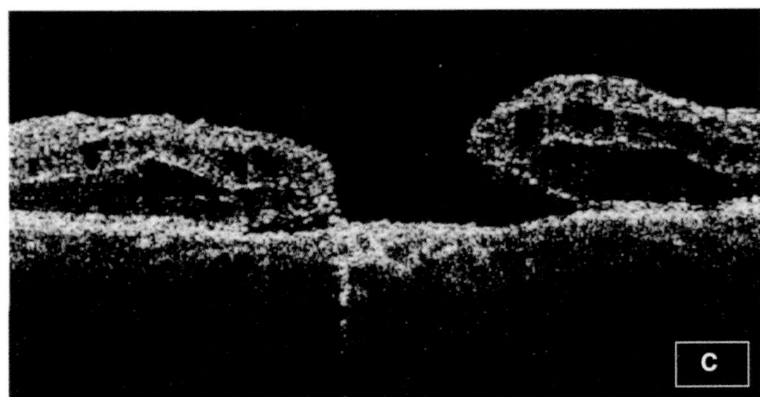

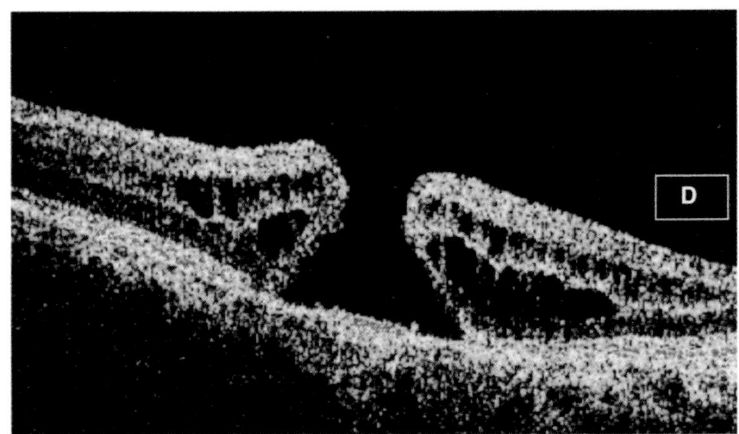

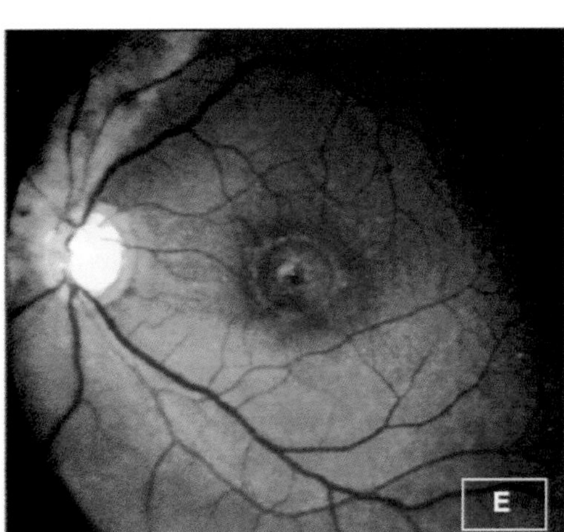

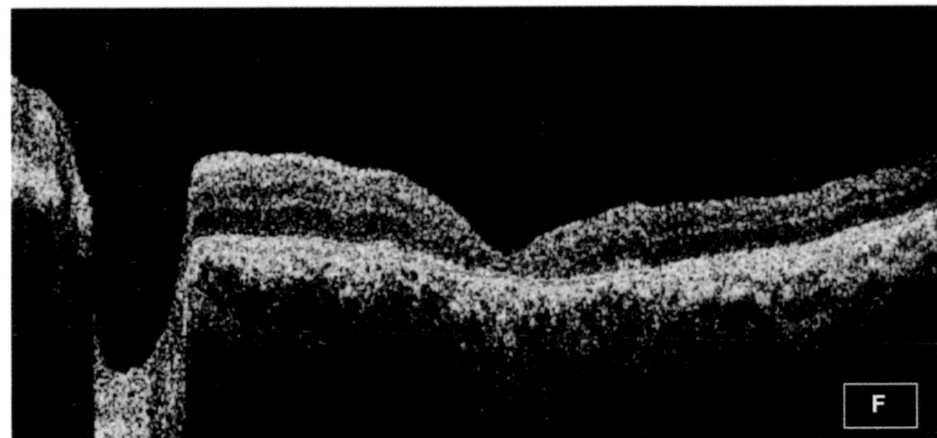

CHOROIDAL RUPTURES

Choroidal ruptures are known to occur following trauma. These are seen as linear, hypopigmented scars and have a risk of developing choroidal neovascularization.

Case 20.5: Traumatic Choroidal Rupture

Case Summary

A 12-year-old male child was seen with juxtafoveal choroidal rupture (arrow) in the left eye following cricket-ball injury (A).

The OCT line scan through the foveal center (B) showed atrophy of neurosensory retina probably due to damage to the underlying retinal pigment epithelium (RPE). The underlying RPE-choroid complex showed thickening that could be reactionary response to trauma.

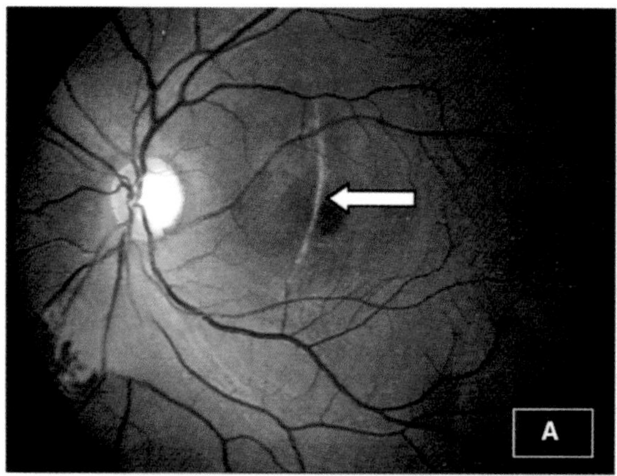

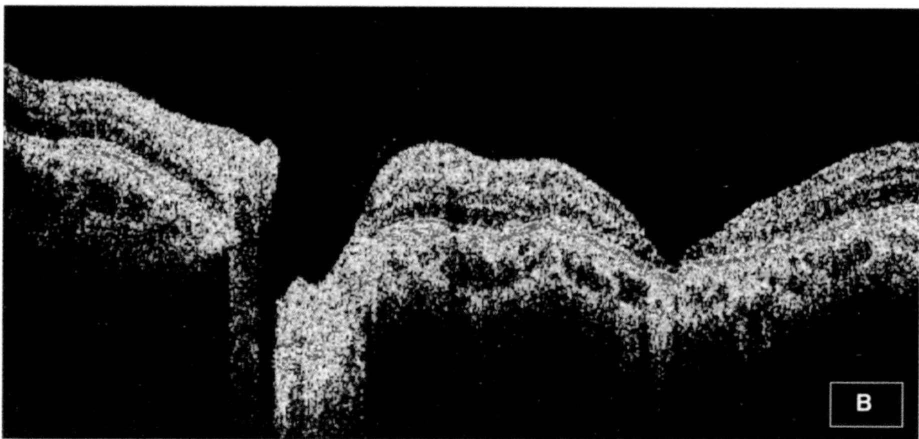

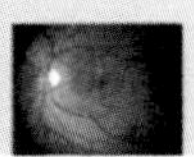

TRAUMATIC RETINAL DETACHMENT

Case 20.6: Traumatic Retinal Detachment

Case Summary

A 13-year-old boy suffered trauma with a stick following which he developed retinal detachment in the right eye (A).

The OCT line scan showed retinal detachment with more fluid accumulation in the temporal retina (B).

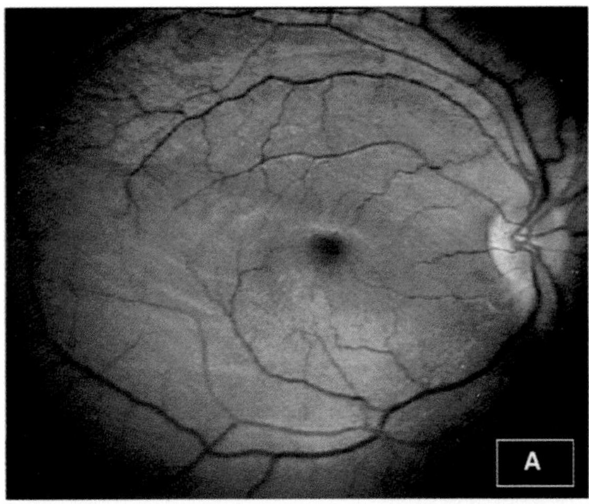

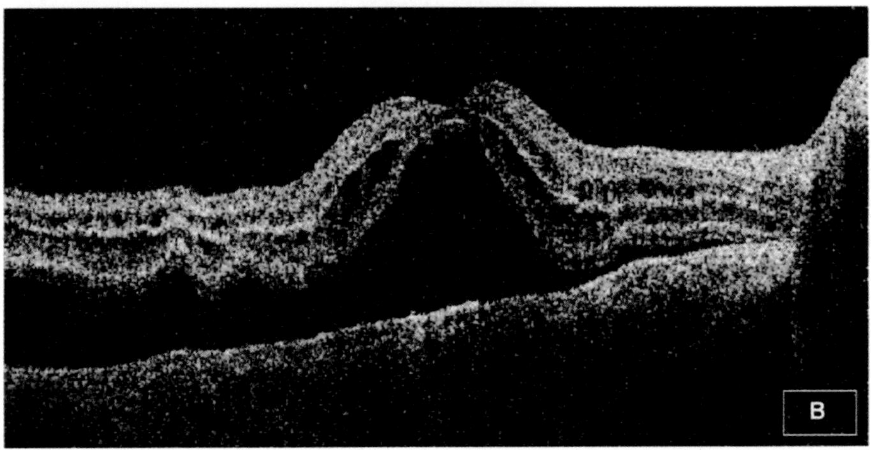

The patient underwent scleral buckle surgery in this eye (C). The repeat OCT showed reattached retina (D).

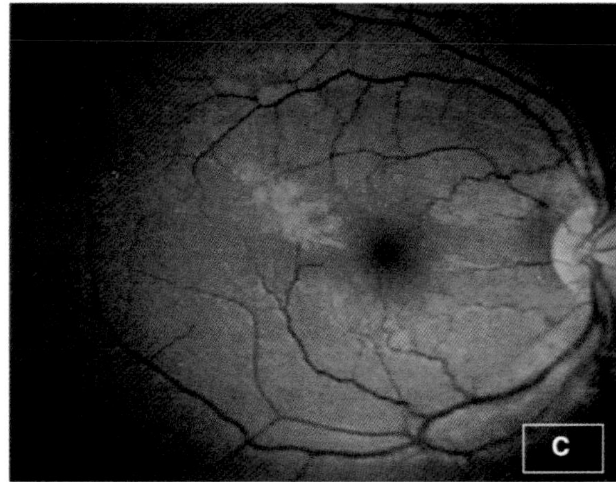

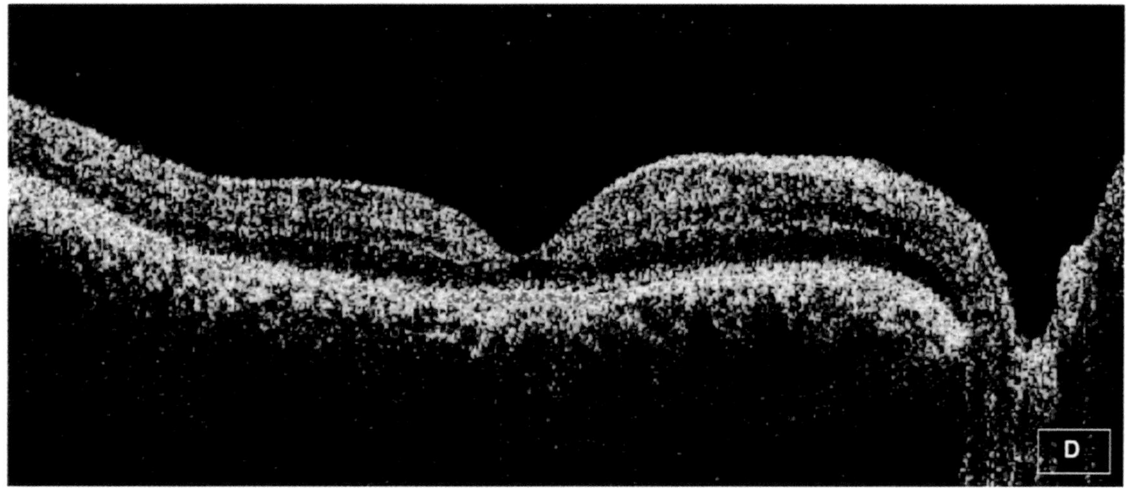

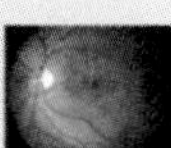

TRAUMATIC CHOROIDOPATHY

Case 20.7: Traumatic choroidopathy

Case Summary

A 21-year-old man was seen with maculopathy and choroidopathy that showed transmission hyperfluorescence on fluorescein angiography (A).

The OCT line scan through the center of the fovea (B) showed atrophy of neurosensory retina with increased hyper-reflectivity from the underlying choroid. The line scan from the area of choroidopathy just above the optic disc (C) showed moderate hyper-reflectivity from the choroid. The overlying retina was normal.

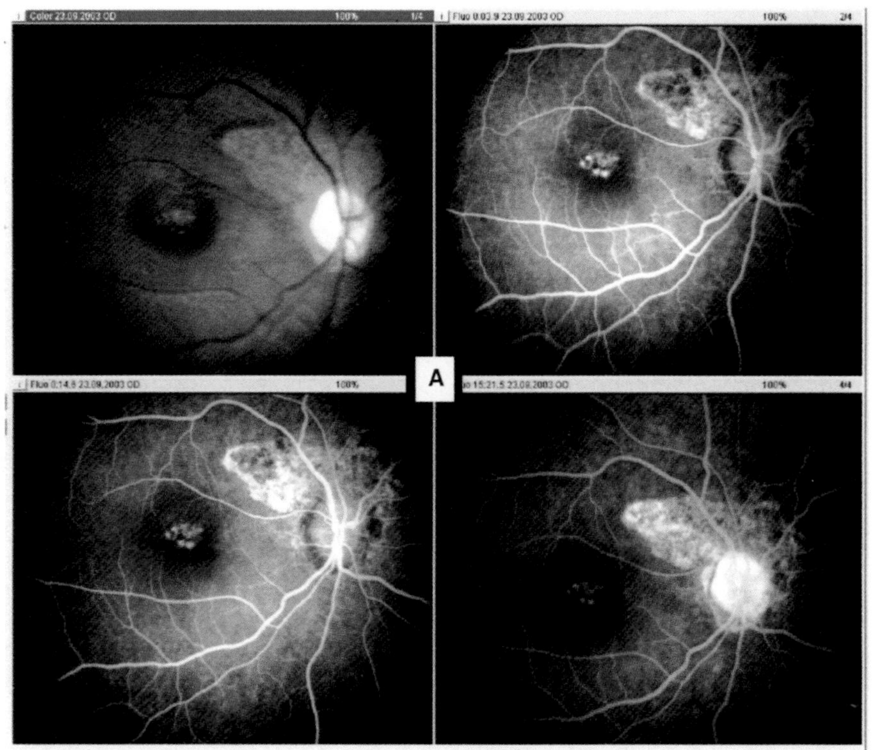

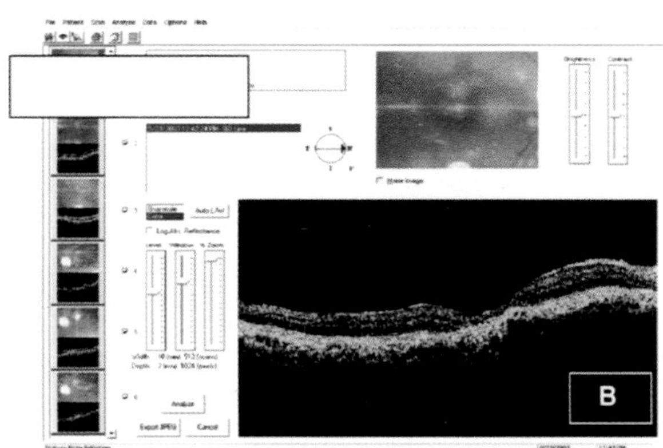

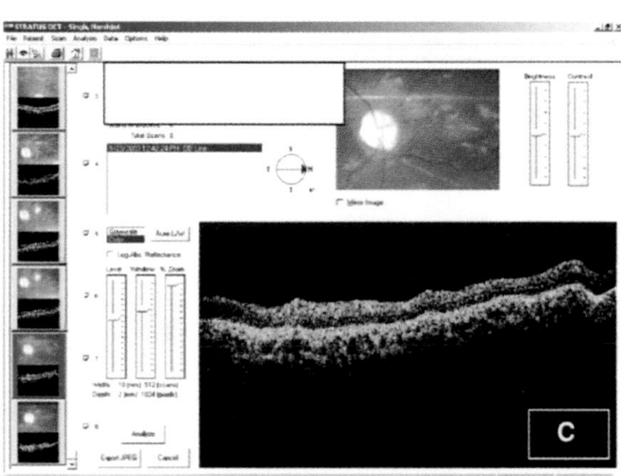

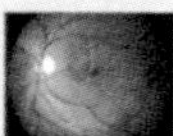

CHOROIDAL NEOVASCULARIZATION

Case 20.8: Traumatic Subretinal Hemorrhage with Choroidal Neovascular Membrane

Case Summary

A 26-year-old man was seen with left eye subfoveal hemorrhage following trauma with a stick (A). His best-corrected visual acuity was 20/200. The fluorescein angiography showed hyperfluorescence suggesting the presence of an underlying CNVM.

The OCT line scan showed a hyporeflective area under the fovea corresponding to blood with an area of moderately increased hyper-reflectivity suggestive of choroidal neovascular membrane.

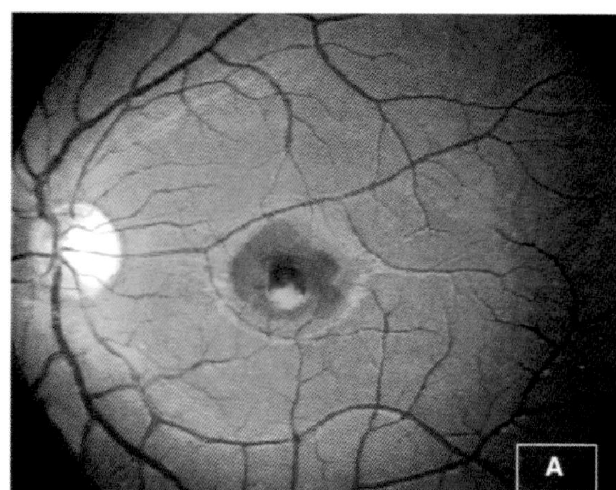

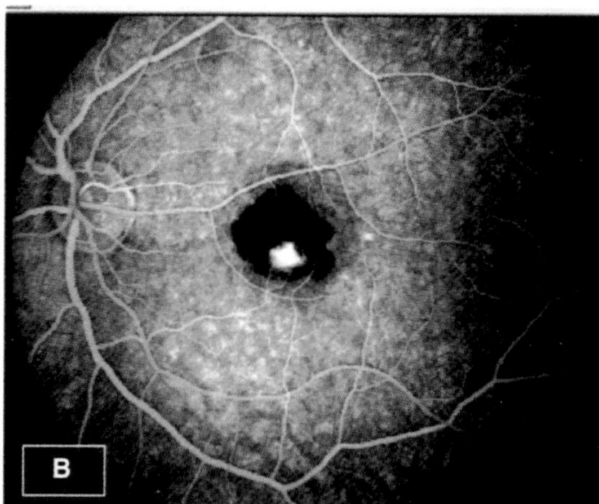

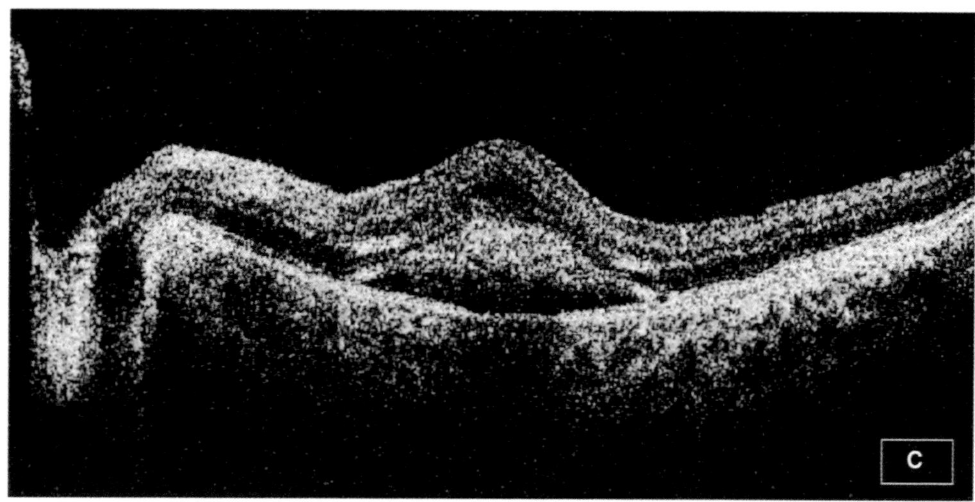

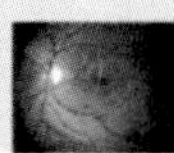

Three weeks later, visual acuity of the left eye was reduced further. The extent of subretinal hemorrhage had increased than before (D). Repeat OCT scan (E) showed further increase in the foveal thickness with increase in the height of fibrovascular complex suggesting further increase in the size of the membrane. The patient refused any intervention.

The choroidal neovascular membrane showed further increase in size with subretinal hemorrhage (F). Note the increase in the area of hyperfluorescence seen on fluorescein angiography (G).

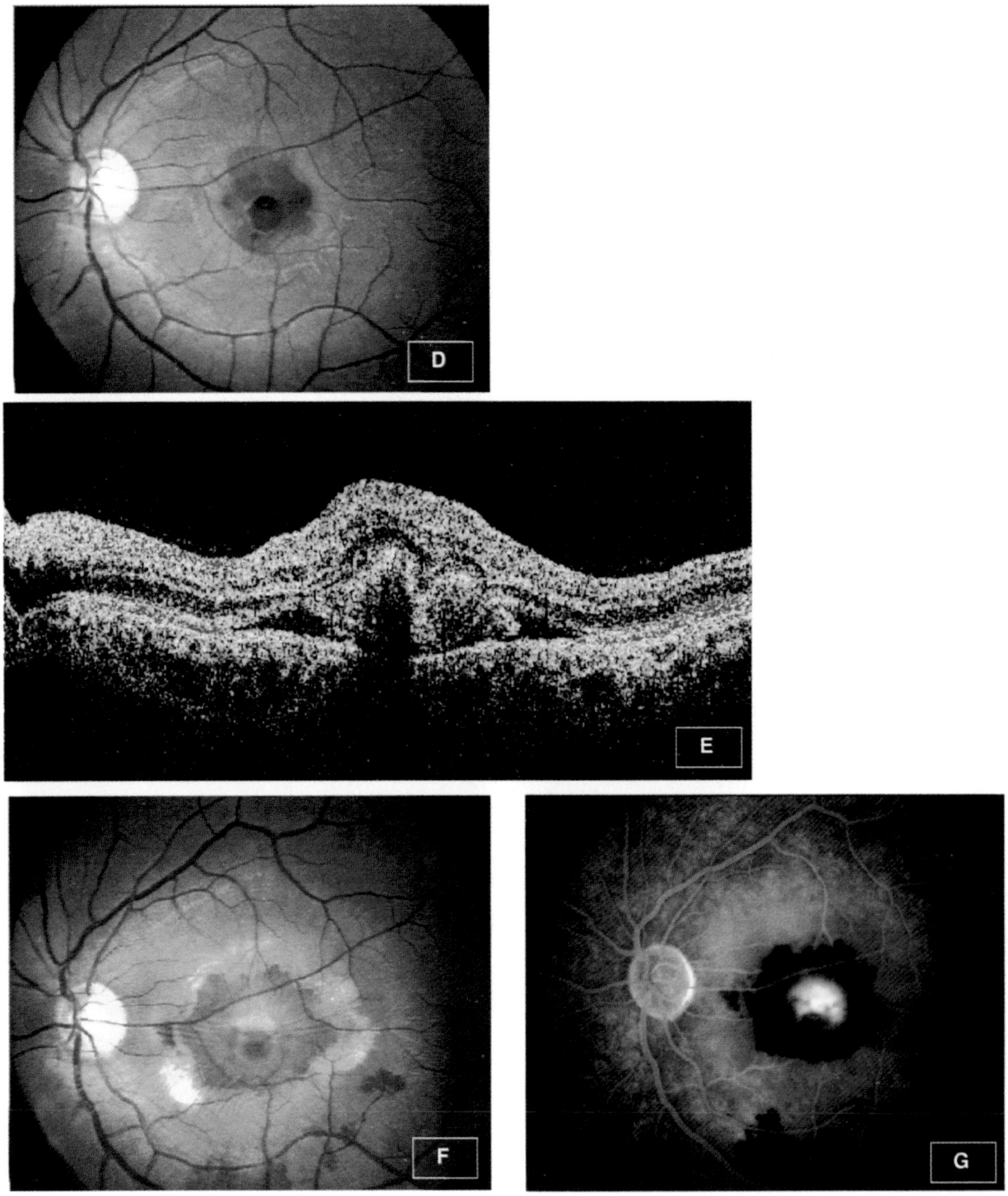

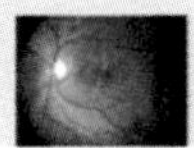

The repeat OCT scan (H) showed an increase in the hyporeflective area under the choroidal neovascular membrane consistent with the increase in subretinal blood seen clinically.

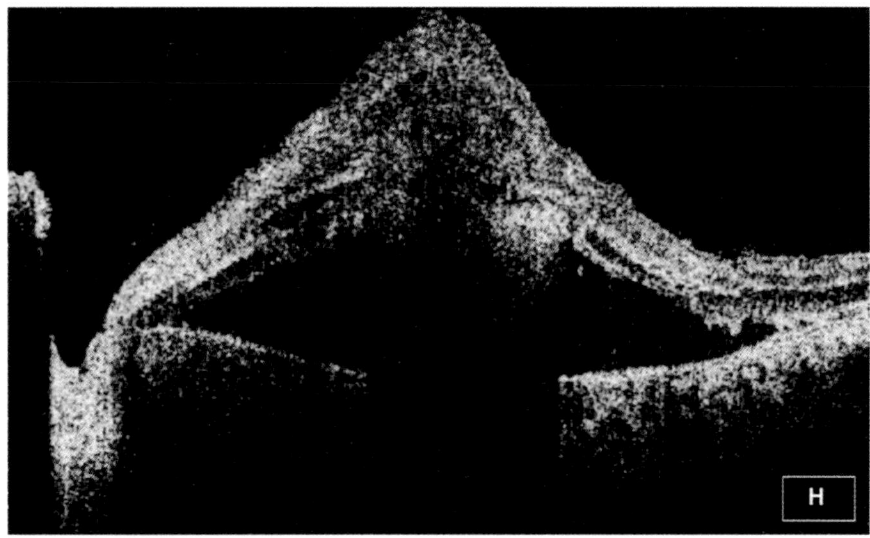

CONCLUSIONS

1. In Commotio retinae, OCT provides the information regarding the changes occurring at the ultrastructural level. These changes were not seen on fluorescein angiography.
2. OCT is very useful in monitoring the development, progression and course as well as response to treatment in macular holes following trauma.
3. OCT can diagnose associated secondary changes including cystoid macular edema, retinal detachment, neurosensory atrophy, epiretinal membranes, subretinal fibrosis etc.

SUGGESTED READINGS

1. Mansour AM, Green WR,Hogge C. Histopathology of commotio retinae. Retina 1992 ; 12:24-28.
2. Hilton GF. Late serosanguinous detachment of the macula after traumatic choroidal rupture. Am J Ophthalmol. 1975 ; 79 : 997-1000.
3. Yamada H, Sakai A, Yamada E et al. Spontaneous closure of traumatic macular hole. Am J Ophthalmol 2002 ; 134 : 340-47.

Chapter 21

Macular Evaluation following Retinal Detachment Surgery

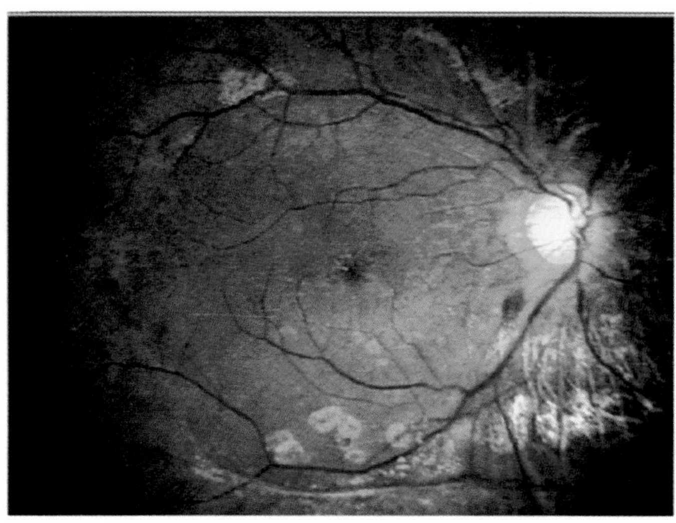

POST RETINAL DETACHMENT SURGERY

Following successful retinal reattachment surgery many a times, the vision does not improve or takes long time to improve. The retina seems reattached and fluorescein angiography too may not show any abnormality. OCT is useful in assessing the status of macula in these eyes in the following ways:

1. It has been found that the eyes with retinal detachment and spared macula preoperatively tend to show subretinal fluid accumulation under the fovea following successful scleral buckle surgery.
2. In eyes with preoperative macular detachment, the retinal detachment persists under the fovea and may take upto an year to resolve. This explains the delayed visual recovery in these eyes.
3. Intraretinal separation of detached retina seen preoperatively is associated with poor visual recovery.
4. OCT helps in diagnosing other causes of poor postoperative visual gain. These include neurosensory retinal atrophy, cystoid macular edema , epiretinal and subretinal fibrosis.

Case 21.1: Macula Post Scleral Buckling Surgery

Case Summary

A 27-year-old man underwent retinal reattachment surgery in his right eye. His best-corrected visual acuity was 20/200 in the right eye. The retina was attached clinically (A) and fluorescein angiogram was normal (B).

Optical Coherence Tomography

OCT line scan through the foveal center showed the presence of small serous retinal detachment under the fovea (C). This serous detachment was not seen clinically or angiographically. When seen a month later, the detachment had become smaller (D).

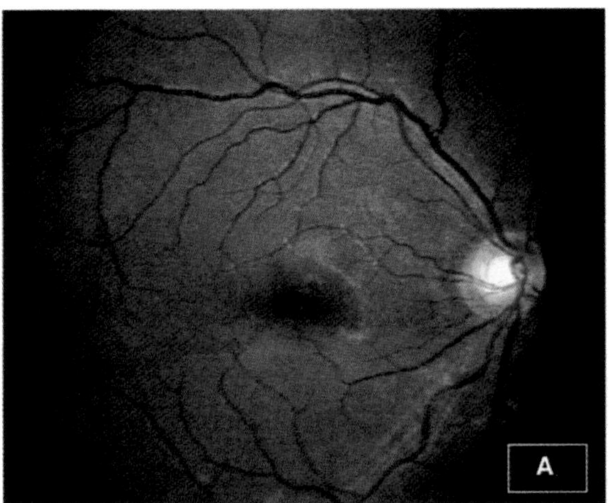

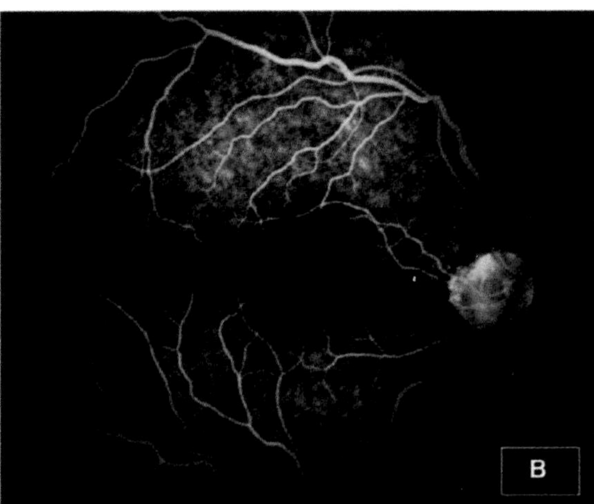

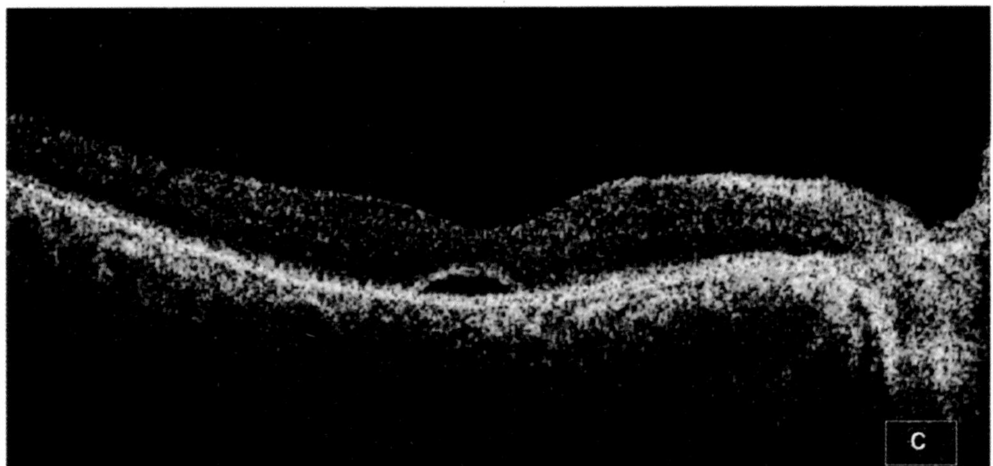

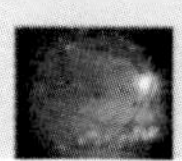

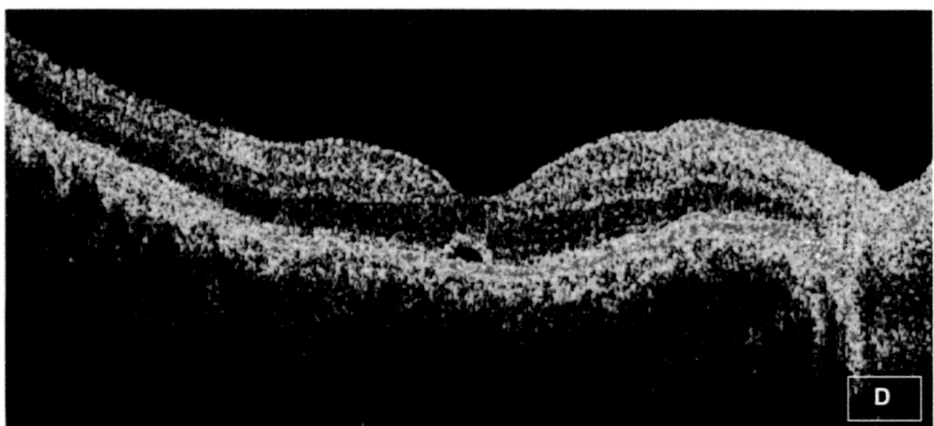

Three months later, his visual acuity had improved to 20/40 (E). Repeat OCT scan (F) showed resolution of serous foveal detachment.

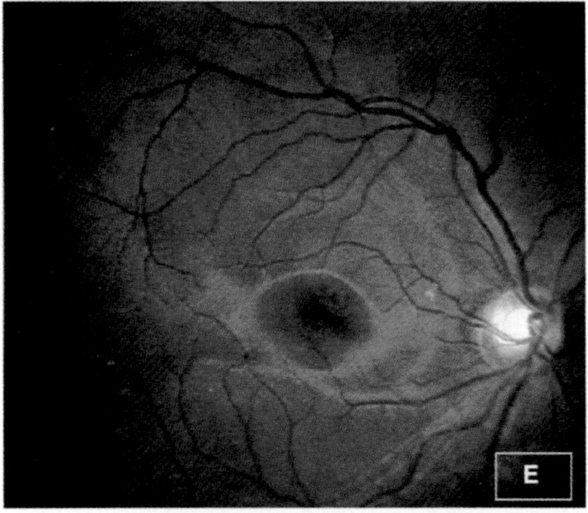

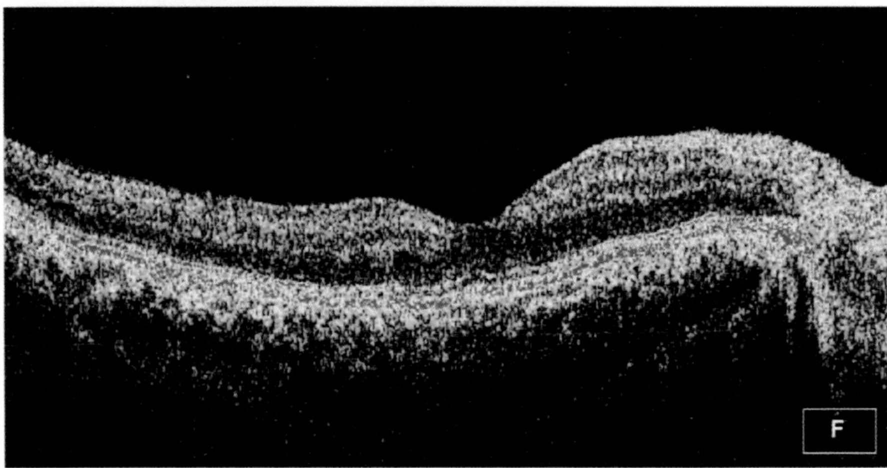

Case 21.2: Neurosensory Retinal Atrophy following Pars Plana Vitrectomy for Retinal Detachment

Case Summary

A 45-year-old woman underwent pars plana vitrectomy for retinal detachment with proliferative vitreoretinopathy (PVR) grade C2. Three months later, her visual acuity was counting fingers. She had developed a fibrous scar in the fovea that was hyperfluorescent on fluorescein angiography (A).

Optical Coherence Tomography

The vertical line scan through the fovea (B) showed the absence of neurosensory retina in the region of fovea suggesting the presence of a hole that healed with neurosensory defect. The underlying RPE-choroid showed increased hyper-reflectivity that could be due to the absence of overlying layers. This patient is unlikely to show any visual improvement ever.

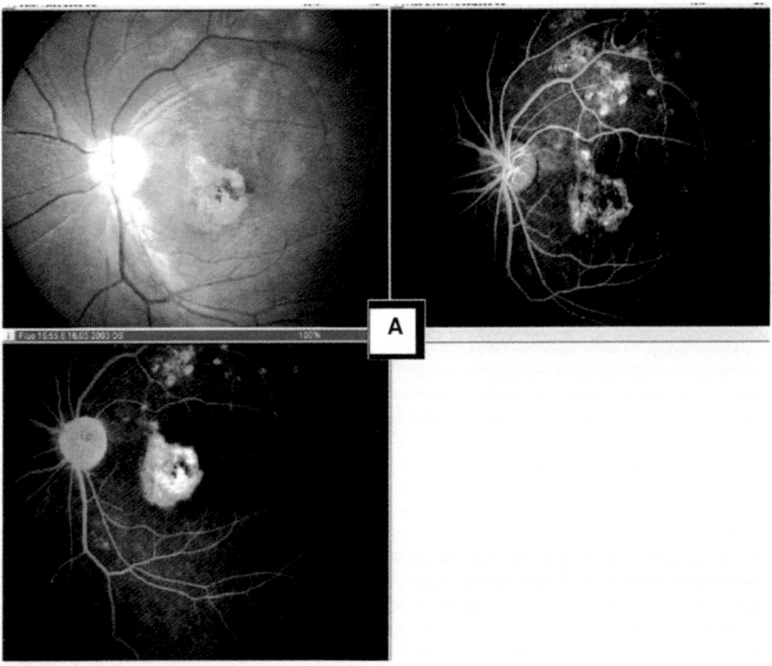

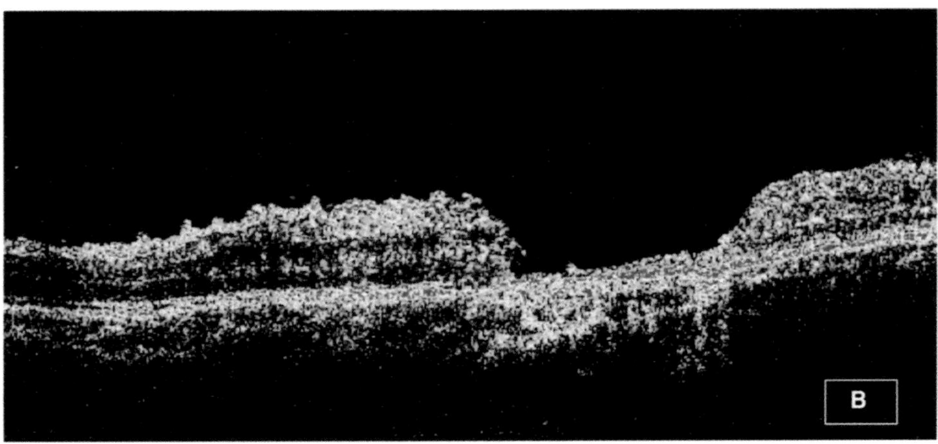

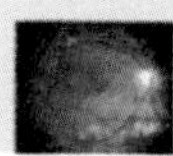

Case 21.3: Cystoid Macular Edema following Pars Plana Vitrectomy for Giant Retinal Tear

Case Summary

A 20-year-old boy underwent pars plana vitrectomy for retinal detachment associated with giant retinal tear following trauma. Four months later, his best-corrected visual acuity was 20/100 in this eye (A). Fluorescein angiography of the right eye showed cystoid macular edema grade IV (B).

Optical Coherence Tomography

OCT line scan through the foveal center (C) showed hyporeflective area under the fovea suggesting intraretinal fluid accumulation. Also seen were small cystic spaces in the overlying retina. The patient was given posterior subtenon triamcinolone acetonide 20 mg to which he responded.

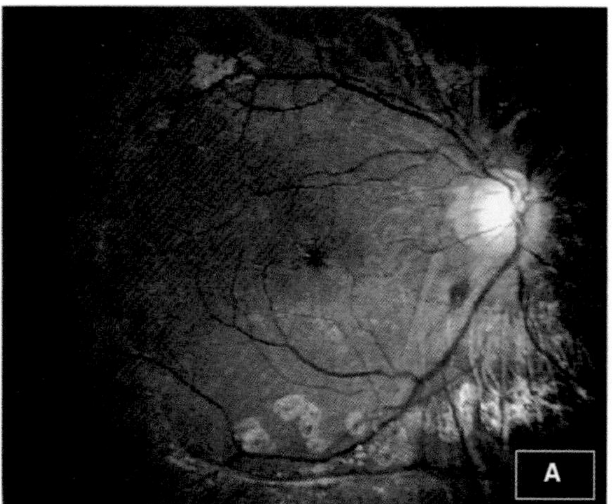

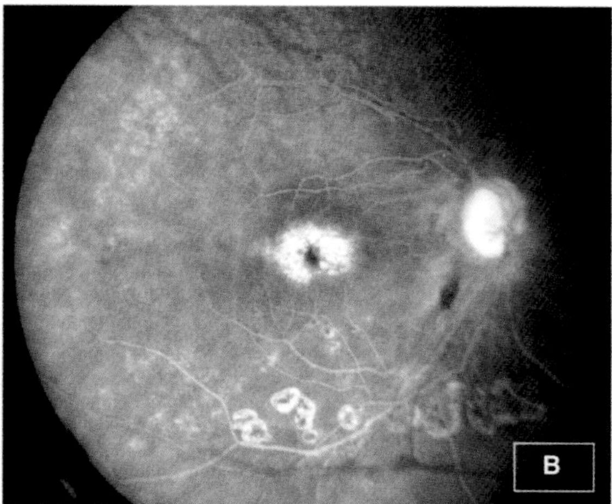

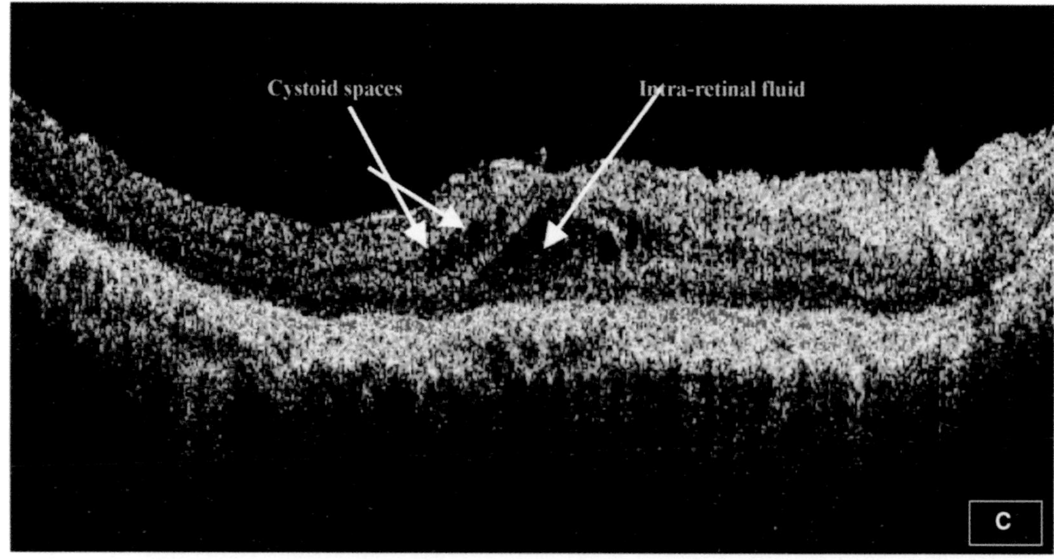

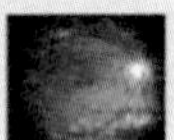

Case 21.4 : Retinal Pigment Epithelial Irregularity following Scleral Buckling Surgery

Case Summary

A 54-year-old woman underwent scleral buckle surgery in the left eye for pseudophakic retinal detachment. Her best-corrected visual acuity in this eye was counting fingers. The retina was reattached (A). Fluorescein angiography was non-contributory (B, C).

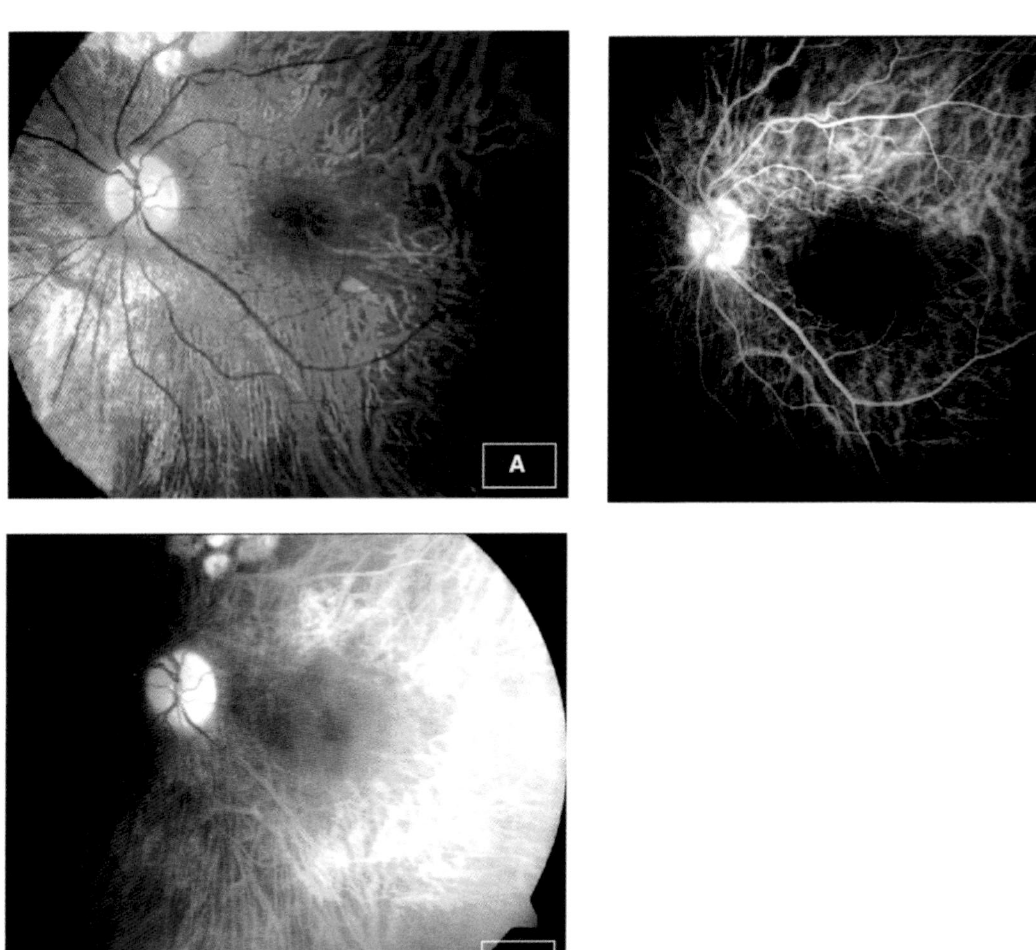

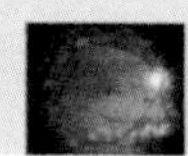

Optical Coherence Tomography

OCT line scan showed irregularity of retinal pigment epithelium (RPE) (D).

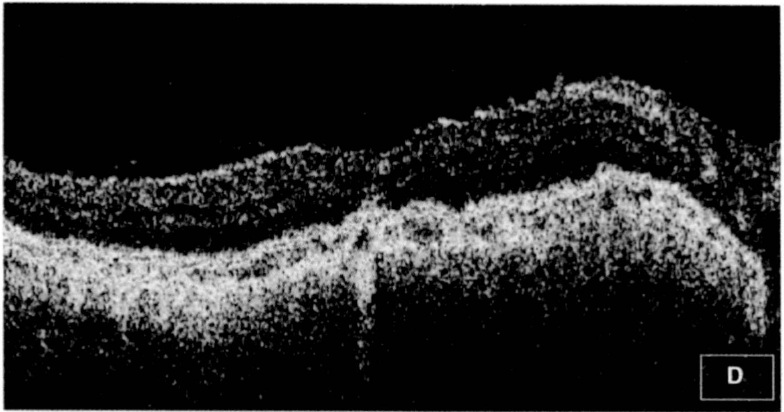

Case 21.5: Neurosensory Atrophy following Scleral Buckling Surgery

Case Summary

A 34-year-old man underwent scleral buckle surgery for post-traumatic retinal detachment. The macula showed atrophic changes in the fovea (A).

Optical Coherence Tomography

OCT line scan through the fovea (B) showed neurosensory atrophy with central foveal thickness measuring 76 microns. This patient is unlikely to improve vision.

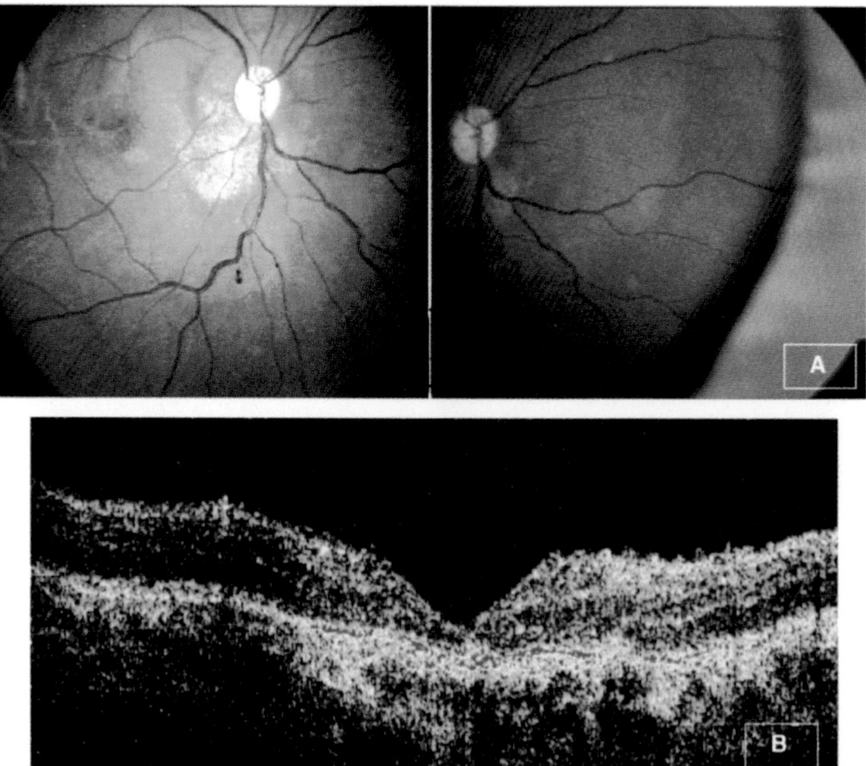

Case 21.6: Retinal Pigment Epithelium Hyperplasia following Pars Plana Vitrectomy for Retinal Detachment

Case Summary

A 27-year-old man had retinal detachment following trauma (A,B) for which he underwent pars plana vitrectomy. Two months later, his visual acuity was 20/200 and macula showed pigmentary changes (C)

Optical Coherence Tomography

OCT line scan through the fovea showed heaped-up retinal pigment epithelium under the fovea (D).

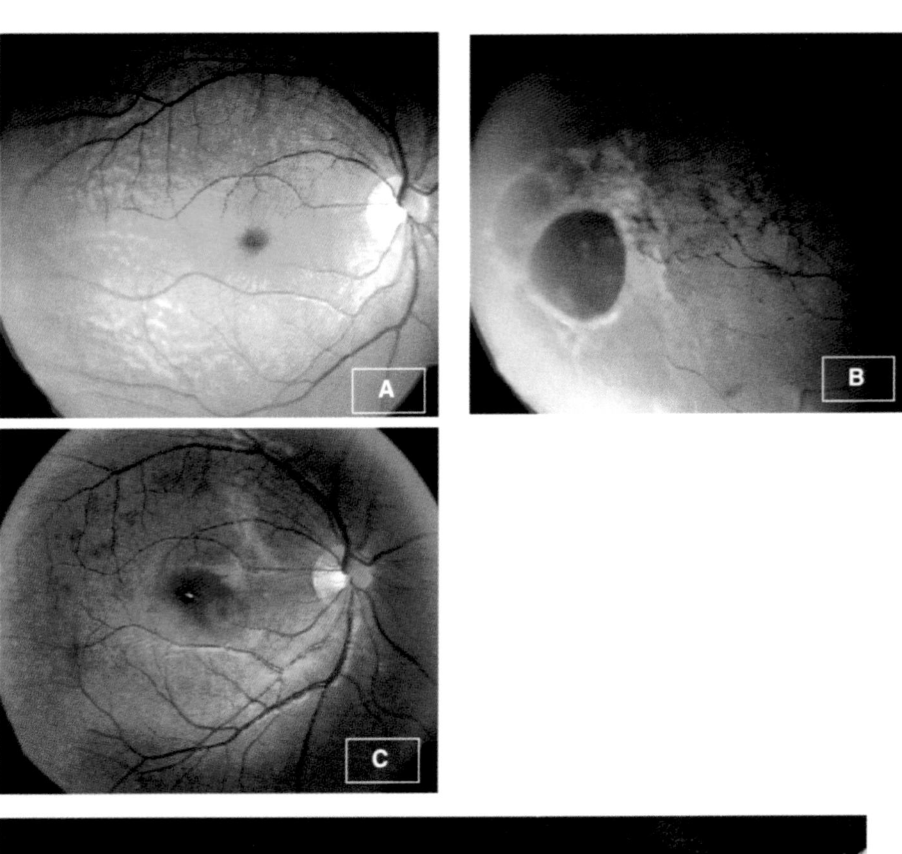

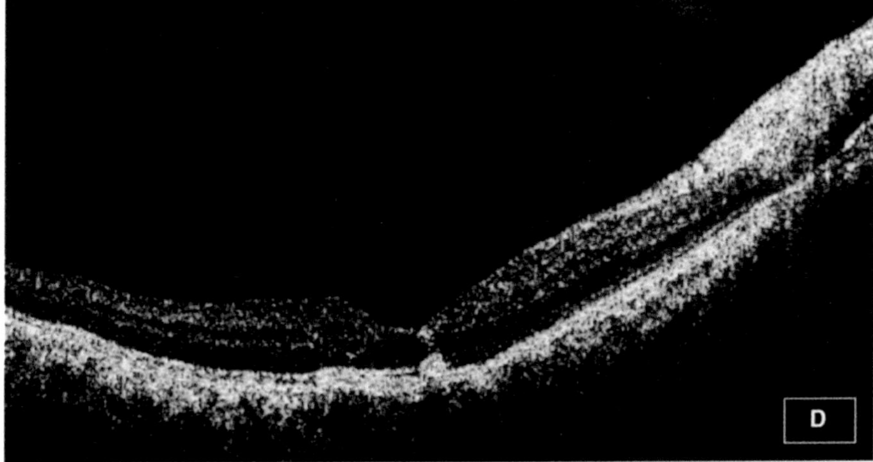

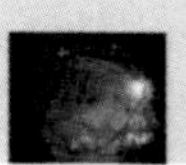

CONCLUSIONS

OCT was found to be a very useful tool in determining the causes of poor postoperative visual gain following successful retinal detachment surgery. The serous detachment under the fovea is so subtle that it is not seen clinically or even on fluorescein angiography. OCT can diagnose the presence of subretinal fluid under the fovea and also monitor its resolution over a period of time. The presence of subretinal fluid under the fovea carries a good prognosis as the patients regain vision once this fluid absorbs. OCT can also help in diagnosing irreversible causes of poor postoperative visual gain, namely, subretinal fibrosis and atrophy of neurosensory retina.

SUGGESTED READINGS

1. Theodossiadis PG, Georgalas IG, Emfietzoglou J, Kyriaki TE, Pantelia E, Gogas PS, Moschos MN, Theodossiadis GP.Optical coherence tomography findings in the macula after treatment of rhegmatogenous retinal detachments with spared macula preoperatively Retina 2003;23:69-75.
2. Hagimura N, Iida T, Suto K, Kishi S.Persistent foveal retinal detachment after successful rhegmatogenous retinal detachment surgery.Am J Ophthalmol 2002 ; 133 : 516-20.
3. Wolfensberger TJ, Gonvers M. Optical coherence tomography in the evaluation of incomplete visual acuity recovery after macula-off retinal detachments. Graefes Arch Clin Exp Ophthalmol 2002;240:85-9.
4. Hagimura N, Suto K, Iida T, Kishi S. Optical coherence tomography of the neurosensory retina in rhegmatogenous retinal detachment. Am J Ophthalmol 2000;129:186-90.

Chapter 22

Intraocular Metastasis

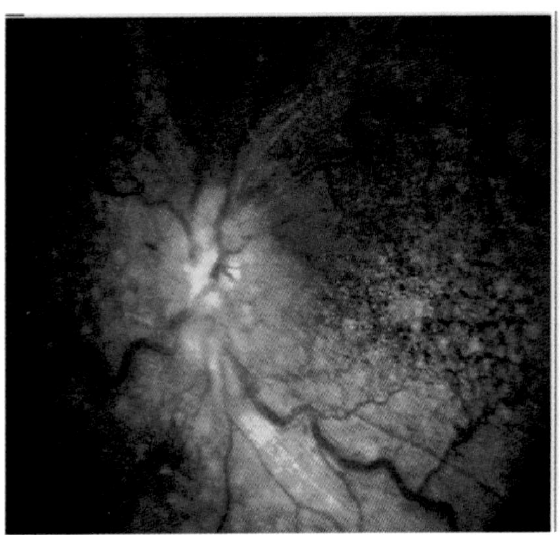

Case 22.1: Chronic Myeloid Leukemia

Case Summary

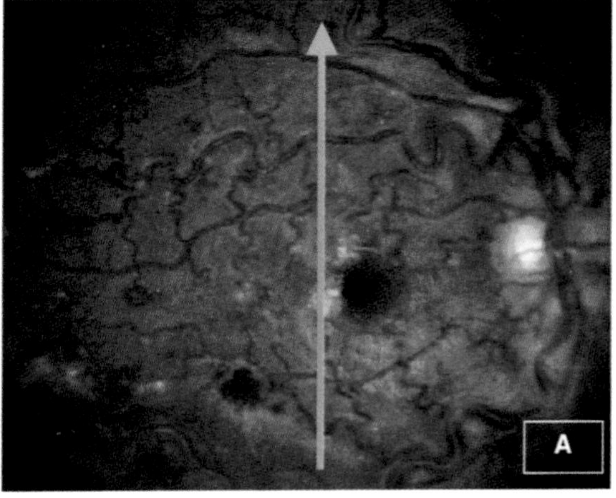

An 18-year-old boy with a diagnosis of chronic myeloid leukemia was seen with visual acuity of 20/80 in the right eye. Fundoscopy (A) showed dilated tortuous veins, retinal hemorrhages and exudates. Fluorescein angiography (B) showed dilated veins.

Optical Coherence Tomography

Vertical OCT line scan (C) showed few hyper-reflective areas in the inner-retinal layers probably representing retinal leukemic infiltrates.

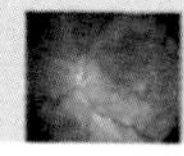

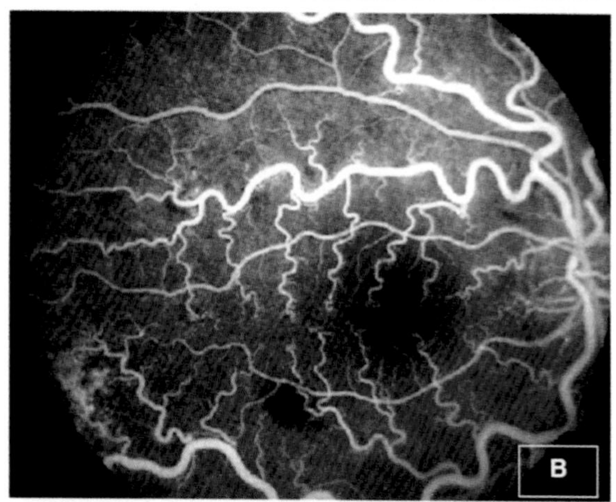

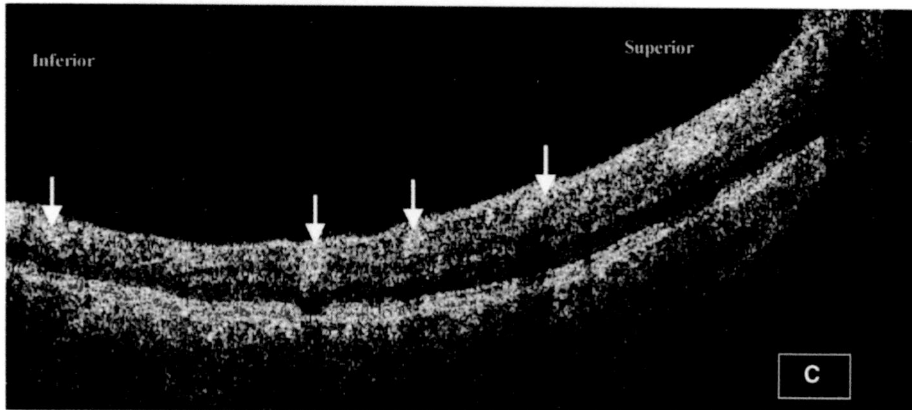

The patient had no light perception in the left eye, which showed multiple deep yellow colored subretinal infiltrates scattered throughout the fundus (D). The optic disc showed hyperfluorescence (E).

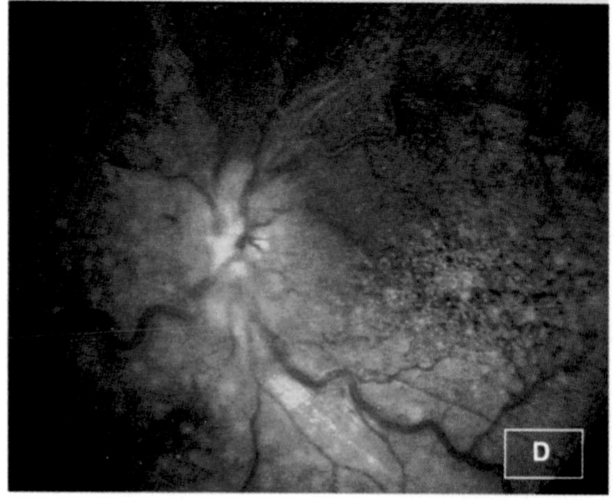

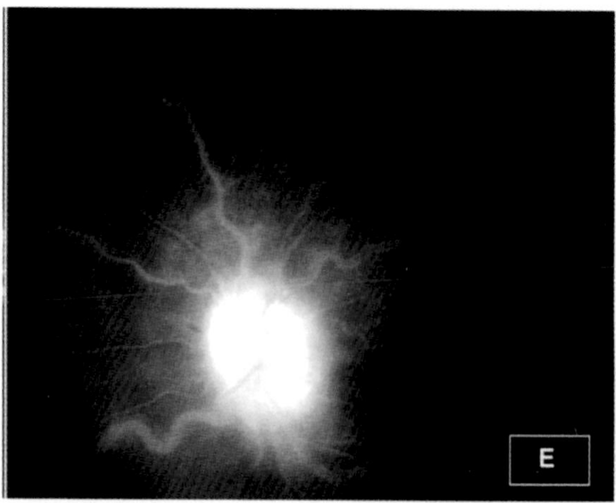

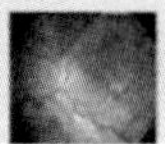

Optical Coherence Tomography

OCT line scan showed atrophy of neurosensory retina. The choroidal infiltrates could not be appreciated (F).

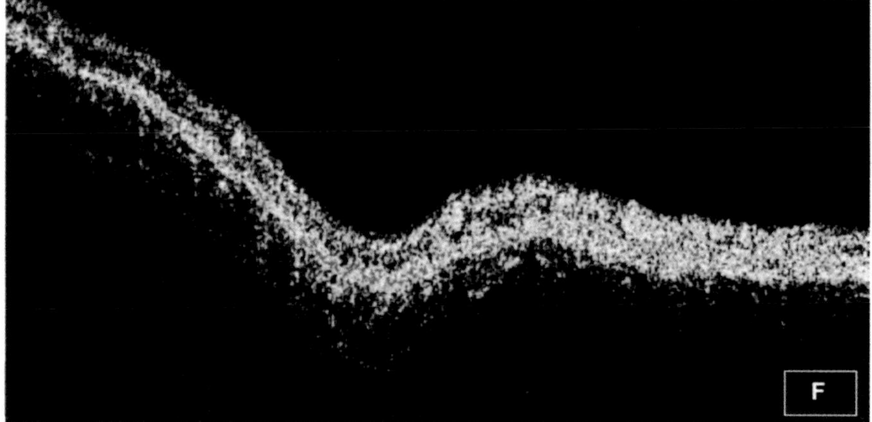

Case 22.2: Metastasis from Breast Carcinoma

Case Summary

A 57-year-old-woman with carcinoma breast was seen with peripapillary subretinal Infiltrates (A).

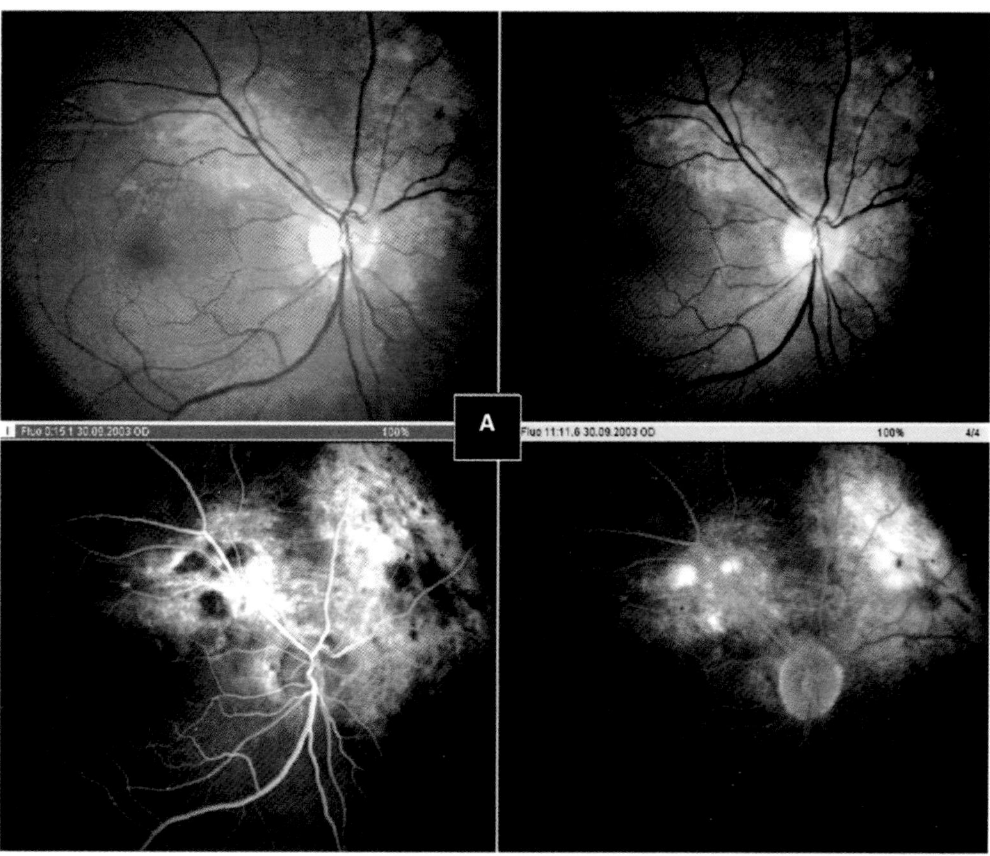

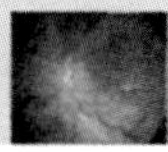

The horizontal (B) and vertical (C) line scans through the areas of infiltrate showed hyper-reflective areas from the choroid (white arrows) and overlying retina (yellow arrows)

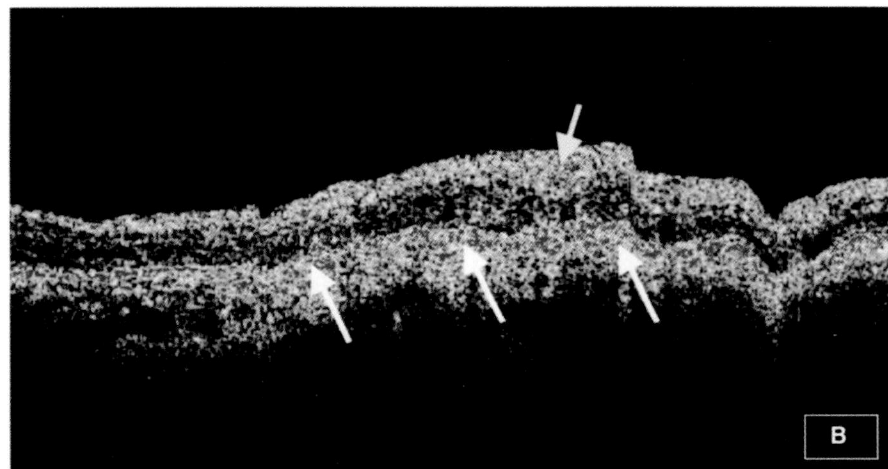

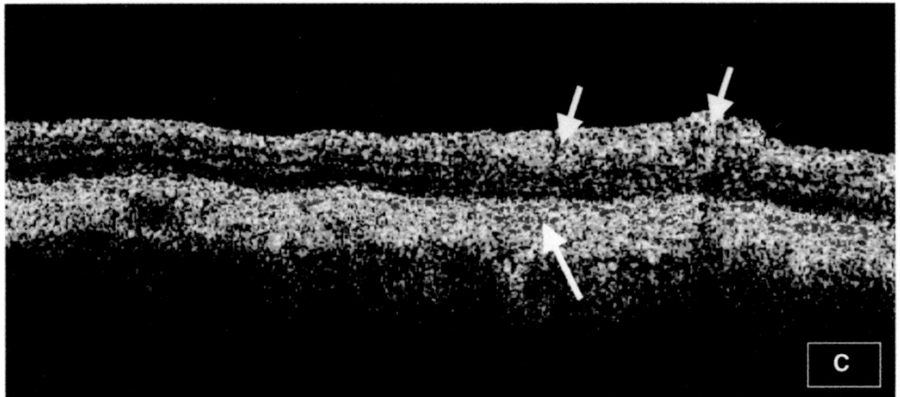

CONCLUSIONS

OCT was useful in localizing the site of metastatic deposits and might help in monitoring response to the therapy.

Index

P

R

T

T - #1059 - 101024 - C318 - 280/216/15 [17] - CB - 9781841844688 - Gloss Lamination